STRETCH

Explore, Explain, Persuade

STRETCH

Explore, Explain, Persuade

Randall A. Wells
Coastal Carolina University

Prentice Hall, Upper Saddle River, New Jersey 07458

Library of Congress Cataloging-in-Publication Data

Wells, Randall A.
    Stretch : explore, explain, persuade / Randall A. Wells.
        p.   cm.
    Includes bibliographical references and index.
    ISBN 0-13-617903-7 (pbk.)
    1. English language—Rhetoric.   2. College readers.   3. Report
writing.   I. Title.
PE1408.W495 1998
808¹.0427—dc21   97-36535
                                                             CIP

Acquisitions editor: Leah Jewell
Editorial/production supervision: Alison D. Gnerre
Interior design: Lisa Delgado
Cover design: Pat Wosczyk
Cover photo: David Madison/David Madison Sports Images
Manufacturing buyer: Mary Ann Gloriande

Acknowledgements appear on page 303, which constitutes a continuation of the copyright page.

© 1998 by Prentice-Hall, Inc.
Simon & Schuster /A Viacom Company
Upper Saddle River, New Jersey 07458

Printed in the United States of America

10 9 8 7 6 5 4 3 2 1

ISBN 0-13-617903-7

Prentice-Hall International (UK) Limited, London
Prentice-Hall of Australia Pty. Limited, Sydney
Prentice-Hall Canada Inc., Toronto
Prentice-Hall Hispanoamericana, S.A., Mexico
Prentice-Hall of India Private Limited, New Delhi
Prentice-Hall of Japan, Inc., Tokyo
Simon & Schuster Asia Pte Ltd., Singapore
Editora Prentice-Hall do Brasil, Ltda., Rio de Janeiro

To
Marjory B. Wells

Contents

Chapter 3   The Informal Essay   63

PART II:
EXPLAIN   83

PART III:
PERSUADE   151

✳ ▬▬▬▬▬▬▬▬▬▬

Chapter 6   Direct Persuasion   163

Additional Readings   215

Acknowledgments

"Why don't you write your own book?"

This challenge, issued by Gerald Groves in response to my grumbling about a rhetoric text, eventually produced *Stretch: Explore, Explain, Persuade.* Gerald agreed to collaborate with me on a book, then after many months graciously let me continue the project alone.

I am also pleased to thank many other colleagues as well as friends, family, editors, and others who are not named in the book. (More people are acknowledged in the Instructor's Manual.)

For reading parts or all of the manuscript as it grew and underwent constant mutation over the years, I thank Glenda Sweet, Jill Sessoms, Ted Walkup, Linda Hollandsworth, Richard Collin, Karlene Rudolph, Ann Roam, Don Samson, Andrea Wells, and Beth Havens.

For using some version of the manuscript in class, I thank Ray Moye, Hyde Abbott, their students, and mine.

For all the power tools—computer, photocopier, telephone, fax machine, and printer—as well as mail privileges, I thank the School of Humanities and Fine Arts, John Durrell, Dean.

For secretarial and computer support, and for leavening competence with wit, I thank Shirell Mishoe, Marie Lovero, and Stephanie Hyland.

For help in locating student papers around the country, I am grateful to Norma C. Wilson, Eva Fuchs, Roland Hinojosa-Smith, and Thomas Gasque.

I thank these people for giving me some of the books, magazines, or newspapers used in *Stretch:* Dudley E. Wells, Laura Peterson, Bill Schaefer, Katie Wells, Bill Irvin, S. Paul Rice, and Dale Collins.

And I appreciate these detectives employed by Kimbel Library: Sallie Clarkson, Jeri Traw, Michael Lackey, Margaret Fain, and Peggy Bates.

For special expertise I thank Pam Duncan, Janie Gardner, Carrie Canniff, Sharon Thompson, Steve Hamelman, Veronica Gerald, Seth Funderburk, Paul Olsen, Patricia Candal, Susan Shepherd, Jeanne Turner, and Abdallah Haddad.

I am indebted to Erika Lindemann for handing a draft of the "Stretch" manuscript to Mary Jo Southern of Prentice Hall.

For the pink telephone-message on my office door, I thank Mary Jo Southern, whose enthusiastic backing I will forever appreciate.

For their valuable perspectives—educational, temperamental, and geographical—I thank the following reviewers: Barbara H. Loush, Oakland Community College, Royal Oak Campus; Ted McFerrin, Collin County Community College; Susan Miller, University of Utah; Marshall Myers, Eastern Kentucky University; Deborah Quirey, Northern Oklahoma College; and James C. Rumple, Jr., Catawba Valley Community College.

To my editor, Harriett Prentiss, someone I have never met but regard like a war buddy, I extend gratitude for directing the Revision Offensive of winter '96–'97. By express mail, telephone, fax, and e-mail, she helped me follow textbook conventions, hew to comments of reviewers, and expand, shift, or clarify material. I appreciate her wide-ranging expertise, encouragement, and company.

To Alison Gnerre, production editor at Prentice Hall, I express my thanks—with a tincture of sympathy for holding down that spot between author and compositor and fielding "MNs," late additions, floating visuals, and what-I-meants.

I apologize to my family for working so long on a book that talks so much about the family. I am especially grateful for the interest, inspiration, discernment, patience, and finally just endurance of my wife, Marjory, who spoke the truth: "You're always in the study with the door closed and I'm runnin' the household."

Randall A. Wells

Your Workout—Why and How

Like an exercise program that flexes and strengthens all the tendons, ligaments, and muscles in your body from neck to ankles—by having you rotate, bend, spread, arch, extend, lunge, jump, swing, rock, tilt, kick, twist, lift, push, reach, squat, and shrug—Stretch will help limber you up as a writer. It will expand your range of motion by inviting you to try a variety of aims, forms, strategies, and even media.

THREE AIMS

The chapters of *Stretch* will take you through an invigorating workout with several basic aims:

Explore

Explain

Persuade

How do these differ? Here is a brief definition of each:

A writer may *explore* his or her experience (as in a story, meditation, or informal essay) by trying to understand its significance through the power of words. Or a writer may emphasize the interaction between his or her unique mind and the subject, whether personal or not. Writing is exploratory when it delays a feeling of certainty in the reader and prolongs curiosity, when it shares with the reader the writer's process of discovery.

When a writer tries to *explain,* by contrast, as in a set of instructions or an objective report, he or she transfers information with the main goal of clarity. The writer may connect the explanation with the reader's needs, announce its purpose and even its outline, and complete the details.

A writer who wants to *persuade,* whether directly or indirectly, tries primarily to affect attitudes or motivate behavior. The writer makes a judgment, interpretation, or recommendation, and supports it.

In writing, although one of these basic aims usually dominates, they often overlap and reinforce each other. So an exploratory essay or story might have a persuasive edge; or an argument might rely heavily on explanation—or even create an exploratory air by its tentative, questioning approach. In *Stretch,* however, you will concentrate on each purpose separately just as you would isolate one group of muscles to build it up most effectively.

Your workout will help prepare you for the diversity of writing opportunities to be encountered during college and afterward. For example, *Stretch* gives you practice with stating a clear thesis (i.e., opinion), then supporting it adequately and systematically, perhaps the most valuable skill you can have as a writer. The book encourages versatility, however, by inviting you to

* tell a story that may or may not declare its significance explicitly
* explore an idea, controversy, person, or place to evoke understanding while writing
* declare an explanatory *purpose* to be accomplished rather than a persuasive thesis to be supported
* explain or persuade with the help of illustrations and visual emphasis techniques such as headings and vertical lists
* support a thesis with a variety of strategies
* lead up to a thesis that may be expressed near the end

This book will stress basic *methods of development*—ways of thinking about a subject and elaborating on it. Here are many of the traditional methods discussed: example, definition, comparison and contrast, division and classification, cause and effect, narration, description, process analysis, testimony, and analogy.

A writer uses these techniques not as ends in themselves but as means to reach an ultimate goal such as exploration, explanation, or persuasion. So any one method can be used for any purpose. The technique of description, for example, can be used in your own "workout" to make a story more vivid, to begin a meditation concretely, to root an essay in the world of the senses, to clarify instructions or other kinds of exposition, or to reinforce a persuasive point.

USING THIS BOOK

Your teacher might assign any or all of the chapters, and in the order he or she judges most helpful.

Each chapter has the same format. After a brief introduction to one type of writing, it invites you to **Warm Up First** to get the ink circulating.

Next it presents models of writing, one by a professional and then two by students in freshman composition (or sometimes advanced composition). The first piece will be annotated in the margin to help you appreciate its features while you read it.

These examples lead to the main writing assignment, which is called the **STR-R-ETCH.** This section includes abundant guidelines for the paper, and most of the chapters offer **Ten + Topics,** suggestions for writing; these often address one of the recurrent themes of the book (introduced below). You also get some pointers for revision.

In a physical workout, after taking a rest "it is a good idea to stretch just a bit farther to better develop your flexibility" (Nieman 319). Likewise, in *Stretch* you can try an **Extra Challenge.** These writing possibilities invite you to extend your versatility even more.

And each chapter concludes with a **Poem** or song lyrics—a further illustration of the main writing concept. The poem in turn inspires a few **Tips for Prose.**

Here and there within each chapter you will also find references to a collection of **Additional Readings** at the end of the book. This writing, done by students and professionals, includes some unexpected formats that will bring fresh oxygen to your imagination. The book's chapters often refer to these readings to illustrate various aims, techniques, and themes.

RECURRING THEMES

In the chapters and in the Additional Readings you will notice that certain subjects reappear, sometimes in surprising contexts, sometimes in combination. Each of these themes is woven through the book so as to highlight the different types of writing that any one subject can produce. And each offers a springboard for your own writing. These main concerns reverberate in your daily life, personally and socially:

Columbus & Co. "At dawn we saw naked people. . . . " Thus begins the first recorded sighting of a native by a European (*The Log of Christopher Columbus,* 75). Like one major geological plate grinding against another, Europeans and indigenous peoples of North and South America encountered each other. The aftershocks persist among social groups and even within individuals.

This theme raises broader questions about the conflicts between groups, the extent to which an individual is defined by a group, and the gains and losses of cross-cultural influences.

The Family. This unit of society seems to be changing in the United States. Single-parent families, the most obvious example, are no longer the exception. What does the family mean to the individual? To society? How does a family stick together? When do family members support each other, when hinder? What kinds of families are there—nuclear, extended, those made up of friends or co-workers? Can the physical world itself be considered part of a family? *Stretch* takes a special interest in one member of the nuclear family, whether he is present or absent: the father.

Communicating. People communicate through a wealth of means, media, and channels. What different powers are enjoyed by communication both verbal (with words) and nonverbal (without words)? How does writing differ from speaking? How can writing work in partnership with the spoken word, or with images either still or moving?

In *Stretch* you will find communication in the form of a letter from a stolen child, an electron micrograph, a sketch, a movie poster, a video script, Daddy's scent, a president's voice, an orphan's dirty face, a fierce wooden mask, a squawking seagull, a gown on a guy, "someone dressed in a military uniform," a wart on a miller's nose, a tatoo on a thigh, and more.

Music. Overlapping with communication, music reaches the emotions right through the ears. With instruments alone, or together with words, images, or dance—how many times have you heard music this week? What does it mean to your life? How much variation can the term "music" cover? When do these invisible vibrations of air make groups more cohesive, in war or peace, through ritual or rap? When does music reflect disharmony between groups? How can music interact with writing?

World War II. The most important event of the twentieth century, World War II began in Europe on September 1, 1939, when the Nazi war machine rolled into Poland. The United States became involved when Japan sent an invitation by airmail on December 7, 1941.

During this six-year attempt at conquest, perhaps fifty million people were killed, many of them your age, often in a military or concentration camp uniform. *Stretch* can only hint at the war's toll on families. An educated person should know what this struggle revealed about human beings and their potential for evil and good.

These five themes will challenge you in an abundance of areas—history, ethics, communication, religion, sociology, geography, psychology, and empathy.

PAPERS WITH RESEARCH

Library research enriches *any* kind of writing, whether for a course, a job, a community or religious activity, or any other purpose. When writing the framework for an extemporaneous speech (one delivered from notes), you can do research to enhance your presentation. Even stories and informal essays can benefit from some unobtrusive background material:

Although ice skating originated approximately 1600 years ago in Scandinavia, for me it all began in 1974 in Canada at the tender age of three years.

Charlene Slugoski

To discover ideas, test them, and support them, there is nothing like a trip to the library. Its reference section alone holds an astonishing variety of general and specialized works, from the staid *Encyclopaedia Britannica* to *Rock On: The Illustrated Encyclopedia of Rock'n Roll*. Its audiovisual materials, books, journals, magazines, newspapers, government documents, and pamphlets help writers get beyond their own experience for background information, details, statistics, facts, quotations, interpretations, and contrasting views.

This material is accessible through on-line catalogues, CD-ROM indexes, printed resources, and the Internet. It comes in a variety of formats, from paper to microfilm, microfiche, or a downloaded disk. Reader-printers, photocopiers, VCRs, and personal computers let users carry material home.

FOUR POUNDS OF WORDS

The most frequent stretch you should make is to reach for a dictionary. You should own a college edition dictionary, up-to-date and hardbound. Indispensable for expressing yourself as a writer or speaker, it will also help you understand the verbal symbols of others as you read or listen.

For a contrast between verbal and nonverbal communication, starting with a "Singles Seeking" ad, read the next section of *Stretch*.

Works Cited

Columbus, Christopher. *The Log of Christopher Columbus*. Trans. Robert H. Fuson. Camden, ME: International Marine, 1987.

Nieman, David. *Fitness & Your Health*. Palo Alto, CA: Bull, 1993.

Why Write?

CUBAN AMERICAN

S ingle professional, 27, 5′9″, 155 lbs, moustache, beard, easygoing,
non-smoker, from Dade, seeks adventurous, educated SF to explore
South Florida's places and events on Harley-Davidson. Enjoys div-
ing, conversation, playing guitar, reggae, salsa.

In the "Singles Seeking" part of a newspaper, the writer hopes to
attract a companion. Using words, he describes his physical attributes
of gender, age, height, weight, facial appearance, and tobacco-free status. Each of these attributes, if encountered in person, would be conveyed to the senses, nonverbally. With words and without words: How
do these two types of communication differ? What are their unique
domains?

VERBAL VERSUS NONVERBAL POWERS

What exactly does *verbal* mean? In regular usage it indicates that something is spoken as opposed to written—such as an agreement confirmed by a handshake rather than a signature. However, the term also
has the special linguistic meaning of *communicated by words,* whether

✴ **1**

orally or in writing. (In fact, the word "verbal" comes from the Latin *verbum,* or "word.")

Nonverbal communication works by gestures, facial expressions, physique, skin color or tint, clothing and cosmetics, objects worn or handled (or ridden, like a motorcycle), distance between speakers, and vocal characteristics such as volume, tone, silence, and laughter. (See Figure 1 for a piercing example.) The physical setting, too, influences communication by suggesting what is appropriate or not.

Verbal and nonverbal communication often work together, as when people speak, so the two modes may be hard to differentiate. Here is one way to approach the distinction: Imagine yourself immersed in a rock concert with its rich appeal to the senses. Then, one by one, take away each stimulus that communicates something by means other than the symbolism of the words being sung.

First, remove the crowd. No more pleasurable subordination to the mass—to its motion, body heat, attention-getting dress, noise, and odors of beer, sweat, cigarette smoke, and perfume. Like a warm-up band, these ingredients all enhance the reception of the singers.

Then, remove the stage. Switch off the lighting that flashes from polished instruments and drenches the performers in color. Then unplug the electronic amplification; then stop all the music that vibrates from guitars, bass, drums, keyboard, and voices. Banish the band. Gone are the hairdos, earrings, and costumes; the skin colors or tints; the intense facial expressions; the hand gestures; the gripping, tilting, or waving of the microphone; the locomotion around the stage; the supercharged voices and unusual accents.

Now stand alone in the hall and read the lyrics silently. If you can ignore the imagined sound of your own unique vocal characteristics, you have pretty much reached the bare **verbal** part of the show. This is the meaning conveyed only by the words themselves: *Put-your-hands-together.*

For Better or For Worse®   by Lynn Johnston

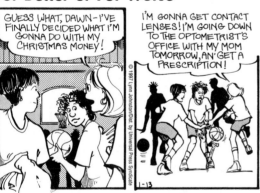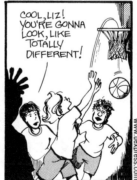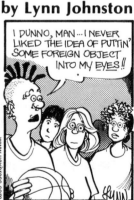

Fig. 1 ✳ NONVERBAL COMMUNICATION

Verbal messages are sent by a code. Known as language, its complicated rules of sound, vocabulary, and grammar allow users to manipulate experience symbolically. Language works by abstractions. These are concepts, like "reggae" or even "hair," which have no equivalent in the sensory world. Yes, they may represent physical things (such as hair) but the words are not the actual things. You can't comb the concept "hair."

Although you can ride a *particular* Harley—598 pounds in weight, patriot red pearl in color, with a 13400 cc. engine, leather saddlebags, 39,043 on the odometer, and a scratch on the back fender—you can't get far on the *abstraction* Harley-Davidson. It is imaginary. The abstraction is constructed by separating out features common to individual objects—Harleys that a person has encountered as opposed to other motorcycles—and creating an abstract category that does not exist in the sensory world. You cannot see the chrome, hear the rumble, grip the handlebars, smell the leather, or push the heavy weight of such a notion because it exists in the intellect as a symbolic representation.

In speaking, abstract ideas are represented to the ear by sounds. These are vibrations of the air caused by breath modified as it passes through the larynx, throat, mouth cavity, and nasal cavity and is shaped by the teeth and tongue. These vibrations have no intrinsic connection with the idea they represent. *Words* are not *things,* any more than the sounds *b-r-d* can fly. Spoken words—acoustic symbols—can in turn be represented to the eye by written marks. You started learning this visual code in grade school.

You have certain magical areas of your brain, generally in the left hemisphere, that can convert sound waves or visual squiggles to meaningful inner symbols. When you hear the sounds *b-r-d* or see the letters *bird,* you convert them to an idea. These neural centers can also generate spoken or written words from inner abstractions. So beginning with the stored concept of a feathered, winged animal, you can express it by the sounds *b-r-d* or by the marks *bird*.

Human beings can manipulate these symbols—by interpreting or generating them—like an expert on the abacus whose fingers can flick tokens around quicker than the eye can keep up. We use symbols to organize experience. Symbols, and the concepts they stand for, allow the motorcyclist at the beginning of the chapter to pass the time by remembering, ruminating, and reading signs. In "Dirty Little Faces," Robert D. Peterson may enjoy the Honduran orphans without understanding their Spanish (see Chapter 1), but he needs language to explore his trip's significance for himself as well as to communicate its significance to others.

Another way to think about language is to imagine a political map of the world. It draws arbitrary lines all over the seamless continents and then fills the many irregular shapes with different colors to define countries and states. For example, the country of Honduras is separated from other countries in Central America—Guatemala, El Salvador, and Nicaragua—by lines that nature does not know. Although like a jigsaw puzzle on paper, in an aerial photograph the shapes of these countries do not appear. In this rather capricious way language imposes borders on reality, which would otherwise be as undifferentiated as the middle of the Pacific Ocean.

Language imposes rules on the way its users see and interpret the world. That is, speakers agree to consider the colored-in shapes as reality. A language organizes experience into innumerable categories, and your map for English is your dictionary. So to a great extent our world is words.

We can sense the human origin of our own symbolic "reality" when we encounter a different map of the same terrain—that is, another language. For example, English speakers will assume that the concept of "liking" something or someone is a reflection of reality; Spanish speakers, however, search their verbal latitudes and longitudes in vain for such a concept. For in Spanish, people don't like something, *it pleases them.* The whole notion of the person as active agent in such a case does not exist. Conversely, where English stakes out part of the landscape with the single concept *bird,* Spanish uses two symbols to subdivide that territory into *el pájaro* (an everyday creature) and *el ave* (a rather scientific and literary one).

During World War II utterly incompatible language systems were put to work over the airwaves when Navajos communicated secret military information simply by speaking their native tongue, for the Japanese could not break this ready-made code.

A warning: Words vary in meaning even among speakers of the same language. Speakers may share only a core of a word's significance while they diverge as to the associations the word evokes. Why? Because of different temperaments, upbringing, and experiences. A tourist at the beach will more likely have positive associations with the word "seagull" than will the owner of an inland parking lot where the birds flock together to scavenge. The more controversial the notion, moreover, the less overlap of meaning among the users of the language. Was the Western Hemisphere "discovered" by Columbus? Does the term "Ireland" mean an island-country? Or an island that comprises two different social and political entities? (For this question, see Martin's paper on the I.R.A., Chapter 7.) What might the concept "baby" mean to those who wish to outlaw induced abortions? To those who wish to keep the procedure legal?

People disagree not only about word-borders but even about the very existence of many a word-place. Is there such a thing as the "master race" so vaunted by the Nazis—that is, an Aryan, non-Semitic, and non-Negroid race? Is there even such a thing as race? (Some recent studies show no genetic basis in traditional distinctions.) Is there really such a thing as attention deficit disorder? As sociobiological behavior (inborn social tendencies that have enabled animal species to survive)? As "hell"?

Words: Ghostly when compared to sensory nonverbal signals, arbitrary as to how they divide up the world, and slippery as to what they mean. Yet despite all these liabilities, verbal communication has clout:

Precision. It can be much more exact than nonverbal. Nonverbal signals can be easily misinterpreted, so the motorcyclist is more likely to be a dentist than a marauder. (In fact, a person's life can depend on misread appearances. See Salomea Kape's true story in the Additional Readings.) And words can handle more complex material: For all their unreliability, verbal abstractions allow the motorcyclist to work out an itinerary with his companion, study the guidelines for a new dental anesthetic, or compose a "singles" ad.

Consciousness. Another strength of the verbal: Words generally have some conscious purpose and can be more tightly controlled, whereas nonverbal signals are often given off unintentionally and are radiated at all times. In the dental office the motorcyclist hopes that his clothing, posture, speech, gestures, and facial expressions help to convey the impression of competence, but he cannot stop his nonverbal behavior or even fully monitor it. When Lacretia stands alone by the fence at recess (see Greene in Additional Readings), she has no choice but to give off nonverbal information about her social status.

Independence. And verbal symbols, unlike nonverbal, don't always depend on a physical context. In Chapter 2 a fellow makes a nonverbal statement that requires makeup, gown, and the presence of an audience. But words can deal with something that is out of sight and with someone who is out of the picture. The motorcyclist can ask directions to Tucson or, when he arrives, send a postcard to a friend, and even direct a "singles" ad to a person he doesn't know.

Complex material sooner or later comes down to those densely packed information-carriers known as words, whether written or spoken. Even videotape productions require a script, and on the Internet, pictures, colors, music, and animated graphics can go only so far.

WRITING VERSUS SPEAKING

Then if words are so powerful, what are the advantages of the written word over the spoken?

For one thing, the writer and reader don't have to be in the same room or on the same telephone line. And the written word usually allows people more time to compose a message than the spoken. Writing "spells it out," literally and figuratively, by organizing ideas, drawing on a wider vocabulary, and using a tighter, more varied grammar. It also uses uniform conventions of grammar to avoid distracting the reader with regional or other variations. And it uses paragraphing to help signal a change of idea. For more on the contrast between speaking and writing, please read the sidebar.

Another advantage of writing: It tends to make greater use of imaginative imagery than does speaking, which tolerates cliches like "the whole ball of wax" and "To make a long story short." And writing stays safely on the page, in the filing cabinet, on the bulletin board, on the disk or hard drive, or on the marble monument, when the sound waves produced by the voice have long since faded away like last year's fireworks.

A reader, furthermore, unlike a listener, can set his or her own pace so as to speed up or poke along. As you know from studying textbooks, a reader can

Doonesbury

BY GARRY TRUDEAU

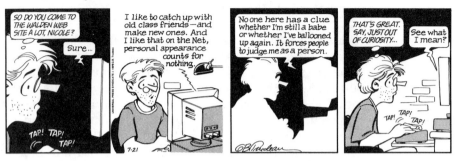

Fig. 2 ✳

also go back over material and even highlight or annotate it. No rewinding necessary.

Finally, for you as a writer, the keyboard or pen can go beyond the mere recording of thought to the generating of thought. This power is magnified by research and revision.

Granted, writing can be tedious. This second code—invented not for the ear but for the eye, like the grids and circles of a musical score—requires that you master a whole set of visual conventions: letters, spelling, punctuation, mechanics, and paragraphing.

But suppose you look at writing in another way. It allows you to fashion marks that stand for speech, without a sound and even without the presence of a sender. It is almost occult in its power. Existing for only about 8,000 years, writing is fairly new to *homo sapiens,* the only species able to use it. Even now millions of people around the world, far from being able to create these meaningful scribbles, look on them with no more comprehension than the blind.

So with its power to generate and articulate thought, its range of vocabulary, grammar, and imagery, its convenience and endurance, what can really rock-'n-roll but the written word.

FATHER'S HOMEMADE HOG FEED

Here is an excerpt from a tape-recorded interview that has been transcribed. The subject is an eighty-five-year-old former nurse and midwife, Ms. Janie Johnson, who was born in 1906. Answering a question, she speaks with admiration about her father, a successful African-American farmer. Notice how her everyday speech—like everybody's—is spontaneous, tentative, and loosely connected:

He would cook his feed that he would feed his hogs with. He would cook his—put sweet potatoes, corn, and peas together. And then he would put so much syrup in. He'd put it in a big containerlike—barrel, and he would feed his hogs like—he would feed 'em through the year. Then at a certain time, be November, maybe, or first of December, he would kill his hogs for, you know, meat for the next year. A cow was the same way. And I know the time that he would butcher cows, and you could hang 'em up in the smokehouse and dry it. But you hang up somethin' now. . . .

Notice that Ms. Johnson relies heavily on coordination—sentences that repeat the same subject ("He. . . . He") as well as clauses connected by the conjunction "and." Speakers tend to favor this principle more than writers, who use more frequent subordination to help to indicate logical relationships.

And everyday speech tends to overlook fuzzy connections between pronouns and what they stand for, as in the phrases "put it" (sentence 4) and "dry it" (next-to-last sentence), where the word *it* has vague antecedents.

To illustrate another quality of the spoken word: The last sentence relies on the intonation of voice as much as its verbal content to get its implication across.

Here is a version of Ms. Johnson's response that is meant to be read. Tightened up in various ways, it shifts emphasis from her authentic, impromptu way of speaking to her historical information:

He would cook the feed that he gave to his hogs. To make it he would combine sweet potatoes, corn, and peas, then add a certain amount of syrup. He'd put the mixture in a large barrel from which he would feed his hogs throughout the year.

Then at a certain time, perhaps November or the first of December, he would kill his hogs for the next year's meat. He did the same with his cows. In those days, when you butchered cows, you could hang the meat up in the smokehouse to dry. But if you were to do so now, you might get into trouble with the law.

Although some of the charm has disappeared from the original, there are no distractions from the remembered information. Writing is a promise to be more careful than speaking. Unlike speech, which must have some human spontaneity, writing can sound like a book. It can please by making departures from everyday speech: its grammar artfully varied for emphasis and variety, its vocabulary right from the SAT practice guide, its thought more studied than spontaneous. Here, for example, is a more highly crafted version of Ms. Johnson's account:

He would cook a feed for his hogs made from sweet potatoes, corn, peas—and just so much syrup. This concoction he would put in a large barrel from which he would supply the animals, vegetarians all, throughout the year. Then in late November or early December he would slaughter his hogs, along with his cows, for the next year's meat. In those days a person could hang the meat up in the smokehouse to dry; today, such a practice would be regarded with a jaundiced eye by the health inspector.

A footnote: Writing can often please with speechlike echoes, such as asking questions, addressing the reader, moving to a new paragraph by a surprising association of ideas, and using a zingy sentence fragment.

Work Cited

Johnson, Janie B. Interview. Bayboro, SC, 25 October 1991. Horry County Oral History Project.

Work Consulted

Knapp, Mark L. *Essentials of Nonverbal Communication.* New York: Holt, 1980.

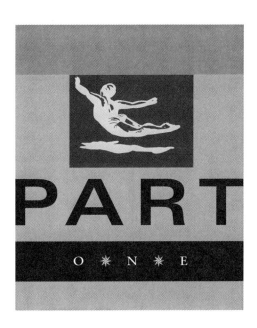

Explore

Exploratory writing, as defined in this book, shares the writer's firsthand experience; or it emphasizes the writer's personality in the process of interacting with a subject; or it does both. You may have tried this type of writing in journals and in freewriting exercises. This part of *Stretch* includes three more kinds, "The Story," "The Meditation," and "The Informal Essay."

Any act of writing evokes thought: Word by word, sometimes tentatively, sometimes surely, the unknown becomes filled in, ordered, shaped. Although a revision looks as if it came off the pen without labor, a draft is a process of trial and error. Research can make a "discovery draft" even more time-consuming, substantial, and stimulating.

But sometimes a writer wants to preserve a sense of this exploration in the finished product. He or she tries to give readers the impression that they are involved in the very process of creation rather than presented with a map already drawn. Here is an extreme example of ideas being generated, a nonstop list of *I Don't Likes*:

I don't like trigonometry, taking notes, not knowing anyone in my class, people who are rude to me, my steak well-done, lobster with no butter, my car, waiting, Pythagorean identities, losing an earring, not having a tan, holes in my socks, ex-boyfriends, grime along the door of my shower, forgetting to shave my legs, criticism, writer's block, getting home early, having no money, being blackballed, losing friends, drunk drivers, suicide, big guns, atomic bombs, peace signs, flower children, Vietnam, champagne, tequila, Canadian beer, hot beer, the food in Spain, the dirty people in France, being broke in London, the Greek alphabet, the fact that ALPHA-BETA comes from Greek, guys with bleached hair, rednecks, getting up early, not having the nerve to get to know someone better, running out of time on the challenge course, being cold, not having someone to warm me up, writing on the last line of my paper, cleaning my room, waiting for the phone to ring, being shuffled by a computer, posers, losing things, missing out, being finished, taking out the garbage, doing the dishes, feeling incompetent, fighting with my parents, mosquitos, insects in general, the threat of war, the boulevard, my curfew, getting caught, brown, orange, my freckles, baseball, no, car insurance payments, being held back, being pushed too hard, term papers, staying after school, misprints, plaids, being embarrassed, not being able to see the chalkboard, "Fergie" bows, getting yelled at, water in my ears. ◆

Michele Paddy

If this series holds some charm for you, can you tell why? In its sequence? In its substance?

Unlike singing and swallowing, writing and exploring can happen at the same time. Whether you want to trace the coastline of a subject or probe inland on the canoe of thought, a ballpoint or keyboard offers a paddle.

Exploratory does not mean dreamy. The following excerpt, for example, comes from a reminiscence about friends who spent summer hours climbing a tree to a swing and dropping into the water. The passage helps to recapture details of the happy experience by precise technical description:

The treehouse over the Waccamaw River was roughly constructed of lumber that had been "found" after Hurricane Hugo. At the height of its glory there were six separate decks: the main deck, the outhouse deck (complete with privacy curtain), the boat deck, and three levels from which to swing, the highest towering twenty feet into the muggy air. The decks wound around and through the edge of a cypress swamp, creating a cool haven on any ninety-degree day. From a distance it looked like a glorified treehouse. The actual swing was a two-and-a-half foot long iron trapeze-bar clamped to an inch-wide cable. The cable hung from the bough of a cypress tree, which was at least a century older than any of the Huck Finn wannabes swinging from its limbs, and which extended about fifteen feet over the water. From the top level, the peak of your outward swoop would be thirty to forty feet above the water. ◆

Amy C. Weaver

Amy tried several times to get the measurements right and the details complete, and her work paid off because the abundance of objective information complements her charming stylistic touches.

Light can be thrown on exploratory writing by contrast with a workaday form called the business memorandum. Used by all kinds of business, professional, and governmental organizations, the memo is a package. It comes tightly wrapped with four strands of tape: **DATE:, TO:, FROM:,** and **SUBJECT:.** The memo concisely expresses something the writer has settled upon. Downplaying the sender's personality, it addresses some practical matter.

Exploratory writing, on the other hand, values the personal over the impersonal, the leisurely over the efficient, the unfolding process over the finished product.

Nevertheless, despite its differences in aim and style, the memo can illuminate exploratory writing if its four components are applied to the topic:

> **DATE:** Exploratory writing may try to make sense of today—that is, of some current event, situation, or issue. Or it may use today's perspective to revisit the past for more understanding.

> **TO:** Exploratory writing is intended for a reader who, by temperament or circumstance, values a little entertainment. The reader does not look for strictly functional information, a solution to a problem, or one side of an issue. The reader tolerates some uncertainty in the writer, values some personality, and expects some artistry.

> **FROM:** The writer wants to emphasize his or her uniqueness—in experience, personality, process of thought, talent. His or her purpose is to share an experience—or the experience of discovery—more than to transfer information or carry a point.

> **SUBJECT:** In exploratory writing, the writer may speak about himself or herself, but he or she need not do so as long as a portrait emerges of an individual engaged with the world. So SUBJECT overlaps with FROM. The writer makes little pretense of objectivity. ◆

You should realize that when writing outside of the academic situation, you will generally enjoy a clearer sense of an audience. Such a limitation will actually help you develop ideas that will be appropriate and effective for the circumstances.

What are some ways to discover topics and approaches for an exploratory paper? Here is a list of heuristic techniques. Many of them will also help you generate ideas for the other kinds of writing discussed in *Stretch*.

Read. To get outside of your own experience and outlook, do some reading in print or pixel. Looking at an article in a general or specialized encyclopedia will enrich your understanding of a topic and suggest ideas for focusing on one manageable aspect. A book of quotations on a subject is a jewelry box full of glittering insights and phrasings. Look through articles, reports, essays, editorials, laws, documents, diaries, pamphlets, statistical tables, maps, and photographs.

You might also read the brief treatise on methods of development on p. 93. And you might scan Chapter 2, "The Meditation," for help with moving from particulars to significance.

Write. For ten minutes or so, write down everything that comes to mind about a subject in sentences and phrases. Don't stop moving the pen because you want to encourage fluency of thought. Look back at what you have written: If you find something that seems to offer special promise, narrow to that aspect and freewrite about it for ten more minutes.

Or start at an inviting access point: something that most appeals to you, puzzles you, bothers you, surprises you.

Generate a list like the one at the beginning of this preface. Try for variety and abundance, an overflowing horn of plenty.

Write a scratch outline that divides up a subject into its most important parts. For an example, see the Web page on p. 154. Should you narrow your topic to one of the subdivisions? In turn, perhaps break this part down into subdivisions?

Write the points you would want to cover in a Web site, including a few links to related material.

Write a double-voice piece on the subject like Melissa Bjorklund's in the Additional Readings. Two points of view will help to move you off center by revealing complexity and stimulating thought.

Write a dialogue. Create two people who explore a topic or debate it. (For an example, see the excerpt from Plato in the Additional Readings.) The two characters can even be aspects of yourself.

Write a letter. This technique gives you a reader to visualize who will therefore prompt you as to what to say.

Talk. "Nobody ever learned anything by talking." This maxim, intended to vaunt the power of listening, is inaccurate. Like writing, talking forces us to articulate our ideas about a subject through verbal symbols. Talking can generate more precise and more profound thought.

So if you discuss a subject with other people, you will understand it better just by formulating words about it.

You might "talk" with other people in a chat room on the World Wide Web. Remember, though, that anonymity offers them extra incentive either to lie or to tell the truth.

You might even talk into a tape recorder. It's an audience of sorts that enables you to think out loud.

Listen. Your ears will enrich your paper. You may be surprised as people share their experiences, outlooks, and associations with you. You might also ask for their comments on your first draft.

Perhaps conduct an interview: Come informed about the subject through background reading so you can ask profitable questions and follow them up. Talk only enough to keep goodwill and encourage responses.

Ask for more details if the speaker abandons a profitable line of thought, and don't be afraid to cut off rambling (tactfully). Get the correct spelling of names. Let the interviewee check your final product for accuracy.

Watch. An ever-growing collection of audiovisual material may be threatening to burst its corner of the library. Take a look at the range of videotapes available and watch one on your topic. Not long ago, this enjoyable way of learning was unavailable to students.

Cube. Please see the sidebar on cubing.

Imagine. Imagine how your topic could be viewed by two widely different people. A related question: How would you develop your topic differently for two different audiences?

Let a sharp image come to mind and explore its significance to your topic. It may concretely suggest important values. Try another image and ponder its importance to the whole.

What sounds come to your memory as you think of this topic? What kind of musical score would you use for a film on this topic? (This question might help you determine the most desirable tone for your paper.) If you were to direct such a film, what would its main focus be? Its opening sequence? Its most powerful scenes?

Think of your subject as a board game. What does the board look like? What is the goal? What are the rules? Who are the players? What are the risks, the lucky and bad breaks, the strategies? Or think of it as a game show on television and ask the equivalent questions.

Imagine a painting—a still life, landscape, outdoor or indoor scene, or portrait: What would capture something of importance to the subject to inspire writing? What would you paint on a mural?

Create a mental montage. Arrange a variety of images or items (or both) characteristic of the subject in a way to explore its complex identity.

Dance is a basic human form of expression; imagine one that helps to explore a subject. Specify the dancers, costumes, music, groupings, and movements.

Whenever you write about one vital aspect of experience—people—you may want to call to mind their unique style of nonverbal communication. Paradoxically, words have great power to describe the *nonverbal*. Writing can select details, present them vividly to the senses, imply significance, evoke emotional nuances. A novel is a nonverbal encyclopedia. (For more help on this subject, see "Why Write?")

Cluster. Please see Figure 6.1. This technique of generating ideas with radiating lines and circles can help you find a topic or develop one. It can work by logical division or by psychological association. For example, a topic such as "Guitars" can be formally divided into acoustic and electric, then further subdivided as to types (six-string versus twelve-string, etc.); or the topic can be expanded by personal associations such as taking guitar lessons, playing in the youth group at a church or synagogue, even hitchhiking more successfully with an empty guitar case.

Write. Get a first draft down on paper or screen. Don't worry about starting it with a perfect introduction because the evolving material will probably cause you to go back to modify your beginning.

Quit. Give your brain a rest. Have a good night's sleep and come back refreshed to your preliminary notes, rough draft, or final draft (if you plan to revise it). A little vacation will help you with precise thought, effective organization, and forceful style.

CUBING

Cubing is a process of looking at a topic as if it were a die being turned over to reveal each of its six sides. Instead of dots, each side has a suggestion. This method can be illustrated most easily with a concrete subject like a musical instrument. Let's try the acoustic guitar:

Describe It. Technically: measurements, weight, materials. Aesthetically: to the eye, a pleasing synthesis of line, form, volume, texture, and color. To the ear, a mellow twang, sometimes punctuated with raps on the side.

Compare or Contrast It. To items in same or similar class: lute, electric guitar, piano; cheaper versus more expensive models. To unlike classes: gourd, front-strapped papoose, lover.

Free Associate It. See above.

Analyze It. Into parts: neck, pegs, strings, resonance chamber, and so on. Or into processes: of making sounds; of learning to play step by step; of building a guitar; its history.

Argue For or Against. Portable (unlike piano). Good solo instrument. Two can play guitars together easily. Players can sing while strumming. Good for popular, folk, or classical music. Can learn basics quickly.

Apply or Use It. Good for parties, solo company, family time.

Exploratory writing, as with every aim and type discussed in *Stretch*, can blend with others. (For example, read Michael H. Robinson's meditative-narrative-explanatory-argumentative piece about bird-brains in the Additional Readings.) An author may seek an air of spontaneity, ask questions, delay stating a point, or move unpredictably from one phase to the next, perhaps more by psychological association than by rigorous logic. So the next few chapters not only will give you experience with altogether exploratory pieces but will offer you techniques that can grace other writing with touches of spontaneity and personality.

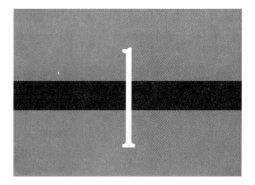

The Story

"**W**hat happened next?"

With its insistent forward-moving appeal to readers or listeners, the story explores the world for vividness and significance. A good story gets attention, builds interest, stirs the feelings, and enlarges understanding. Typically it works by narrowing the events to be covered, defining the characters and setting, and ordering the presentation of events so as to bring about an intended impact.

But like language itself, the story has a problematic relationship to reality: Depending on one's perspective, it can be true, false, or fictional. It can both reflect life and affect it. A dramatic example of all these qualities is furnished by the group of myths that surround Quetzalcóatl, the Feathered Serpent, who was priest-king of the Toltecs in Mexico:

He never offered human victims, only snakes, birds, and butterflies. But the god of the night sky, Tezcatlipoca . . . , expelled him from Tula [capital of the Toltecs] by performing feats of black magic. Quetzalcóatl wandered down to the coast of the "divine water" (the Atlantic Ocean) and then immolated himself on a pyre, emerging as the planet Venus. According to another version, he embarked upon a raft made of snakes and disappeared beyond the eastern horizon.

The legend of the victory of Tezcatlipoca over the Feathered Serpent probably reflects historical fact. . . . [Quetzalcóatl's] sea voyage to the east should probably be connected with the invasion of Yucatán by the Itzá. . . . Quetzalcóatl's calendar name was Ce Acatl (One Reed). The belief that he would return from the east in a One Reed year led the Aztec sovereign Montezuma II to regard the Spanish conqueror Hernán Cortés and his comrades as divine envoys, because 1519, the year in which they landed on the Mexican gulf coast, was a One Reed year.

"Quetzalcóatl" 855

To the Aztecs this story, in one version or another, told the truth about a god-like, animal-like figure whom most people of the present day would regard as fictional. Yet there does seem to be historical fact perceptible through the distorting lens of myth. Moreover, the story then affected historical events by making Montezuma II more receptive to the conquistadors, who unwittingly disembarked during one of Quetzalcóatl's special years.

Like the myths of the Feathered Serpent, stories can be traditional in the sense that they arise anonymously and circulate orally from one generation to another. Of course, narrative is often the basis of carefully researched historiography—the writing of history. Stories can not only explain but preserve: Laurie Ann Occhipinti's account of her grandparents during World War II (Chapter 5) keeps alive family memories. Stories can also give bite to an argument, like Jing Dai's personal testimony against tracking in school (Chapter 6).

Stories can be realistic, highly imaginative, even allegorical—having a systematic correspondence between surface details and concepts. For example, in *The Pilgrim's Progress,* by John Bunyon, the main character, Christian, treks toward the Celestial City, along the way encountering places like the Slough of Despond and characters like the Giant Despair. Such physical entities represent theological ideas (Part 1, 1678). As with *Pilgrim's Progress,* stories can blend sharp, everyday details with unworldly fantasy.

A story can make use of prose or verse. It can be *narrated* (i.e., told, as in "Once upon a time"), whether by speaking, writing, chanting, or singing. Or it can be *dramatized*—acted out—whether by humans, puppets, or animated characters. It can be wholly sung (as in an opera) or partly sung (as in a stage musical). It can be read aloud, as the phenomenon of books-on-tape can attest.

Stories can be told without words. They can be carved into marble, expressed by a series of drawings, or conveyed by masked dancers, as in the poem that ends Chapter 2. (For the account of a dance that portrays the conflict between Disease and the medicine man, see Jeffery Gilbert's story in the Additional Readings.) Stories can even be pantomimed by ice skaters whirling atop a four-layer surface of the kind illustrated on p. 116.

A story can draw emotional power from background music, like the television series *Victory at Sea,* which began in 1952 and featured a score by Richard Rodgers. It can even be expressed by music alone, like Moussorgsky's *A Night on Bare Mountain,* a symphonic version of a Russian legend.

Fig. 1.1 ✳ POSTER FOR MOVIE *SANTA*, 1931

Starring Lupita Tovar. Directed by Antonio Moreno. Black and white. "This movie served as the cornerstone of the Mexican sound-film industry" (program note).

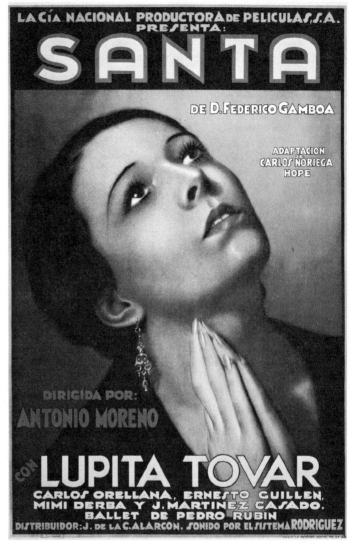

A story can be retold in different versions, so that depending on which myth was believed, Quetzalcóatl met his demise on either a pyre or a raft. Medieval England's Chaucer usually took earlier tales and combined or otherwise rewrote them. So robust are stories, with their conflicts, characters, scenes, surprises, and insights, that many have been adapted successfully from one mode to another. *A Night on Bare Mountain* was illustrated by an animated cartoon in Walt Disney's movie *Fantasia*. A story by Federico Gamboa was transformed into the movie *Santa* (*Saint*):

This tale of a small-town girl, fated to become the star attraction of a Mexico City brothel, solidly established in the cinema a preoccupation of Mexican literature and culture—that of the young woman, seduced and abandoned, then left to her own devices in a society that rejects "used" women.

Program note.

For a poster of this film, see Figure 1.1.

As another example of adaptation, one probably closer to your moviegoing experience, Louisa May Alcott's novel *Little Women,* published in 1869, enjoyed its most recent movie version in 1994. The screenplay for this music was in turn transformed back into a novel—a brief, simplified tale directed to young people. You might read an excerpt from Alcott's book in Additional Readings and then read a scene from it that has been rewritten by two students, Gary Walker and Diana Jo Wilson, also in Additional Readings.

In whatever version or mode of presentation, what is a story? How does it command attention and keep interest? To help you write an engaging story, take a look at the sidebar for a helpful structure.

CLASSIC STORY STRUCTURE

Your story should seek its own most effective shape rather than follow a preconceived formula. The basic pattern of many stories, however, can be approximated by the following graph. Take from it what helps, diverge from it when necessary:

Here is a brief explanation of these phases.

First the background is established—geographical, social, psychological. Then something complicates the status quo by triggering a conflict or problem. Suspense rises as the characters grapple with some force, and their conflict may result in one or more crises—times when great pressure forces a revelation, decision, action, or the like. At the highest stage of interest, the climax, the pressure is greatest and the outcome is determined. Finally the resolution, a falling-off of tension, reveals the outcome.

For more helpful theory, see **Tips for Prose** at the end of this chapter.

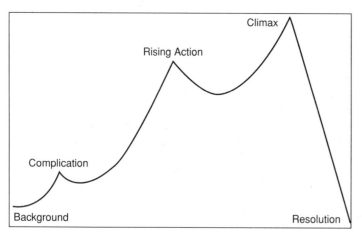

BACKGROUND, COMPLICATION, RISING ACTION, CLIMAX, RESOLUTION

By yourself—or working with a classmate or two—take another look at the "Singles Seeking" ad that begins the previous section of this book. Then imagine the first uncertain meeting of the motorcyclist with his adventurous SF, continuing to do so as you write. Include description and dialogue.

PUBLISHED STORY

This narrative comprises Chapter 21 of *Andele, the Mexican-Kiowa Captive: A Story of Real Life among the Indians,* published in 1899. The biography was written by Rev. J. J. Methvin, evidently on the basis of interviews with Andele—in modern parlance, "as told to" the author.

The author served as superintendent of Methvin Institute, a missionary school for Indians in Anadarko, Oklahoma Territory. There he encountered Andele who, as a boy named Andrés, had been kidnapped from New Mexico by members of one tribe and then traded to another. Andele had lived as a Kiowa (rhymes with Iowa) for almost twenty years, until the time of this account.

Comments in the margin are meant to help you appreciate the unfolding nature of the storytelling. Feel free to come back later to read these notes.

LIGHT DAWNING

✳

J. J. Methvin

This chapter evidently has a theme that interprets the events as an awakening of some kind.

Andele had for years lived a veritable Indian. Yet, as the years rolled by, he saw the wretchedness of the Indian life and became disgusted with it. Nevertheless some of the Indian ways had become his fixed habit, and any effort to change them by others offended him.

The background is given in summary form. The protagonist is frustrated: On the one hand he feels disgust at Indian ways, and on the other he resists changing them out of pride and habit.

But light was beginning to dawn upon him. He could see as far as he had been brought into contact with them, the strength and thrift of the white men, and he had gone at one time with an Indian wagon train two hundred miles away to Caddo, and had seen there a railroad train. It set him to thinking that there must be something better for him than wandering in blanket and wild robe over the prairies like the wild buffalo. The buffalo were fast being killed out by the restless, aggressive white man, and it was probable that the Indian would go likewise, unless there was a change; for the white man seemed as glad to kill an Indian as a buffalo.

A "one day" narration is more fully dramatized and relates a turning point: Andele resolves to work like a white man, however out of place he looks.

One day he heard the United States agent, George Hunt, talking to the Indians through an interpreter. He said:

"The Great Father at Washington wants all your young men to learn how to work, so that they may make money and have homes and be peaceable."

That same day he took an interpreter to the agent and explained what he wanted, and asked for work. He was put into the government blacksmith shop to learn that trade. He was a wild looking spectacle, and awkward enough in a blacksmith shop with all his Indian paraphernalia on, full rigged and ornamented. But he was honest and earnest in his purpose to learn, and soon began to show progress.

In a surprising turn, Andele is introduced to another custom of Europeans, writing. This phenomenon works as a catalyst for further awakening, this time to his Hispanic past.

New things were constantly opening to him as he was brought more directly in contact with the whites, when one day he happened to be in the store of an Indian trader where a post office had been established. He had seen people trading with the merchants, receiving goods over the counter for which they paid money, but he noticed now the merchant seemed to be handing out things for which the people paid nothing. He could not understand it, and his curiosity was so much excited, that he asked the blacksmith, under whom he worked, what it meant. The blacksmith answered that the people were getting messages from their friends; that people could talk on paper to one another although they were a long distance apart. He said no more, but it awakened a hope and set him to thinking, and thus he soliloquized:

"Long years ago, I was stolen from my home. The Apaches stole me. Now, as I think of it, it all comes fresh to my memory. The Indians call me Andele, but my name is Andrés. My father, who was he?"

This crisis leads to a more poignant turning point when he remembers a key word. Suspense continues: Will he be reunited with his original family?

He sat straining his memory, going back, back, over the wild scenes of his Indian life, through the years since he was stolen by the Mescaleros in the little vega [meadow] where he tended the cows.

"Who was my father?" and occasionally memory would almost catch back the long forgotten name, but then—

"Now I have it!" he exclaimed. "I remember now, it is Martínez. Martínez, Martínez; yes, that is it," and he continued to pronounce it, lest it should slip from him again.

It was night, and he went to his bed and lay down, but could not sleep. His mind was full of thoughts of home, mother, the scenes of his childhood. Memories long since dead were revived. He lay there wondering, and the more he thought, the more wide awake and restless he became. Hope began to spring up in his heart, and he arose and made his way at that late hour to the sleeping apartment of the United States physician, Dr. Hugh Tobin. He rapped at the door, when Dr. Tobin bade him come in; for although it was late, he had not yet retired.

Methvin goes into detail about Andele's emotional and physical turmoil, evoking sympathy from the reader. He continues to emphasize the importance of this day, which began at the trader's store, by using plenty of dialogue to dramatize Andele's visit to Dr. Tobin.

"Why, what brings you here at this late hour, Andele? Anybody sick?" asked Dr. Tobin, in the Comanche dialect; for he and Andele both had some knowledge of that language.

"I am come," replied Andele, "to tell you something that disturbs me much, and keeps me from sleeping. I am, as you know, a Mexican captive. I learned today that people may communicate with their friends on paper through the post office. I have been thinking it may be possible for me to find out my people from whom I was stolen long years ago when I was a small child. Do you think I could?" and he looked anxiously and intently into Dr. Tobin's face as he asked the question.

"Do you remember the place where your father lived, and do you remember your father's name?" asked Dr. Tobin.

"I have been lying awake on my bed, thinking, thinking, oh, so hard, and at last my father's name has come to me. It is Martínez, and the place close to our home was Las Vegas, and my oldest brother was named Dionicio. I remember him well, now."

"Well," said Dr. Tobin, "we will write to your brother, because if your father was an old man at the time of your capture, he is probably dead ere this."

"Will you please write now," asked Andele, as his heart beat in ever increasing interest.

"I will," said Dr. Tobin, and he turned to his desk and penned the following brief note:

KIOWA AND COMANCHE U.S. AGENCY,
ANADARKO, IND. TER., JAN. 6, 1883.

DIONICIO MARTÍNEZ,

LAS VEGAS, N.M.

DEAR SIR: Did you have a little brother stolen by the Indians many years ago, by name Andrés? The Indians call him Andele. If so, write me at once. He is here, and we think can be identified fully.

Respectfully,

HUGH TOBIN,

U.S. Physician.

"Now," said Dr. Tobin, "this letter will reach Las Vegas in about ten days, and if your brother is there, he will get it. In thirty days this letter will come back if your brother don't get it. Be patient and we shall hear."

Will the discovery of "talking on paper" lead to the recovery of a lost family? The account of this day in Andele's life comprises more than half of the story. It may be the climax.

Andele went back to his own bed, but he could not sleep. The vague memories of the long ago came flooding his mind and heart, growing more and more distinct, till they stood before him as but the happenings of yesterday. After a month had elapsed, the letter came back, not having been called for at Las Vegas. It was a sore disappointment, for Andele felt confident that it would reach his brother. Dr. Tobin encouraged him to hope, and he wrote the second letter, but it, too, came back after some delay. But Andele seemed more determined to hear from his people, and he continued to send letters for nearly two years, till one day, Dionicio Martínez, who had years before moved with his family to Trinidad, happened to be on a visit to his mother in Las Vegas, and received Andele's letter.

Andele's persistence evokes admiration, sympathy, and suspense.

He did not break the seal of the letter till he reached the house and sat down near his mother. He was so astonished when he read the letter, he could scarcely restrain an outcry; but fearing lest the news should too deeply affect his old white-haired mother, he, with a great effort, tried to conceal his emotions. The quick eye of the mother detected something unusual, and she asked:

"What is it, my son? Is there some evil news in your letter? Is some one sick? Tell me at once, for I see something is wrong."

"No, mother," said Dionicio, "no evil news but good news. I hardly know how to tell you. Will you please nerve yourself to hear something that will surprise you much?"

"Well, tell me quick, for you hold me in suspense."

"Mother, will you be prepared to hear that our little Andrés, whom the Indians stole long years ago, is still living and here is a letter from—"

Although perhaps the climax of the story, this scene is more likely the resolution. However touching, it is less fully developed and more external than the trader-Tobin episode.

But before he could finish the sentence the white-haired mother had swooned away, and was falling from her chair. It was an affecting scene, and here we draw the curtain.

Questions

1. Since Andele and Dr. Tobin do not speak the same language, how do they communicate verbally?

2. What are the major scenes re-created? Why does the author put such emphasis on them?

3. What is the central conflict, if any? Do you observe an important outer conflict, a socioeconomic one? Inner conflict, a psychological and emotional one?

4. Both Andele and the central character of the movie *Santa* find themselves abandoned in one sense or another. But instead of "An Awakening," what does the saint-to-prostitute experience? If you were to draw a graph representing the direction of their lives—saint and Indian—how would the direction of the lines contrast?

5. Where does this story seem to reflect the assumptions of the era? About Native Americans? About narrative style?

The Additional Readings have several pieces that have ties with this story: Read the European Michel de Montaigne's reaction to "these lately discovered nations" back in the 1500s. For the story of a young white man's encounter with a present-day Native American and his tribe, see Jeffery Gilbert's "Conversations with Lehlooskah." And for a letter sent to a lost family member after World War II, see Salomea Kape's "Designer Genes."

Consider the Themes

* How does the theme of the encounter between European and Native American have a twist or two in the whole story of Andrés-Andele-Andrés? (To begin with, can you distinguish between outer and inner encounters?)

* How might a member of Andele's Kiowa tribe tell the story with a different slant?

* Regarding communication, in what ways do personal letters influence the re-Europeanization of Andele-Andrés?

STUDENT NARRATIVE 1

This account of the writer's trip from Rockford, Illinois, to Central America subordinates the question "What will happen next?" to the question "What was the meaning of the experience?"

DIRTY LITTLE FACES
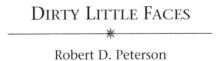

Robert D. Peterson

Staring through the thin wire fence on the roof top, I saw a universe of little lights scaling the hillside. It was a beautiful array of colors and lights. What a false perception the night can give to gullible eyes. When the morning sun arose over the town of Tegucigalpa the hundreds of captivating lights seen the night before were gone only to leave behind a poverty stricken city. How tempting it was for me to turn away from the slums by closing my eyes to see the night lights once more.

Tegucigalpa, the capital of Honduras, was a culture shock that I thought I would never see other than on television specials that I would quickly flip by. I guess I should not have been surprised, seeing that

Honduras is one of the poorest countries in the western hemisphere as well as in Central America. I can still see the faces of young children begging to carry my luggage in hope for some change as I walked out of the airport. The poverty of these people was tremendous. Families lived in houses the size of a one car garage, made out of sheets of metal strapped together. They had enough clothes to cover themselves and plenty of food to survive. It still amazes me that their life expectancy is as high as it is, fifty-six years.

Despite their circumstances the Honduran people still contained a glow that you could always see in their eyes. They possessed a joy that is very hard to find in the prosperous country of the United States. I remember watching a friend of mine teaching a young Honduran boy the game of marbles with some of the few toys the young boy had, rocks. They drew a circle in the dirt and played that game for an hour or more, and I remember the joy that my friend received from the excitement that the little boy had from learning a new game and making a new friend.

The people we met gave us so much more from nothing than we could have ever given them from something. I found this to be true especially at the orphanage we visited, which was one of the most powerful parts of our mission's trip. There were children as old as twelve and others who were just infants. As my group approached the gate, a hundred or so dirty little faces appeared at the bars to greet us with an excitement and happiness I had never seen before. They knew no English and we knew very little Spanish. The few hours we were there we communicated and had fun without the use of words. They had no family, no money, no shoes, a few scraps of clothes, and no realistic future other than a low paying job to live on. Despite their lack of material items, the only thing these children really wanted was to be loved. So for the few hours we were there my group loved these children as much as we could. Many of them just wanted to be held or sit on your lap. Others wanted to wrestle with you like brothers do, but all of them wanted us to stay.

Halfway through our visit we put on a puppet show and passed out cookies. They were amazed at the puppets and devoured the food. The older children tried to hide their food in order to get more than their share. They were trying to get as much as they could, a principle taught to some of them by the streets. Still, they were grateful for what they received and were sorry to see us leave.

I will never forget how hard it was to leave that day. Our group walked slowly to the gates that we had entered, what seemed like just minutes ago. Around the corner came a flash of hands, arms, and feet and the kids literally clung to our arms and legs in a desperate attempt to keep us there. We pulled them off of us and they were called back by their teachers. As soon as everyone from the group had slipped through the gate, those dirty faces ran to the bars of the gate and stretched out their skinny arms—reaching out hoping that we might come back.

I remember the ride back to the missionary school. I don't believe one word was spoken and if it was, I would not have heard it. All I could think of was how much joy those children gave me and how little materially they had. How much do we have and how often do we take the time to thank God for it? How often do we spend time, not materials, on other people? If we have so much shouldn't we have even more joy than those who have nothing, and if so why don't we give some away? It is easier to write a check than give a hug sometimes, but a check is not what's always needed.

So on my flight back to the States, I challenged myself to be grateful for what God has entrusted to me, and to give not only more of my material things, but also more of me to those who I might meet in life. I once heard a saying, "I was mad because I had no shoes until I saw the man with no feet." I no longer pray for shoes, only that I might some day be able to change the life of one little dirty face.

Questions

1. How does Bob Peterson's "culture shock" (paragraph 2) compare with Andele's?
2. What is the climax of this story, if it has one?
3. How is the ending a "resolution" in two senses?
4. In paragraph 2 the writer mentions the life expectancy of Hondurans (a detail added in his second draft after consulting a general encyclopedia). Did his research enrich the essay or distract from it?
5. If you were to walk directly north from Tegucigalpa and then sail directly north toward the United States, you would land on the western part of which state?

Consider the Themes

* The children literally and figuratively reach out to touch the writer. What are some of the nonverbal ways they communicate information to him, whether intended or not?
* How does this encounter between a descendant of Europeans, on the one hand, and native Central Americans, on the other, differ from the meeting described in Paul Rice's poem (Chapter 3)?

STUDENT NARRATIVE 2

Whereas "Dirty Little Faces" draws power from the writer's growth in sympathy and even wisdom, "Laugh, Sherry!" draws power from the ongoing incongruity between the reader's understanding and the central character's lack of it.

LAUGH, SHERRY!

*

Sherry Todd Murrell

I was delighted to see all the relatives in my home. It made me feel warm and happy. I knew they had come for the funeral, but somehow I had not quite understood exactly why everyone was sad or weeping. I tried very hard to imagine not ever seeing Daddy again but I just could not. Grandma kept telling me, "Honey, your Daddy is gone." I could not stand it. I was sure that was not what dying meant. It could not be so, for Daddy and I loved each other too much for him to be gone.

I was soon reminded that it was a solemn occasion. When my brothers Tony and Larry, aged fourteen and twelve, saw me enjoying the company of my cousins, they yelled sarcastically, "Laugh, Sherry!" I saw the grief in their red, swollen eyes and immediately felt ashamed, though for what I was unsure. I wanted to be out of their sight so I ran into the house.

Once inside, my father's sister beckoned me into his bedroom where she began stripping me of my clothing. "It is time you were dressed, the funeral begins at ten o'clock." I did as she bade me and commenced pulling on white lacy anklet socks and my white slip. From the closet she picked the white dress that Daddy had given me last Easter and guided me into it. I held my hair up off of my back while she fastened me. It felt good to be all dressed up in my Sunday clothes. I was content to sit on the side of Daddy's big old bed while my aunt knelt beside me buckling white patent leather shoes onto my feet. "Now sit still," she warned as she stood and checked me over one last time. My hair didn't pass inspection so she grabbed Daddy's hairbrush from the dresser and smoothed my long brown hair. Just as she finished, Grandma came into the room and announced that it was time to go.

I climbed into the front seat of my aunt's car as she and my uncle climbed in on either side of me. My grandparents were in the back seat. We left the driveway and formed a line behind a police car following him the short distance to the church.

The church was already full of people who stood as we filed in two by two. I sat at the end of the second pew next to my aunt. The choir sang for a short while and then Reverend Frye began to preach. His voice rose up and went down and rose up and went down. I began to breathe in time to his rhythmic speaking. My eyes grew very heavy. All of a sudden I heard my name. Reverend Frye was calling for my brothers and me to go stand in front of him. I saw Tony and Larry on the pew ahead of me stand to go up so I hurried to join them.

The three of us stood before Daddy's casket. The bronze was so shiny and the spray of red and white carnations on top went the entire length of the casket. Reverend Frye spoke to us of my father's life. He talked of things I did not understand and I wanted to sit down. He gave us each a little black Bible and a Baptist Hymnal. A quick peek revealed blue ink on the inside cover of each one. I could hardly wait to get back to my seat in order to try to read what had been written. My class in school had just begun studying cursive writing so maybe it would not be too difficult to make it out all by myself. Reverend Frye prayed for the three of us and then sent us back to our seats. I was glad. He returned to the pulpit and continued.

I soon tired of looking at my new books. I was bored. My aunt's knee was touching mine and I noticed her dress. It was navy with red roses stitched on it. In my mind I traced the raised shape of the roses with my finger. I wanted to touch them to see if they felt as I imagined but I was afraid she would not like that.

The organist began to play and everyone except my family stood. Two men in black suits went to the front of the church and began pushing Daddy's casket down the aisle. I could see several members of my family begin to sob and their cries frightened me. I clutched the pew in front of me. My aunt must have noticed for she picked me up and carried me. I was glad.

Once again in the car we formed a line but this time there was a hearse between us and the police car. It was a slow moving convoy and the car was so warm that I lost my battle with sleep. The journey to the cemetery lasted about an hour and a half, for it was in another town. When we arrived and I awoke, I felt as though a whole day had passed since I had fallen asleep. The day was certainly lasting a long time and I was ready for all of this to be over. I did not like all the sorrow that I was seeing and not understanding very well.

We took seats under a tent in much the same order as we had been in the church. Reverend Frye spoke again but was through much sooner this time. He walked down each aisle and shook everyone's hand. People began to leave. Tony and Larry were leaning against the casket each with one arm around the other and one arm flung over the casket. They sobbed openly. An uncle ushered them away and into his car where they could mourn in private. I made my way over to the car and claimed my seat in the front again. Only Granddaddy was inside. He was crying into his handkerchief. I could hear his sobs and they frightened me. Granddaddy tried to comfort me with soothing words and, indeed, he succeeded. Soon everyone was in place and we headed for home. I slept again.

Once at home I tore out of the car and raced into the house all the while pulling my clothes over my head. I scurried around seeking out my play clothes, hurriedly dressing as I found them. I could hardly wait to join my cousins so we could play. The funeral was forgotten for now. By bedtime my only memories of that day were of the fun I had playing with my kin.

After my bath I dressed for bed and jumped into Daddy's bed where I had long ago claimed a spot. I knew that my aunt would join me later so I was not afraid to be alone for a while. I plunged my face into his pillow. How good it smelled, just like Daddy. I felt safe and loved just breathing in his scent. I picked one of his gray hairs from the pillow and held it between my two fingers. My dreams put me in Daddy's arms and blessed me with his smile.

Questions

1. What do you understand throughout the story that young Sherry does not fully appreciate?

2. This mocking incongruity is called *dramatic irony*. Where does such a clash most strongly evoke your sadness and pity? Does this story move you to cherish life more?

3. The narrative has a complicated point of view. Although the events register on Sherry as a nine-year-old, her experience is recounted by Sherry as a college freshman about twenty-three years later. What advantage does a mature narrator bring to the telling? What would be forfeited if the experience had been told by the child in a diary?

4. In this account Sherry favors short sentences that tend to begin with the grammatical subject. Should she vary their length and construction more? Or keep them "as is" to suggest the thought processes of a child?

5. To what extent does the typical story structure pictured in the sidebar on classic story structure illuminate this account?

Consider the Themes

* How many kinds of nonverbal communication can you find in "Laugh, Sherry!"? Why do they tend to have special pertinence to this story, considering the main character's age?

* The story includes only a few instances of dialogue—verbal communication—or at least of spoken words that evoke no spoken response. What is the importance of each quotation?

* Who else is missing from the story besides the father? How does this absence add poignancy? Who are the members of Sherry's family?

* As in the funeral that Sherry describes, the electric organ is a mainstay of many religious services throughout the United States. If you are familiar with a religious group, what kind of musical instruments and styles does it employ, if any? How does the group define itself by its musical choices?

STRETCH:
WRITE A TRUE STORY

Although you will probably recount an experience of your own, you may write about someone else's (as Methvin does with Andele).

In reflecting upon it, ask what the event revealed about yourself, others, or life in general. Possibilities range from the comic to the somber. Your way of telling the story can range from the heavily editorial to the "no comment"—specifically, you can point out the story's significance in the title, in an introduction, in a conclusion, or along the way or imply its significance through your choice of scope, organization, details, point of view, and tone.

Just as when you try to *persuade* a reader, make sure that each aspect of your narrative has the impact you want on the reader's mind and emotions. Here are some guidelines, based on many narratives written by college students, for exploring your experience and then fashioning and polishing your account:

"So What?" Zero in on the Impact

What new understanding or appreciation of life does this story bring? What emotional impact? As you explore the subject with prewriting techniques and a first draft, see what comes to the fore as the aspect of the experience you want to emphasize. Narrow your scope to this essence—and then expand upon it.

For example, one student told of being jailed for disorderly conduct. Her first account covered the trauma from the beginning of the party through her release from jail the next morning. Her second, to emphasize her remorse and suffering, dwelled on the ugly details of the jail and ended with her long night behind bars.

You can let the story's implications speak for themselves, as Sherry Murrell does. Here is another, brief, example:

The bull snorted and wobbled from side to side. Blood poured out of his mouth and nose. The sand around him became a dark hue of red. The noble one touched the bull's head to show his bravery. Within minutes the bull collapsed.

Kathy Coleman

Kathy never terms the bullfight cruel, but she does imply the judgment through *verbal irony:* Her words "noble one" and "bravery" are mocked by the picture of the tottering bull.

The technique of suggesting significance rather than stating it involves the reader more fully in the act of interpretation. It also risks leaving the reader in the woods without a compass.

If you choose to express the significance explicitly, there are any number of ways available. You can announce it beforehand, in an introduction, even in the title—"The Trip to Hell." This way you can front-load the piece as you do when aiming to explain or to persuade directly, by giving the reader a framework for understanding the material to come.

Or you can suggest part of its meaning in the title or introduction and then bring out the full implications later. Of course, like a guide, you can interpret as the story unfolds:

The guys' calls to watch out as they drunkenly stumbled and struggled to carry the blazing couch down the avenue and across the boulevard *were more pathetic than humorous.* We all stood on top of the cars to watch our boys throw their couch into the ocean and lose their safety deposit all in one hurl.

Catherine R. Johstono

As another option you can express the full significance of an event toward the end. Christina Greene moves in this direction when she reports that Lacretia became her friend but continued to endure scorn from others ("Lacretia" in Additional Readings).

Experiment with Sequence

You can always follow the calendar or clock, as in "Light Dawning," "Lacretia," and "Laugh, Sherry!" But "told" does not have to follow the same sequence as "happened." To highlight the "So what?" you can experiment by varying the real-life order of events.

"Titles, Starts, and Stops"(see p. 31) shows a few ways to start off by reshaping chronology to begin the story. In fact, you can begin it with the last phase of an experience. Here is a paragraph that originally concluded a narrative but in the final draft began it:

The scent throughout the gourmet restaurant would make anyone want to eat. I was so hungry but couldn't eat a morsel of food. I had a weird feeling and cold chills running throughout me during my entire lunch break. I couldn't stop thinking how some people could have been so cruel and thoughtless. "Could I have been more helpful?" was the question that kept popping into my head. I had felt so worthless and helpless at that time.

Amy Lang Schaffner

By shifting the conclusion to the beginning, Amy was able to emphasize the incident itself as the climax of the story rather than conclude with its effect on her. In the bargain, she gets a curiosity-raising introduction.

Whatever sequence you adopt, however, guard against revealing something that should surprise. Keep the reader in suspense:

We were just mingling around, laughing and cracking jokes when a quarrel between two fellas started over on the south side of the parking lot.

Compare this sentence to the original phrasing, which jumped ahead and told what the narrator could not yet have known:

We were just mingling around, laughing and cracking jokes when *the confrontation between life and death began to brew.* A quarrel between two fellas started over on the south side of the parking lot.

In another kind of writing, when explanation is the primary aim, you try for everything-up-front clarity. For example, a police report about the parking-lot brawl might list the casualties and then relate the circumstances. But the aim of storytelling is to share the sense of an unfolding experience, so avoid revealing after-the-fact information.

Titles. Does the title do more than label your paper? It should catch interest and hint at significance. "Dirty Little Faces" was a phrase pulled from a first draft and given prominence as the title of Peterson's essay. And the student who wrote about her night in jail drew her title from the words of the policemen who arrested her: "I haven't made up my mind about anyone getting a ticket but *an attitude like that* will help me decide." This title helps her to stress her responsibility for the debacle.

First Sentence. Just as the flavor of a good-tasting food or drink stimulates the tongue immediately, your first sentence should seem fresh rather than warmed over or even freezer-burned. Use some art. Perhaps look at some print advertisements to get ideas for an attention-getting opener.

One possibility is to start with dialogue: "Who's the girl in the red dress?" I asked Hannah . . ." (Salomea Kape's "Designer Genes," in Additional Readings). You could ask a question, make a startling assertion, spin out some vivid description, or just begin narrating with sharp details.

As with all writing, beware of starting out with the words "It is" or "It was" because they lack energy: "It is projected that. . . ." (An exception: "It was the day after a Valentine's Day on which I had neither received nor given any love"—Pippa D. Slover.) Especially at the beginning, favor colorful, active verbs. The infamous first sentence "It was a dark and stormy night" might be improved to "The thunderclaps seemed to chop at the oak tree, which, glimpsed in the flashes of lightning, already leaned dangerously in the wind and rain."

First Paragraph. You might alert the reader to the tone and main emphasis of your story. For example:

Our usual Christmas trip to Philadelphia this year consisted of many amusing and often aggravating episodes. This year we took my grandparents. My grandmother is a motormouth and my grandfather is known for his thriftiness. I knew right then that this was going to be a good trip.

R. J. Loskill, Jr.

To help you narrow the focus, you might condense the background information at the beginning instead of covering it in detail. Notice how the following student first tries to engage the reader's interest and only then works in details about time and place:

Sweat filled my hair and ran down my cheeks. I was not prepared for this Bermuda heat. Even the cool ocean breeze felt warm against my blue shirt.

Now I stood, weak from the stress of competition, on the tee of the sixth hole at the Belmont Country Club, with no desire to continue with my round. My face no doubt painted a picture of disgust as I penciled in my score from the previous hole. After a perfect drive I had carelessly bladed a wedge shot into the front sand bunker resulting in a double-bogey seven. At this moment I hated myself, wanting to be back in Massachusetts. Today was my big chance to prove myself in the world of junior golf. I was playing in my first international golf tournament and in five short holes had already dissipated my chances along with my aggression and competitive edge.

Brett Tyler Wentzell

This way of jump-starting the story keeps the golfer's sense of pressure in the foreground.

Another way to begin: Let the present trigger an association with the past:

As I walked out my front door and down the cool cement sidewalk, I breathed in the warmth of the afternoon. When my bare feet touched the hot blacktop of my driveway I jumped back quickly onto the cement. I could see the heat rising off the pavement. Carefully, so as not to burn my tender feet, I skittered across to the road. By this time I could feel the beads of sweat already beginning to form on my upper lip. I looked down onto the black tar bubbling through the dusty pea-gravel of the road and suddenly I was reminded of my childhood.

Sarah M. Christenson

Conclusion. However you end your story, do so decisively. Beware of going on and on, like a TV in an empty room. Perhaps repeat a phrase from your title, quote some pungent dialogue, point out some irony or overall lesson, or just leave the reader with a dramatic image.

Your conclusion may interpret the account's significance:

Looking back, I can't help but feel guilty about actually wanting a hurricane to come close to a place where my home is and my friends live. The selfish thing was that all I thought about was the waves and not the destruction that was coming with Hugo. Ironically, only one good day of waves came with the storm, which could quite possibly be the last day of surfing here for months. Along with all the garbage and no sand bar, there was, and still is, human waste flowing from damaged sewage lines into the ocean. The city was forced to close the ocean due to health hazards, and according to the public waterworks it could be up to six months before the problem is corrected. One day of surfing and six months without are odds that have caused me to never hope for another hurricane in my life.

Matthew Michael Hayden

Or it might echo the first paragraph:

After one more stop, we finally made it to Philadelphia. I was never more relieved at the sight of William Penn's statue or graffiti painted along every wall. By this time, I knew my grandparents would not be aggravating us much longer. It seemed once we arrived in Philadelphia my grandmother hit the turbo button on her mouth and constantly talked about going here and there. My grandfather was impressed by how cheap gasoline was.

R. L. Loskill, Jr.

Play Time like a Trombone

After you have settled on the order of events, vary the degree to which you expand on them. Be able to slide back and forth from the fully dramatized to the quickly summarized and anywhere in between.

A dramatized narration is very detailed. Like a scene in a play, it retards the forward momentum of events to lavish attention on what is happening now. Dramatized narration gives details that let the reader share the experience: sensory appeals, dialogue, and thoughts.

Be especially careful to do justice to the climax, the most engrossing part of the story:

Months into school now, Chris was on her way from biology to the bathroom. A feeling of disgust crossed over her as she fumbled with pot in her pocket. As her nerves tensed up, her shoulders and neck, eye and hand coordination failed, and the bag landed on the ground. As Chris started to reach for it she noted the reflection of the lights on the floor was not as constant as usual. The silhouette was dressed in a sharp suit from . . . oh, say, 1977. That suit was filled with one hundred and thirty pounds of teacher.

Constance Schlette

The more summarized the account, in contrast, the fewer the details and the more quickly you pass over something. To illustrate, here is a skimmed-over version of the event described in the previous example:

Then one day in school she was walking toward the bathroom to smoke some pot. But she became upset and dropped the bag. Suddenly a teacher appeared.

This sketchy account forfeits the appeal of lived-through drama.

You will, however, need to summarize material to one degree or another whenever it should be subordinate in importance.

Characterize the Teller

Much of the interest of a story can arise from a sense of the narrator's personality, as in Woody Guthrie's "Talking Dust Bowl," the song lyrics at the end of this chapter.

On the other hand, you can characterize the teller as a disinterested reporter by avoiding any self-reference, as Kathy Coleman does in her bullfight account. Or you can talk about yourself but gain a measure of detachment by using the third person singular point of view—"The girl spoke," "Tsutomu looked at his watch"—perhaps even changing your name.

Up the Voltage

Details can intensify everything from the solemn to the comic: "Of course Mom and Dad had to find the best camping spot, which meant that we could see the little girl figure on the ladies' restroom door" (Abby Gants).

Dialogue. Re-create some speech to give a "you are there" effect. What would be lost without the conversations in "Light Dawning"? In "Lacretia," who is the only one to speak?

Sensory Details. Writing itself will help you mine the event for appeals to the senses. A writer who remembered the sound of an experience in one draft added the feel of it in another: "As I moved numbly across the floor something grudgingly gave way beneath my foot, and I heard the dull snap of a potato chip long since stale" (Chester Ligon). As with this last example, by the same student, appeal to the senses of hearing, sight, smell, touch, and taste: "Dishes can be overlooked until one of them is full of tuna fish, smelling up the apartment, fermenting on the couch for a week."

Besides the traditional five senses, remember the sense of one's own bodily movement and position, called kinesthesia. Constance Schlette appeals to this sense, above, when she has Chris fumble for the bag of pot and lose her coordination. And don't overlook the sensation often combined with it, what might be called the perception of physical resistance. The brain receives these signals from receptors that lie in the muscles and tendons whenever we lift, squeeze, throw, catch, climb, hang, stand, pull, or push: "Slamming the file drawer with a hefty bump from the right hip . . ." (Sheila Burgoyne). Even the resistance offered by one's own body-weight can be described, as in the dream recounted by Andrew Karns (see Additional Readings). See Figure 1.2 for the joy of holding a heavy mace.

Amy C. Weaver, who uses verbal carpentry to reconstruct the river treehouse described on p. 10, appeals to the combined senses of kinesthesia and resistance at the peak of her story:

The weight of the bar pulled me forward as it fought to free itself from my clutch. I glided down towards the water and then soared up far above the Waccamaw River.

Amy C. Weaver

Figures of Speech. For power, why not experiment with figurative language. Its meaning is not literal but "so to speak":

First I was late to catch the bus, so I couldn't eat breakfast. Then my family and I weren't getting along too well that morning so that was another bug on the window.

James Ruff

THE FAR SIDE By GARY LARSON

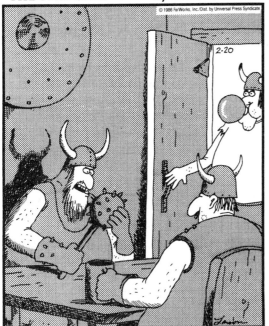

© 1986 FarWorks, Inc./Dist. by Universal Press Syndicate

2-20

"You know, Bjorg, there's something about holding a good, solid mace in your hand—you just look for an excuse to smash something."

Fig. 1.2 ✳ **THE JOY OF HOLDING A HEAVY MACE**

In actuality there is no insect: The writer equates his morning with a smeared windshield. Ruff uses a metaphor here by drawing a term from one category of life (insects) and using it to name a surprisingly different one (his setbacks). Another example: "No, the difficulties of the world could not break through the flowers and the picket fences that surrounded North Olmsted" (Leah Rogalski). Here the writer speaks of the world's problems as a physical intruder, and of the town's gentility as landscaping details.

Here is another example of metaphor:

We drove for many hours in anticipation of what was to come at 7 o'clock in the evening. As we got within a hundred miles of Indiana, we started seeing more followers and many more blue lights. We were pulled over and searched three times, due to the officials' justified suspicion of drug use based on the Grateful Dead stickers on our car. After eighteen long hours, we were there. As we stepped out of the car, we put our feet down on the moon.

Bryan J. Monroe

The concert environment was so unearthly as to be called the lunar surface. For a story that depends on a metaphor for its conclusion, read "Inferno" by Kyle Thrash (Additional Readings).

Grammar. You might try the present tense for an impression of immediacy: "We drive for many hours in anticipation of what is to come." Occasionally you might even vary from the expected punctuation and grammar to gain power. Notice the sentence fragment below:

Why my mother hired her, I have no idea. She needed a full-time babysitter because she worked during the week and needed someone to look after my younger brother and sister and me. The summer months were the worst. *All day long with this woman and she wouldn't even take us to the community pool.*

Amy Helm

These last words add the zing of everyday speech. Contrast the standard grammar with its explicit subject and verb: "*We spent* all day long with this woman and she wouldn't even take us to the community pool."

Check your sentence length. Like cars caught in traffic, do they start only to stop again? If so, you may be presenting a series of subject-verb, subject-verb constructions, one per sentence, which make the reader work too hard. He or she must figure out how the parts relate logically, and what parts should be subordinated to others in importance. So vary the length of your sentences by combining them whenever helpful.

Here is a before-and-after example from a story about the replacement for the old Comiskey Baseball Stadium in Chicago:

Before: The new park looked like a prison. It had unpainted stone walls. There were no windows. The entrance had a chain-link fence around it. The park was surrounded by parking lots. I kept noticing how dark the park was. It seemed lifeless.

After: The new park looked like a prison with its unpainted stone walls with no windows. The entrance, surrounded by parking lots, had a chain-link fence around it. I kept noticing how dark and lifeless the park was.

Kit Kadlec

Notice how the writer has combined the original first three sentences so that the details of "walls" and "windows" are now clearly subordinated to the idea of "prison." (In this case, full sentences have become the prepositional phrases "with X" and "with Z.") He has combined the next two sentences by tucking the "parking lots" detail of the second into the first. And he has combined the last two sentences so as to put both the adjectives "dark" and "lifeless" before "the park."

Ten+ Topics

Here are a few writing possibilities. They may provide a topic or suggest a related one. Many of them invite you to explore your experience with the help of the writing samples in this chapter or of the recurrent themes of *Stretch:*

1. Paradise Lost: A household move or a change forced upon you that seemed to end your happiness.
2. Light Dawning: A slowly emerging realization that had an important effect on your life, perhaps on your very identity.
3. Appearance versus Reality: A lesson about the difference between what *seemed* and what *was*.
4. A Child's View: How you understood something only dimly at the time.
5. An Encounter: How you got to know someone else—a stranger, a date, or even yourself.
6. A Turning Point: A dramatic change in the "graph" of your own life.
7. Music: The reader's ticket to a performance and an experience.
8. The Letter: A little stamp, a little spit, a big effect.
9. A Trip: A journey to remember. Your account could build to a climax or, instead, relate the various incidents to a central theme. (Be sure to engage the reader's interest rather than merely stringing together events.) For a brief travelogue, see Woody Guthrie's poem at the end of this chapter.

    You might even narrate an allegorical journey—that is, *A Freshman's Progress,* the experiences of a typical first-semester college student who meets symbolic characters and places, some helpful, some harmful, on the road toward Success City or wherever.
10. A Family Story: A new stepfamily (or stepparent).

REVISE TO MAKE THAT REACH

With the help of a classmate or two, if possible, go back over your narrative to bring out its potential.

As you rewrite the story, look for places that make the reader juggle too many words for the amount of information they convey. To help keep attention, split up any overlong paragraphs. Any rambling sentences? Shorten or reshape them. Any clauses that should be reduced to a phrase or word? (For example, "The skier *who was* tumbling toward a fir tree *that stood* in his path" should be shortened to "The skier tumbling toward a fir tree.")

Circle all your uses of "is" and other forms of the verb "be": Do they overpopulate your story? If so, you can cut some of them out by changing the grammar to avoid any verb at that point. For example,

My roommate *is* a night owl who *is* always wherever the action *is,* whether in the dorm or in town.

Change to

My roommate, a night owl, always swoops toward the action, whether in the dorm or in town.

To monitor the variety of your sentences, circle all their periods and question marks. Do the sentences tend to run about the same length? Avoid lurching forward bit by bit, or lulling the reader with any recurrent length, varying the norm with a few short sentences and a few long ones.

Avoid yawners such as "It seemed like an eternity," "Then it happened," "I will never forget," and "Words cannot express."

Have you stimulated the reader with firsthand, primary details instead of summarizing? Especially at the climax of your story, try to recapture the way the original sensations impinged on your consciousness before you made some kind of order from them. Here is the key moment of an until-then-tedious family vacation, as the family approaches the hot springs in their swimwear:

We continued on our journey down the path, and when we arrived at the springs I stood frozen, almost hypnotized. To our great surprise, we just happened to be on vacation the same time the nudist colony was having a reunion. I had never seen so many naked people in my life. We weren't quite sure whether to turn around or enjoy the steaming springs.

This writer merely reports her conclusion, "nudist," perhaps understandably. By reliving it, however, she can share her initial sensory perceptions. Here is the same moment expanded to re-create the initial sensory perception of the author:

We continued our journey down the path, and when we arrived at the springs I stood hypnotized by firm, bare butts of nice young men and the hairy sacs in front of the older ones. The sagging breasts and stomachs of the women made me turn my head as I blushed. To our great surprise, we just happened to be on vacation the same time the nudist colony was having a reunion. I had never seen so many naked people in my life. We weren't quite sure whether to turn around or enjoy the steaming springs.

Megan A. Coker

The author also later added a figurative image—a *simile*—that vividly expresses her discomfiture: "Deciding to stay, we sat like Popsicles in the hot springs."

Even though you want to give your reader the same experience you had, don't give out information he or she may want to infer from the context. Not blind, the reader prefers to cross the street unaided. A good story encourages the reader to feel involved and alert, so it does not state the obvious. Applying this principle, would you omit "To our great surprise" in the revised paragraph on nudists, above? What about the first sentence of the last paragraph of "Lacretia"?

Would research extend the significance of your story? For example, one student wrote about the discouragement of working in a homeless shelter in Delaware—a feeling caused by the violence of the surroundings, the overwork, even the political pressures. She presents a statistic that generalizes this phenomenon, that is, expands its relevance from the personal to the national:

One time a tour was due to come through early in the morning. Unfortunately a murder had taken place the night before, and there was a chalk outline on the sidewalk. The "suits" called our janitor to come in and scrub down the sidewalk, so that the visitors would not be offended by the sight. We were so few, and it seemed like there was a never-ending stream that needed help. It was very easy to get to the point where you felt you were not even making a difference. *Seven out of every ten social workers burn out because of this stress.*

Michele A. Robertson

(For this figure the writer credits Kathleen Elgin, *The Forgotten People,* White Plains, NY: Longman, 1991, p. 31.)

Watch your story's tone to avoid a misinference on the part of the reader. Don't let the reader wonder if tragedy will strike in a narrative that you want to seem entertaining, and don't let the reader expect cheerfulness to continue in a narrative of traumatic events. Films can use musical scores to help evoke an atmosphere ranging from the ominous to the whimsical (see John Horn's discussion of such music in the Additional Readings); but writing can only use words to clue in the reader. Your title offers help toward this end.

ORAL VERSUS WRITTEN STORY-TELLING

In oral storytelling there is dramatic interplay between the speaker's words and his or her nonverbal signals: Voice, facial expressions, eye contact, gestures (whether descriptive or emphatic), body movement, and appearance—including clothes, age, race, body type, and attractiveness.

In actual oral history interviews, for example, one person leans forward suddenly at the climax of his story about mule-trading; another remembers his childhood experience of going down a well in a bucket, his monotone voice offset by a sparkle in his eye; the daughter of a Confederate veteran, recalling an event ninety years earlier, declares, "I wasn't spoiled, but I was *bad*"—holds a frown for a moment and then breaks out into wrinkled laughter.

A raconteur (storyteller) in writing has to compensate for the absence of such body language. You can't enlist your unique "voiceprint," or your regional accent, or the dramatic effect of a varied tone, speed, volume, or pitch. So you must take care that an effective "voice" emerges from your written words. Moreover, since you cannot monitor the readers' own nonverbal responses, you have to imagine where their interest might wane and then try to maintain it.

Your challenge is to cast a spell on the reader with tiny black shapes. Or even better, to entice the reader into becoming a co-creator, one who transforms your letters and punctuation marks into symbols—one who helps to keep your canoe from tipping as two paddles slice into the lake of imagination.

EXTRA CHALLENGE

In your journal or in a separate paper, try another stimulating experiment. You might collaborate with someone.

1. Recount a vivid dream with all its non sequiturs. For a precedent, see Andrew S. Karns's piece in the Additional Readings. Or make up a dream with a partner.

2. Rewrite your own narrative in a way that stimulates your creativity. Perhaps adapt it, or part of it, to a rough two-column video script. (For a model, see the explanation in Chapter 4.) Or tell it backwards, or as a stream of consciousness, or in one long sentence, or in the style of the King James Bible, or as an unrhymed poem, or as fiction arising from some other point of view. For a scrambled story, see the revision that follows "The Mistake," by Brian Goshow (Additional Readings).

3. Rewrite Jesus' parable of the Good Samaritan (Luke 10:30–35) or of the Prodigal Son (Luke 15:11–32). Vary the original in a striking way.
   Or rewrite part of a published story; for an example, read the expanded and warmed-up scene from *Little Women* by students Gary E. Walker and Diana Jo Wilson (Additional Readings).
   Or adapt part of a published story to film, giving instructions as to camera work, sound, and scene.
   (Possibilities: a segment of the *Andele* excerpt "Light Dawning"; the excerpt from *Little Women* in the Additional Readings.)

4. Write, or begin writing, a fictional story. Perhaps tell it twice, from two points of view. You could even tell it through the double-entry format used by Melissa Bjorklund in "Catholic School" (Additional Readings). Or tell it by letters sent by two or three people, as in an epistolary novel like Samuel Richardson's *Clarissa*.

5. Tell the story of Mr. Dallan Fairchild. According to the anonymous chain letter in Additional Readings, he refused to believe the letter, threw it away, and died nine days afterward. In full detail have him read his own name; then tell his reaction and fate.

SONG LYRICS: CALIFORNIA OR DUST

Many songs tell stories. The following lyrics tell about a father who leads his family out of drought and Depression.
   "Talking Dust Bowl" was written by Woody Guthrie (1912–1967). According to the *Dictionary of American Pop/Rock,* Guthrie grew up in Oklahoma surrounded by folk music sung by his family as well as by his

black and Indian neighbors (Shaw 154). Guthrie published over a thousand compositions. He was a major influence on Bob Dylan, who on his first album imitated Guthrie's "talking" style.

Instead of singing, Guthrie intones the words to this song in a rhythmic counterpoint to his guitar. Can these printed words stand on their own as poetry? Or do they seem as thin as the family's "'tater stew" without Guthrie's picking, strumming, and gently ironic twang?

TALKING DUST BOWL
(Talking Dust Blues)

Woody Guthrie

Back in nineteen twenty-seven
I had a little farm and I called that heaven.
Well, the price was up and the rain came down
and I hauled my crops all in to town.
I got the money,
bought clothes and groceries,
Fed the kids and raised a family.

Rain quit and the wind got high,
And a black old dust storm filled the sky,
And I swapped my farm for a Ford machine,
And I poured it full of this gasoline.
And I started–rocking and a-rolling–
Over the mountains out towards the old peach bowl.

Way up yonder on a mountain road,
I had a hot motor and a heavy load,
I was going pretty fast, I wasn't even stopping,
A-bouncing up and down like a popcorn popping.
Had a breakdown—a sort of a nervous bust-down
of some kind.
There was a fellow there, a mechanic fellow,
said it was engine trouble.

Way up yonder on a mountain curve,
It was way up yonder in the piney woods,
And I give that rolling Ford a shove,
And I was going to coast as far as I could.
Commenced coasting; picking up speed;
(there) was a hairpin turn; I . . . didn't make it.

Man alive, I'm a-telling you
The fiddles and the guitars really flew.
That Ford took off like a flying squirrel

And it flew halfway around the world
Scattered wives and childrens
All over the side of that mountain.

We got out to the West Coast broke,
So dad gum hungry I thought I'd croak,
And I bummed up a spud or two,
And my wife fixed up a 'tater stew.
We poured the kids full of it. Mighty thin stew,
though;
You could read a magazine right through it.
Always have figured that if it had been
just a little bit thinner some of
these here politicians could have seen
through it.

TIPS FOR PROSE

This poem, in miniature, illustrates phases and characteristics that are typically found in longer narratives.

Like many literary terms, the ones listed here can overlap, and their meaning can be complicated and debatable. But a brief working definition of each will give you a start.

NARRATOR: The teller. In this case it is one of the characters, the father. His narration is told in the first person (*I*). Many stories are told in the third person (*he, she, they*).

TONE: The attitude that seems to emerge from the telling. The narrator's personality helps to create this story's mixed tone of bantering seriousness.

EXPOSITION: The background. On the Eden-like farm, a family thrives in the harmony of weather and income.

COMPLICATION: A new stimulus that triggers unrest. A dust storm threatens paradise.

CONFLICT: Often a clash of values between people or within them, or between people and nature.

CRISIS: A phase of great pressure that forces a decision. As with Andele, the man's way of life is gone with the wind. Unlike Methvin's story, this account skips over the father's inner turmoil. The narrator decides to leave, like the Joad family in Steinbeck's novel *Grapes of Wrath*. (Notice the alliteration of "farm" and "Ford" that emphasizes the switch from stability to mobility, from a secure homeland to a machine.)

SUSPENSE: A pleasurable anxiety about what will happen. Will the family escape in its overloaded car?

SURPRISE: An unexpected turn of events. First the engine trouble, then the hairpin turn and the out-of-control vehicle.

CLIMAX: The phase of greatest interest that determines the outcome. In this story, the wreck. The "mountain road" account, like that of Andele's long day and night, comprises about half the words of the song.

IRONY: A mocking incongruity between what someone believes or expects, on the one hand, and reality on the other. The family, once sowers of seed, is itself scattered upon hard ground.

PATHOS: A feeling of sadness and pity aroused in the reader. Expelled from their home, the family is now thrown from their car. The narrator, however, treats the incident lightly. How? The similes are playful—"like a popcorn popping," "like a flying squirrel." So is the exaggeration: "halfway around the world," "wives" so scattered that a single wife becomes multiplied. Injuries are ignored.

RESOLUTION OR DENOUEMENT: The outcome. This refugee family reaches the West Coast—an anticlimax, a letdown, because the farmer, instead of making a profitable new start, must borrow potatoes. The wretchedness of the family, however, is offset by the bantering narrator. Don't miss the triple assonance of "bummed up a spud"—the repeated vowel sound *uh*. Note his wry soup-metaphor about politicians and their lack of vision.

Works Cited

Guthrie, Woody. "Talking Dust Bowl" ("Talking Dust Blues"). Words and Music by Woody Guthrie. TRO © Copyright 1960 (Renewed) 1963 (Renewed) Ludlow Music Inc., New York, New York. Used by Permission. Copyright 1960 Ludlow Music, Inc.

Methvin, J. J. *Andele, the Mexican-Kiowa Captive: A Story of Real Life among the Indians.* Originally published as *Andele, or, The Mexican-Kiowa Captive.* Louisville, KY: Pentecostal Herald Press, 1899. Rpt. University of New Mexico Press, 1996. Introduction by James F. Brooks.

Program note in the Pacific Film Archive Series, "Classic Mexican Cinema," *University Art Museum and Pacific Film Archive Calendar,* January/February 1994; University of California at Berkeley; copyright Regents of the University of California.

Shaw, Harold. *Dictionary of American Pop/Rock.* New York: Schirmer (a division of Macmillan), 1982.

"Quetzalcóatl." *Encyclopaedia Britannica. Micropaedia* 9: (1990) 855–56.

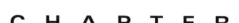

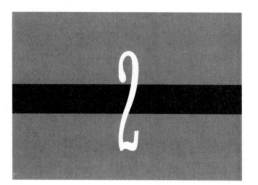

The Meditation

Speeding down the highway, the solitary motorcyclist described in "Why Write?" is fleeing from crowded Miami on a weekend jaunt. He enjoys watching the mangrove swamps turn from dense thickets up ahead to blurs alongside. A connoisseur, he appreciates the expensive rumble of the Harley as it blends with the wind and the vibrations of the road.

But accompanying this outer stimulation is inner reverie. Thanks to the human ability to manipulate verbal symbols, this lone biker can be good company to himself as he muses upon events, lets his mind sort things out, semiconsciously reflects on a problem at work (perhaps a new computer billing system), finds significance in the life he's coming from or going to.

How much has your education encouraged a silent flow of ideas? Or would you agree with Theodore R. Sizer, the author of books on the American high school, that in that institution "a low premium is placed on reflection and repose"? That savoring knowledge seems out of place, "nor is such meditation really much admired" (338)?

Perhaps you were asked to keep an informal journal that invited rumination on events, people, reading, and so on. If so, you have a head start in understanding the meditation, which begins with the specific—places, objects, people, events, situations—and ends up in the realm of the abstract, that is, of intangible significance.

Originally a religious exercise, the meditation, like the narration, encourages you to explore life through writing. And like the typical story, it works chronologically. It has three specific phases:

the composition of place, in which the writer describes a setting in rich detail; this phase gives rise to

the internal colloquy, in which the writer asks questions and invites associations; this phase leads to

the resolution, in which the writer arrives at some insight or new idea

Instead of stating a point in an introduction and supporting it, as much writing does, the meditation progresses from a concrete situation to inquiry to illumination. Rather than package ideas already arrived at, these phases help to *generate* new understanding. The analogy of baking bread may help you understand this concept: The writer measures out some flour from life, adds the yeast of thought, kneads it with questions, and lets it rise in the warm silence of reflection.

The meditation values the spontaneous while shunning the mechanical. Although physically it appears to involve only the typing fingers, it recalls the discipline of yoga, in which one attains a position of some difficulty and then uses his or her breathing to relax the tightened muscles, a process that can encourage introspection and spirituality.

This threefold meditation sequence will increase your versatility as a writer in several ways. First, you can use it as a complete writing task, a self-contained contemplation, like John Donne's meditation on a church bell tolling for someone who has died (see the Additional Readings). Or you can incorporate features of it in other kinds of writing. In a description, for instance, you might ruminate on a place; in a narration, on an event or person. In an explanatory or persuasive effort, a single paragraph or a series of paragraphs might engage a reader with a tone of inquiry.

By writing a meditation you can also recognize and appreciate its features in the discourse of others, whether written or spoken. For example, Robert Frost's poem "Mending Wall" is partly meditative, partly narrative, and partly argumentative (see Additional Readings).

WARM UP FIRST

The meandering of the human brain when left to its own unguided self is often called stream of consciousness. This flow of thoughts, sensations, memories, associations, and feelings helps to carry the meditation along. Re-read the biker's self-description in "Why Write?" and then record his flow of consciousness for one motorcycle mile. To accentuate the impression of a flow, you might even present the details with little or no punctuation in one very long sentence; see Michele Paddy's tumbling-forth list of "I Don't Likes" on p. 9.

MEDITATION-IN-PROGRESS

To give you an idea of how a meditation progresses, the author of this text-book will try his hand while commenting on the experience. I'll label the three stages so you can see how each is different, although each gives rise to the next without a heading, organically, as a plant grows by seeking its own shape. In fact, the unique shape may be reached when its phases overlap each other or repeat themselves.

THE COMPOSITION OF PLACE

Phase one of a meditation re-creates a scene. Its sensory nature engages the reader and provides the rich material for thought. I choose to write about a little household drama.

As I punch letters of the alphabet on the keyboard, more details come to me about this morning's playlet.

Phase one is not an introduction to a predetermined point you want to make. Instead it invites the reader's curiosity and the writer's exploration. So this phase both introduces and produces. The reader accompanies the writer from the known circumstances to the unknown significance.

A little while ago my family split off into four directions. The two children went off toward Monday morning carpools, one daughter on her way to a friend's, the other on foot to the neighbor's. After a spat with my wife about the fluorescent light bulbs in the kitchen, I sat here by the computer with its familiar key-clacking and humming while she prepared to go off to work.

Even before we all dispersed, hardly anybody sat down together except in the automobile. Paths crossed in bathrooms and kitchen, but almost as many words were directed to the pet guinea pig as to each other: "Could you iron this?" "Do you want some toast?" "I like your earrings—they match your eyes." "If somebody irons something for you, don't leave it in a ball on the counter." "It's 7:50." "I dit'n do it." "There is no such word as 'dit'n.'"

One of us tried to prepare food and stood right in front of the drawer that another must open so as to deposit the clean silverware. One child, always on time with homework completed, got me to drive her to a friend's house but had little appreciation for the lift, judging from the single syllable, "Bye." One spouse switched off a light to save money and reduce glare while the other, who had just recently driven to a different town for the new 70-inch-long fluorescent bulbs (and then driven back to exchange one of them) protested at having to get coffee in the dark.

THE INTERNAL COLLOQUY

In the second phase the writer asks questions about the scene just described.

Writing elicits more reflection. I even do a little research in *The International Thesaurus of Quotations* spurring thought.

Thanks to the spontaneous chemistry of the mind, an image presents itself of the weekend just past.

Unexpectedly, the family situation connects with the topic of dance.

One question arises from another.

The internal questioning continues to expand the meditation.

I am struck by the mixture of helping and hindering, of cooperation and discord. Does the tension between them define a family? Does a family share the same roof and the same blood yet constantly test its own limits?

"The family," declared Aristotle, "is the association established by nature for the supply of everyday wants." But "a family," asserted Alexander Pope as if in reply, "is but too often a commonwealth of malignants." When does a family start hurting each other more than it helps? Is there a family glue that keeps it together despite troubles?

The last few jammed days—what light do they throw on our family? We tried to "self-actualize" everybody by fulfilling their potential. On behalf of one daughter we hosted a fellow from Germany for several nights. His visit drew her into parties, a dance, and an excursion to the beach. The younger child had to attend a dress rehearsal, and both daughters as well as a visiting cousin took part in a dance recital in two long segments. My wife herself attended a dance workshop for six hours and the next day took part in a liturgical dance. I drove the "taxi," did desk-work, ran errands, applauded, gave permission, and enforced quiet time. Not to forget a party one evening for the adults and, for a daughter, the Blue Crab Festival: "I've got to go—my favorite band is The Mullets!"

What about all this dancing? Does it not make some kind of parallel to this morning's interaction and separation?

I remember the auditorium filled with tap, jazz, and ballet, as well as the long, dark grass on Sunday morning pressed by the bare feet of a dozen dancers: While sweeping big cloths of red, green, blue or yellow they filed in, then circled with hands clasped, met at the center with raised banners, whirled capes separately like technicolor tornadoes, then circled again in a sort of "clothesline step" with fabric held outward and oblong.

Maybe this morning was the parody of a dance. But at its best, shouldn't the family, Aristotle's special "association," give its members the pleasure of unity-amid-variety? A pleasure that comes from hard practice, trial and error, physical contact, cooperation, even creation?

But at times doesn't every family become a disorderly, colliding, sometimes dangerous inversion of grace in movement?

The so-called dysfunctional family, one whose relationships are destructive—could its members be called anti-dancers? Yesterday one strutter fell during a performance; in a dysfunctional family she might have been pushed. But art does not require happy subjects, so could dance tell the story of a destructive family?

Given the tendency of families to fragment, why did this weekend go so well? I realize that our most important activities—the visit of the exchange student and the dance performances—were collaborative.

THE RESOLUTION

—✳—

The family members did not simply use each other for goods and services but took part in the various activities. One parent enjoyed testing out half-forgotten German on the poor guest. The whole family went to the welcoming party for the student visitors. Both parents sat through the gamut of dance numbers from "Doggy in the Window" to "Hit the Road, Jack" to "A Midsummer Night's Dream." The other family members (as well as the drafted exchange student) watched proudly while Mom did her grass-&-fabric routine on Sunday morning.

Yet despite all this joining in, I notice, each person got time away from the whole group. Parents also got time away from children and vice versa. This is part of the dance, for not everyone should be on stage at all times.

On a few occasions people tried to jam too much in at the expense of everyone's composure. Dad made daughter take an orange poncho to the festival and ended up retrieving it from a bush. In fact, now I suspect that today's somewhat chilly start may have been a result of over-doing the weekend. Sore muscles. Perhaps this type of up-and-down itself is part of a family's rhythm.

I come to see the family as a half-trained, half-willing dance troupe.

Each member shares something of daily rhythms with the others, and many of these actions, including cross-purposed ones, could even be choreographed and performed at the next recital, such as morning preparations, meal times, chores, and other routines.

But family life, of course, abounds with improvisation. No member follows a step-by-step group plan beyond the next ring of the phone.

The challenge is to find the balance between cooperation and individuality. When our family traveled abroad, I would exhort the children, only half facetiously: "Subordinate yourselves to the needs of the group!" In families, it's the troupe. But one dancer sometimes trips another by accident or design, or fails to show up, or arrives drunk, or dances without luster, or refuses to do the steps, or leaves early, or doesn't like the music, or has a hissing fit with another, or otherwise diverts attention from the task at hand.

What is the task? To supply the everyday wants of its members, yes. But isn't one of these wants the very need to belong rather than to dance solo?

Granted, family members are not *cast* members. They do not perform, they do not subordinate themselves completely to a rehearsed group effect.

The family is for *them* more than they are for the family (at least in the individualistic United States). Nevertheless, they should not give up trying to enjoy—or perhaps just salvage—a hint of the dance with its grace, sweating and touching closeness, rhythm, variety, and unity.

* * *

This meditation generates electricity between its two poles, the initial one of specifics and its final one of abstraction. First reporting on a place in detail, it then explored its implications, which in turn helped the writer discover a little wisdom.

Remember as you write that the meditation offers you possibilities within possibilities. Donald C. Stewart, a pioneer in using the form in college writing, calls it "a *flexible* and highly problematic structure, capable of many variations and possessing considerable power to generate new concepts as you work with it" (157). Suppose, for instance, that the dance analogy had come to me immediately after describing the morning scene. I still could have slowly and artfully led up to it. Stewart allows for such an after-the-fact progression:

It is possible, as you think and write, that your mind will leap ahead from a composition of place to a particular internal colloquy and resolution. The writing of the meditation will then only represent a process of thought already completed." (154)

Or while writing I might have judged the "dance" metaphor to be a dud (like the fluorescent light bulb) and replaced it. Instead I might have pursued the subject of family glue: What is its source? What renders it useless? How is it replenished? Or I might let this idea drop as an unproductive tangent and shift to another: For example, what can a family offer a member that nothing else can? How does a family compensate for the loss of one of its members? When is a family stronger with one parent in the house than with two?

For your own meditation *Stretch* will envite you to take the form's possibilities even further than Stewart does. Instead of beginning with a place, you may begin with anything rich in concretes—an event, situation, object, even a reading selection—that gives rise to an internal colloquy and a resolution. No matter where the flow of thought begins or carries you, like a good meditation as defined by Stewart, it "approximates the way the mind works associationally" (148).

Questions

1. What does this piece have in common with a story? Where does it diverge from narration? Why?

2. Is there a better analogy for your family than a somewhat raggedy dance troupe? What analogy would you use to define your stepfamily, double-family, odd family, extended family, or quasi-family?

3. How would you title this piece? A clear forecast such as "Family as Troupe" would have what advantage? What corollary disadvantage?

4. One authority on reading, Frank Smith, observes that a writer can intentionally manipulate the reader's predictions about upcoming content (171). Much writing tries to help the reader accurately predict upcoming ideas. Would you agree that an effective meditation works to *resist* such predictions?

5. How much meditative effort goes on behind the scenes in any kind of writing that you do?

Consider the Themes

* Has music enhanced your family's harmony? Lessened it?

* When can one individual's effort to reach his or her potential start to erode the quality of family life?

* How well do people in your family communicate verbally? What are the characteristic ways they use to communicate *non*verbally?

VOICE AND MASK IN WRITING

Like every piece of writing, a meditation has a "voice"—a metaphor based on speech. Readers, like actors, do a sort of oral interpretation of writing by imagining its vocal quality, tone, speed, volume, and pitch based on the written symbols. The inferred voice in writing can seem wrought up, wry, dry, genial, bland, or even computer-generated like those in the airport subways that tell people, "Move-back-from-the-doors."

Changing the metaphor from sound to sight, one may also say that writers wear *masks*. They do this not so much to conceal their true selves as to accentuate one attitude and de-emphasize others. The usual term for this phenomenon is the writer's "persona"—a Latin word for "mask."

Just as mentally healthy people present themselves in various ways depending on circumstances, writers adjust their "expressions." For example, Paul Rice wears a mask of righteous anger in his poem "Dear Christopher" (Chapter 3); it may help him to project just one side of his ambivalent feelings about the conquest of America. Sherry Murrell in "Laugh, Sherry!" (Chapter 1) seems detached when telling a story about her young self, although she may have wept while writing it, and as a result, the details evoke more authentic emotion in the reader.

In an article entitled "The Healthy, Happy Human Being Wears Many Masks (*Psychology Today*, May 1972, pp. 31–35+), Kenneth J. Gergan writes:

Taken together, our experiments document the remarkable flexibility of the self. We are made of soft plastic, and molded by social circumstances. But we should not conclude that all of our relationships are fake: subjects in our studies generally believed in the masks that they wore. Once donned, mask becomes reality. (64)

One student in Business/Professional English offers her testimony:

If you were to ask a few people at my work what type of person I am, you would get different answers, because my personality and manner are dictated by the person I'm dealing with at the time. When talking to my boss, my attitude and tone become very friendly: I sometimes ask questions about his family and friends. When negotiating and dealing with contractors or suppliers my personality becomes very aggressive and hard-nosed. One of my lazy employees might describe my personality as authoritarian and demanding. On the other hand a good employee might say I have a very laid-back and friendly personality. These employees produce more and better work when I deal with them more personally.

Paula Davis

Like versatile human beings, the effective writer has many masks available to suit his or her purpose, meet the reader's expectations, and adjust to the general circumstances.

STUDENT MEDITATION 1

For this writer, a family troupe becomes a source of anguish when one member dons the wrong costume.

ISN'T SHE LOVELY?

✳

Anonymous

"Well, what do you think?" he asked, half smiling, half frowning with his forehead crinkled. The fear shone readily in his eyes. I had never seen him dressed this way, and I was shocked at the sight.

He stood in front of me gracefully poised wearing a red and silver sequined gown, velvet pumps, and silver jewelry. The wig he wore was shoulder length, and the soft blond curls fell gently around his face. The pink blush and lipstick he wore brought out the natural beauty in his skin, and his eyes were immaculately made up. He obviously knew how to apply his makeup better than I did. His walk was also more graceful than mine, even though I'd been a ballet dancer for fifteen years and had taken a modeling class. He had practiced going up and down the stairs for hours to get the walk perfect and it was.

I watched him in the bar that night. The role of a woman seemed so natural for him, and yet he was so masculine, too. I laughed at some of his actions because they were so cute. But at the same time I felt a knot in the pit of my stomach growing strong. I had to bury my feelings deep inside of me because I did not want him to see me crying, and I knew how important it was to him that I accept him this way. It had taken him three years to tell me he was gay because he was afraid I would not love him anymore. I felt let down because he was a different person than I thought he was, hurt because he had not told me sooner, embarrassed because of my actions, angry because he had lied to me, and afraid because of my religious teachings.

Is homosexuality wrong in God's eyes? Is it a sin? The gay people say, "That's just the way we feel, and we can't help it!" Is that true? Or can they control it if they tried? The prophets throughout the Bible say homosexuality is wrong and that it is unclean in God's eyes. Are the prophets wrong? Is there something about homosexuality God withheld from the prophets' understanding? Will all homosexuals go to hell? If it is not wrong in God's eyes, then why did he make two sexes? He made a man and a woman's bodies to fit together; therefore, weren't they meant to be attracted to each other, also? The church I belong to teaches that homosexuality is wrong, and anyone who practices it will be excommunicated. Is it unfair for the church to do this, or is it fair?

What causes people to be homosexual? Recent studies indicate it can be caused by chromosomal damage, or it can be caused by severe hormonal imbalances. Are these studies correct? If so, and homosexual people will always be that way, then can God hold them responsible for their actions and send them to hell? Is there another reason for homosexuality that has not yet been thought of? Is it possible that God would allow female spirits into male bodies? Or is there a possibility that we choose our own sex before we are born?

My church believes that all families must be bound for eternity, that we live together in the next life as a family, that homosexuals will not be able to live with their families because of their grievous sins, and they will go to hell. If the church is right, then I must face the fact that I will lose a member of my family. The heartache that thought brings is too painful to bear when you love someone. While I cannot say the prophets of God are wrong, there have been other issues in the Bible where God makes statements that are contradictory.

The evidence that recent medical research brings cannot be denied. I have read documented case histories where men and women report that while their hormones were off balance they felt "intense feelings of homosexual arousal that were insatiable, and those intense feelings would last for several days at a time." One woman relates these feelings to a hormonal imbalance caused by an extensive infection. When the infection began to clear and her hormones began to balance, those insatiable feelings went away. Other homosexuals report that they still have those intense feelings once their hormones are in balance. There is also further evidence linking homosexuality to chromosome damage. An old theory is that homosexuals are psychologically ill. There are some who are ill, in my opinion, but it is proven that most are not.

All of my questions can only be answered by God. The differing opinions between the Bible, the churches, and recent medical evidence is confusing to me and produces anxiety. How can the opinions differ so much? The only way I can deal with the confusion is to use the facts from medical research as hope that God will not send a member of my family to hell. And I let my heart ache because I love him and fear the prophets are right.

Questions

1. Would you agree that, to the author, what's at stake is even higher than life and death?

2. There seem to be two conflicts revealed by the internal colloquy. One is love versus fear, and another, related to the first, is religious authority versus other evidence. What kinds of challenges does she perceive to the teachings of her church?

3. Where exactly does Jewish or Christian scripture condemn homosexuality? In a revision, should the author quote from "the prophets"?

4. Do most homosexuals cross-dress? Are most transvestites homosexuals? Where can objective information be found?

5. To what extent does the writer resolve her painful exploration at the end?

Consider the Themes

* At the writer's Composition of Place, where does she describe these nonverbal signals: Facial expressions? Clothing? Artifacts? Motion? Where does she report having to suppress her own nonverbal communication?

* Would you consider the transvestite's makeup a kind of mask? If so, what is its relationship to reality? If not, why?

* How do you feel about the notion of legal marriage between homosexuals? Does it strengthen or weaken the family unit? Or both at once?

* Can you name three major religions that, unlike Native American religions, base their teachings on the written word? For which one of these three are letters (usually called "epistles") the earliest known documents?

STUDENT MEDITATION 2

Like the writer above, Krause reflects on the nonverbal communication of a fellow patron.

THE LITTLE BIRD THAT COULD

* * *

Daniel J. Krause

Sunny as the day was, a trip to McDonald's seemed to be in order. As I pulled up to the drive-through in my pickup truck, I took notice of the flock of seagulls in the parking area ahead. There must have been a thousand or so, I thought, as I received my Number Two Combo, which consisted of two plain cheeseburgers, large fries, and a large Coke.

After receiving my order, I slowly pulled around to the parking area where I would have a clear view of the seagulls I was observing earlier. Slowly they scampered around and got out of my way so I could roll down my window, turn up my radio, and enjoy my lunch in my car on a crisp, clear, South Carolina day.

As I pulled into a parking space most of the birds scattered and flew off. I glanced to the left of my car window and noticed one stray little fellow. He was about five inches long with a grayish, white color to him. The seagull oddly had a larger body than the others. His back had a pinkish cast and he had an expression that just seemed to say "Hello, I'm a happy bird." As I studied the bird a little closer I noticed he was making loud, boisterous noises. The cawing he was doing let out a firm, confident tone; however, a seemingly begging tone was mixed in. I listened to it for a little bit and realized he was hungry and was not going to shut his beak unless I donated to the cause and gave him some hamburger bun.

I tore off a piece of bread and made sure it was small enough for the bird to eat so he wouldn't choke on it. A few more pieces were thrown until I noticed my hamburger bun was slowly disappearing. It became obvious to me that soon enough, all I would have left was a piece of fried burger and a slab of cheese. As I continued to eat my lunch, my mind wandered astray from the bird for a while as I listened to my music. A few minutes later I heard this loud squawking noise from the same exact bird that was standing there before, looking up at my window standing on one leg. It was probably the most adorable sight I'd ever seen. I continued to throw more bread to him until he was full. Somebody might ask me how I would know he was full? After I tossed this little guy enough, he turned in circles and made a different kind of squawking, as if he was calling his friends to inform them that there was a free meal going on at McDonald's.

All of a sudden, tons of birds started flying in and landing everywhere. Two of the birds even landed on the hood of my car. The gobs of birds were there for about ten minutes until another car drove by and scared them off. All but that one bird, presumably their leader. He continued to stand there with his one leg up, begging for me to throw more food.

As I pulled out and began to leave, I watched curiously as the bird turned his dainty body and watched me. We sort of watched each other. There was this look of despair to him, as if he was watching a friend leave.

Waiting for the traffic at the exit sign I started thinking of the seriousness of this little episode and the impact and representations of life it gave to me. As the little bird begged for food, it reminded me of people's attitudes these days. People feel everything should be handed to them on a silver platter. What happened to the old theory that people should have to work for their food? Animals have to work for their food, but now it's been proven to me that the animals don't even have to work anymore.

It's as if McDonald's is a welfare system for these birds and the one lone bird is a welfare advocate.

As I continued to get myself all worked up, I had to think things aren't the same anymore; times are different. As Bill Clinton said, "The rising tide is not lifting all boats." And it makes sense. As the wilderness becomes demolished for new roads and subdivisions, these birds have to resort to the fast food era. These birds here are stuck on welfare and they have no programs to get them off of it. As the Myrtle Beach area grows and land disappears, I see no alternative for the birds. They will soon begin to die off and a population will quickly diminish. Wildlife is worth protecting.

This bird was in a way pleading for help and a chance to make it in his world—a one-of-a-kind in his aspect, considering his friends weren't willing to work the system and survive off it. I feel it would be of value for ourselves and our friends in nature to protect the wetlands and expand on the national park system. If we protect nature, all people and nature can live in harmony with each other. Hunters will have ample hunting due to ample species population, and species will not be endangered. People and the land, together, is my dream thanks to a little knowledge I gained from the help of a little bird in despair, but surviving at McDonald's.

Questions

1. Can you trace the writer's changing impression of the seagull? The question in paragraph 7—"What happened to the old theory that people should have to work for their food?"—evokes what further thought in the next paragraph?

2. Does the resolution of this piece seem to grow naturally and convincingly from the composition of place?

For a brief treatise on the intelligence of birds, read Michael H. Robinson's "Phenomena, Comment and Notes" in the Additional Readings. The piece starts like a meditation, then develops into a technical explanation in the service of persuasion.

For more examples of the meditation, see the Additional Readings: Ellen Goodman's "Planning on the Luxury of Rest" seems to have been written in a hammock. Jamie L. Stanton's "Falling Short" is triggered by the pain of a racquetball injury.

Consider the Themes

* To what extent does the success of the seagull's nonverbal communication depend on a physical context?
* To what extent do you think animals can understand verbal symbols? Do you know of any research being conducted on primates?

STRETCH:
WRITE A MEDITATION

Let the givens of life, vividly described, arouse questions that reach implications.

Start with something richly concrete and particular—a place, an event, a situation, an object. Allow your mind to wonder about it, to interact with it, to be uncertain and questioning rather than certain and controlling. See if your exploration leads to discovery around a bend of the river.

Here are a few tips for consciously expanding the phases of your meditation. Remember that each phase may repeat itself, so that questioning can lead to understanding, which in turn can provoke more questioning.

Composition of Place

What might a camera record? A tape recorder? Have you appealed to as many senses as possible? Can you add details to sentences? Sentences between sentences? Another paragraph? Do you assume that the reader shares your familiarity with the place, situation, event, whatever, rather than providing enough details for him or her to do so? Imagine that the reader is trying to paint the scene with a brush: Where could you offer help with details?

Internal Colloquy

Don't try too hard. Come back to it in several stages. Exploring is not like cruising on the *Carnival* line, so perhaps imagine that you are probing an unknown coast in a small boat: "What will I find if I turn up this river or follow that creek, or drag it onto that beach and poke around in the jungle? Welcome any dissonance that might arise between your ideas; although exploration can evoke confusion in the writer, bewilderment can help you to press for even more inquiry and arrive at more insight.

What associations come to mind? Implications? Doubts, uncertainties, fears, funny memories, conflicts, concerns, conversations, and images? Don't forget the old standbys of who, what, when, where, why, and how. Enjoy the mind's power to explore through verbal symbols. You might review the heuristic techniques described on p. 11.

Resolution

Make Socrates happy by graduating from the sensory to the philosophical. What general understanding can you reach about yourself or life in general? Can you satisfy the reader's need to have the world ordered or somehow illuminated? Have you stopped prematurely, or should you press this last phase to broader implications?

A meditation does not have to be sobersides. Your "mask" can be light-hearted, mischievous, or whatever seems most true to the attitude you wish to project. In any case, to please the reader, can you heighten the unpredictable, associative nature of the whole process? As if writing a piece of music, surprise the reader; even show off your inventiveness.

Ten+ Topics

Here are some possibilities for a meditation:

1. Describe a place that has an abundance of associations for you and let questions percolate. (In the Additional Readings you might read Melissa M. Bjorklund's "Catholic School" and Tracy Graham's "Flirting Nonverbally.") Or go observe someplace firsthand—a dormitory room; a part of the Student Union; a store; a setting for a party, job, family, or religious ceremony.

2. Describe a typical activity in your school, family, job, or elsewhere and see where the images lead you.

3. *Briefly* narrate a particular event that stirs your interest—for example, coming to college. Then ask questions about it in hopes that they lead toward a resolution. Do *not* let your paper become a story.

4. Reflect on something suggested by what you have read in *Stretch* (in this chapter, in others, or in the Additional Readings). Possibilities: dance; personal letters; a family or family member; birds or other animals; rituals; clothing or other nonverbal communication; masks; song lyrics; motorcycles; people and the land.

5. Take part in a "chat room" via the Internet and mull over the experience.

6. Ruminate upon the "Singles Seeking" pages of a newspaper. Or upon the issue of a newspaper printed on the day you were born or a hundred years earlier. Or upon an issue of a newspaper printed during World War II. Or upon the "Indian Removal Act" in the Additional Readings.

7. Explain something provocative that you learned in another course and explore its implications.

8. Turn on the television and do some research by watching a few soap operas, or music videos, or situation comedies, or other genres. Capture details and wax philosophical.

9. Meditate on the subject of drought, rainy days, or snowy days.

10. Do a little reading (or videotape watching) on the arrival of Christopher Columbus or one of his fellow Europeans. In sharp detail, report or imagine some encounter he had with the native people; then let physical events evoke mental ones.

REVISE TO MAKE THAT REACH

When you compose your meditation, be sure to allow yourself enough time to avoid forcing thought.

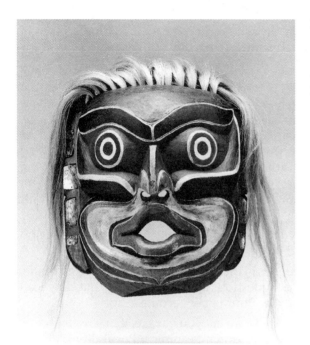

Fig. 2.1 ✳ WOODEN MASK WITH ABALONE INLAY. FT. RUPERT. KWAKIUTL TRIBE (NORTHWEST COAST)

Acquired by Emmons in 1929. H 41.6 cm. W 30.5 cm. (c) Steve Myers 1988 AMNH, 16.1/1872.

Be sure to start off as concretely as possible at the beginning by stating vivid details rather than summarizing things so they come to the reader secondhand. An example of an engaging composition of place is Ellen Goodman's column on vacationing (see Additional Readings). Sent to Boston from Maine, it begins with a poetic description of the season:

CASCO BAY, Maine—The light has already changed. The soft airbrushed quality of August has lifted and everything—the prematurely red branch of the sumac, the wilting jewel weed, the overripe rosehips—is outlined in September clarity.

How much more appeal to the senses these details have than something like "Autumn is coming"! Share as many specifics as you can with the reader at the beginning to emphasize your modulation from concrete life to abstract thought.

Your first draft will itself serve you well as a basis for further exploration. Why not take some time off to let your unconscious do its mysterious work? As with an unaccustomed stretch of the body, easy does it.

EXTRA CHALLENGE
✳ ▬▬▬▬▬▬▬▬▬▬

1. Since the meditation form was originally a spiritual exercise, try writing a three-phase religious meditation. See Louis L. Martz, *The Poetry of Meditation: A Study in English Religious Literature of the Seventeenth*

Century (New Haven, CT: Yale University Press, 1954). You can adapt the Christian theology of the original exercise to another religion.

2. Write a letter to the author of "Isn't She Lovely?" offering your own meditation on her gracefully poised problem-relative.

3. If you have already studied Chapter 6, "Direct Persuasion," rewrite your meditation by declaring a thesis (an opinion) and supporting it.

POEM: MASKS, MACHIKANESE, AND MYTH

Observing tribal objects with precision and passion, the poet wonders why they should be housed with the bones of long-disappeared animals. What is her resolution?

See the photograph of a Kwakiutl mask in Figure 2.1, page 58. For the use of masks in a Native American dance, see Jeffery Gilbert's "Conversations with Lehlooskah" in the Additional Readings.

REFLECTIONS ON A VISIT TO THE BURKE MUSEUM, UNIVERSITY OF WASHINGTON, SEATTLE

Gail Tremblay

The things live there, held still in glass cases,
set on pedestals, displayed—the masks,
clothing, boxes, baskets, feast bowls, all
made beautiful so the legends could be told
in ceremonial splendor, so raven, killer whale,
bear, and wolf would dance in the circle
of the people to the songs the families possessed.
On those days, masks inlaid with shell of abalone
reflected firelight more subtly than oil
on water makes rainbows in the sun.
Some masks, made to split apart, transformed
characters inside the rhythm of the dance,
a ritual bursting forth that in a moment
altered everything that was. The dancers
dressed in woven aprons and in shawls; cedar
bark ruffs encircled ankles, necks, and wrists
and flapped in wind created by motion contained
inside the vibration of the drums. Song and story
filled the room and beat as steady as the heart
of the people who knew the magic that made
life sacred as it emerged from changer's mind,
who still perform at feasts how things came to be
and know performance is a gift. Even without the people
to move in them, magic resides in these objects.
The vision of the makers informs the eye.

Around the edges of the room are bones
of long dead creatures who bear exotic names:
Allosaurus, Nannippus, Tylosaurus, Tomistoma-
Machikanese, beasts from before the time of man
that no hunter ever killed. These creatures
who have evolved and ceased to have these ancient
forms are mere frames for a past so long dead
we think in awe, in fear, how we could never
fit in such a world. Extinct, they make space
for other bones, for mammoths young enough
to be hunted by ancestors of the makers
of masks and bowls some twelve thousand years
before the carvers had their tools. But bones speak
of death, of things that cannot come to earth again.
Why should they rest next to the works of men
whose grandsons still explain how we did this
in the old days. The carvers and lovers
of this vision still reside among the people
even though the Europeans who took the land
worked laws to make the old ways die.
Those who made the myth Indians would vanish
as surely as the creatures in the corners
and stairwell of this room, put Native works
of art together with these long-gone bones—
the vision of the makers informs the eye.

(194–95)

TIPS FOR PROSE

Tremblay's poem uses no paragraph indentations, so the organic progression of thought is emphasized. To emphasize each shift, nevertheless, put a mark wherever a new paragraph could be started.

Works Cited

Goodman, Ellen. "Vacation's over, but Don't Leave the Leisure Behind." *Boston Globe.* 3rd ed. 5 September 1985: 19.

The International Thesaurus of Quotations. Compiled by Rhoda Thomas Tripp. New York: Crowell, 1970.

Niatum, Duane, ed. *Harper's Anthology of 20th Century Native American Poetry.* San Francisco: Harper & Row, 1988.

Sizer, Theodore R. *Horace's Compromise: The Dilemma of the American High School.* Boston: Houghton Mifflin, 1984.

Smith, Frank. *Understanding Reading: A Psycholinguistic Analysis of Reading and Learning to Read.* 2nd ed. New York: Holt, Rinehart and Winston, 1979.

Stewart, Donald C. "The Meditation." *The Versatile Writer.* Lexington, MA: Heath, 1986. 147–61.

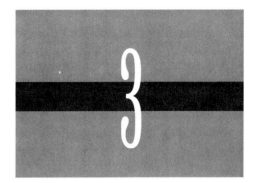

The Informal Essay

Renowned writers of the informal essay (also called the familiar or personal essay) such as Michel de Montaigne, Charles Lamb, E. B. White, and Joan Didion may choose a subject, flip it over and back again, and examine it inside and out, writing as much to entertain the reader as to argue a point. Sometimes they use a subject partly as a pretext to talk about themselves, to tease the reader into sympathy with their idiosyncrasies, to show off their prowess with words. At other times they explore a subject to discover worthy ideas to explain, argue, or touch.

Gerald Groves

Renowned writers certainly avoid mechanistic systems. In other words, they let the essay find its own shape rather than forcing it into a conventional pattern. You may be acquainted with an extreme example of mechanical form, the five-paragraph theme. It imposes a stern arrangement on the writer's material; so different is the informal essay that it may indulge an occasional tangent as the price for not sounding canned.

According to one writer and teacher, Howard C. Brashear, the familiar essay can give readers great aesthetic pleasure because it tries "to catch the kaleidoscope of experience for our wondering gaze." He goes on to contrast this type with more formal and practical writing:

Exposition hopes to fix, to define, to delimit, so that clarity and precision are perfect within a certain scope. Persuasion presses toward assent, conformity, submission, so that force of expression and argument are translated into belief and action. The familiar mode tries to open, to stimulate, to inject multiple overtones, so that insight is expanded and pleasure is aroused. (154–55)

To gain insight into people, your informal essay may capture instances of nonverbal communication. Along with the kinds discussed in "Why Write?" such communication, taken broadly, might include a person's deeds. What might the following actions "say" about some of the people you will encounter in this chapter: A father sending letters to his daughter over the years? A beleaguered mother washing and greasing her children's hair? A young American clutching a handful of Mexican recipes?

WARM UP FIRST

For five or ten minutes, write down associations that come to mind about personal letters. Be receptive to memories, images, events, ideas, feelings. Keep the pen moving or the keys clicking. You could write (1) a list expressed as a single, long sentence such as the "I don't like" passage on p. 9, (2) a vertical list of items, (3) a series of sentences in a paragraph, joined by commas to keep the momentum, or (4) a stream-of-consciousness mixture of sentences, phrases, and single words that make up a full paragraph. (For an example of this last type, see the free-flowing rewrite of McCall's essay in the Additional Readings.)

PUBLISHED ESSAY

The syndicated columns of Ellen Goodman, who writes for *The Boston Globe,* often have a receptive, contemplative air. The following, published in 1985, explores a change in communication forms.

The comments in the margin analyze the essay as a process of discovery. Read them as the essay unfolds rather than afterward or, if these comments distract you, just come back and note them on a second reading.

GENTLE COMMUNICATION

Ellen Goodman

Somewhere, in the boxes that I have moved from one address to another, are small packages of summers past. Letters from my parents. Letters from school friends. Love letters. Private history wrapped neatly in rubber bands.

Most of them are, by now, more than 20 summers old. The datelines remind me of camp, college, trips. They also remind me of my father's humor, the rhythms of my mother's daily life, the code words of adolescent friendships—S.W.A.K., sealed with a kiss—the intimacy of the young.

My friends, my family and I rarely mail our thoughts anymore. The mailman brings more catalogs than correspondence to our homes. The letters that come through our mail slot are mostly addressed in robotype. The stamps we buy are to go on bills.

We direct-dial now. Spoiled by the instant gratification and the ease of the phone, we talk. The telephone call has replaced the letter in our lives nearly as completely as the car has replaced the cart.

When we were kids, I remember, long distance was reserved for announcements. The operator was almost an evil omen. If we had called from camp or campus our parents would have answered the phone with "What's wrong?" Today, our own children, the products of Sesame Street numbers and telephone company technology, have grown up knowing area codes before they knew addition. They bounce intercontinental calls off satellites . . . just to say "Hello."

I am not railing at this progress. A Frequent Dialer with bills to prove it, I often choose the give and take, the immediacy of the phone. I accept charges from children with an uneconomical glee. A friend and I, separated by hundreds of miles, have declared our phone bills "cheaper than therapy." It's good to hear a voice. But it isn't the same.

Sometimes I think that the telephone call is as earthbound as daily dialogue, while a letter is an exchange of gifts. On the telephone you talk; in a letter you tell. There is a pace to letter writing and reading that doesn't come from the telephone company but from our own inner rhythm.

We live mostly in the hi-tech, reach-out-and-touch someone modern world. Communication is an industry. It makes demands of us. We are expected to respond as quickly as computers. A voice asks a question across the ocean in a split second and we are supposed to formulate an answer at this high-speed rate of exchange.

But we can not, blessedly, "interface" by mail. There is leisure and emotional luxury in letter-writing. There are no obvious silences to

Marginal notes:

A recent move sets the writer's thoughts in motion. She notes with regret that letters have become a sort of endangered species in her life, but she does not go so far as to pronounce this change good or bad.

Far from being certain, she feels ambivalent. Perhaps she will come down in favor of letters over telephone calls, for she does imply that something is lost with the shift to dialing.

The phrase "reach out and touch someone" alludes to the current advertising slogan of a major telephone company.

anxiously fill. There are no interruptions to brook. There are no nuances and tones of voice to distract.

The essay has developed into a celebration of letter writing over telephoning. She compares the two as a way to open her mind to further understanding.

A letter doesn't take us by surprise in the middle of dinner, or intrude when we are with other people, or ambush us in the midst of other thoughts. It waits. There is a private space between the give and take for thinking.

I have known lovers, parents and children, husbands and wives, who send each other letters from one room to another simply for the chance to complete a story of events, thoughts, feeling. I have known people who could not "hear" what they could read.

There is this advantage to slowing down the pace of communications. The phone demands a kind of simultaneous satisfaction that is as elusive in words as in sex. It's letters that let us take turns, let us sit and mull and say exactly what we mean.

Today we are supposed to travel light, to live in the moment. The past is, we are told, excess baggage. There is no question that the phone is the tool of these times. As fine and as ephemeral as a good meal.

The "we" has become general in meaning as opposed to the "we" that referred earlier to her family. So the essay expands its insight from personal to public relevance.

But you cannot hold a call in your hands. You cannot put it in a bundle. You cannot show it to your family. Indeed there is nothing to show for it. It doesn't leave a trace. Tell me how can you wrap a lifetime of phone calls in a rubber band for a summer's night when you want to remember?

Questions

1. Does this essay itself have an "inner rhythm" of the kind that Goodman says letters express? If so, can you trace her thought as it explores the contrast?

2. Where does the essay admit the "multiple overtones" that Brashear speaks of? Where, for example, does Goodman seem ambivalent?

3. In the paragraph beginning "But we cannot," why does Goodman put the word "interface" in quotation marks? What is its denotation (i.e., its appropriate dictionary definition)? What are its implied connotations (i.e., its associations, emotional overtones)?

4. In the last paragraph, to whom does the pronoun "you" refer?

5. Write a new first paragraph that will precede the original one. End it with a thesis about letters versus phone calls—in other words declare that one medium is superior to the other—so as to turn this essay into an example of direct persuasion (an aim discussed in Chapter 6). What positive qualities does the change forfeit?

For a letter that tries to connect someone with his family—and with his original identity—read the story "Light Dawning" in Chapter 1.

For an example of a more formal essay, read George F. Will's "Tearing the Social Threads" in the Additional Readings. Although more conventional in structure—with its thesis-and-support approach and tripartite development—and devoid of any personal references, "Threads" has the basic qualities of any true essay, however formal or informal, in contrast to an impersonal report. One is the impression it gives of a unique personality testing its own powers.

Consider the Themes

* You know of *e-mail*, but what about *V-mail?* During World War II, victory-mail was photographically reduced in size to save on space and weight. For an example from someone's treasured bundle, see Figure 3.1. What nonverbal, sensory pleasures would postal mail afford compared to e-mail?

* How could a letter be more gratifying than a phone call, which is able to carry the sound of a person's voice?

STUDENT ESSAY 1
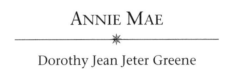

In the following informal essay, Dorothy J. Greene explores her memories of a person. For her inspiration she credits a story that you can find in the Additional Readings.

ANNIE MAE

Dorothy Jean Jeter Greene

Reading the narrative by Dick Gregory inspired me to share a personal experience about myself.

Dick Gregory was an insecure individual. Growing up without a father in the house and being poor were problems that would trouble him.

I was born to Wallace and Annie Mae Jeter on July 9, 1965, in Haw Creek, a small town in Western North Carolina. Having to care for five daughters and nine sons was a job for my parents. My father died when I was in the fourth grade, and I found it hard to accept this while maturing.

Growing up without a father was difficult for Dick Gregory to accept also. Having a father that died can be devastating when you're so young and can't understand why daddy went to heaven so soon.

Annie Mae is a wonderful mother. Mama is a 5'4", 165-pound lady of pure delight. Whenever she smiles, I feel a big glow of sunshine that can brighten any cloudy day. When I was young, Mama would always work hard just to make sure we had a meal and clean bodies.

On Saturday night it was time to start the fire in the big wood burner stove and heat water for baths. There was running water in the house, but a tub we could not use because the house was so cold. We had to take turns going into the woods to find kindling since Mama could only afford to buy coal once a month. The coal man would dump big lumps that were sometimes so heavy it would take two people to lift.

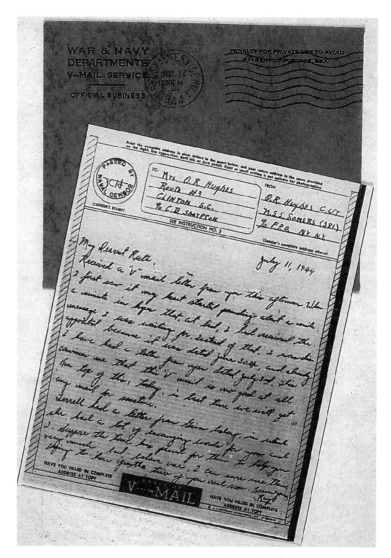

Fig. 3.1 ＊ **V-MAIL LETTER AND ENVELOPE, 1944** (letter size 4¼[w]x5¼[d])
Written by a sailor aboard the U.S.S. *Somers*, a destroyer, and sent from a port
unidentified for security reasons. The writer jokingly hopes to hear from "the two
of you," not knowing that his wife has already given birth to a daughter.
(Courtesy Mrs. O. Ray Hughes.)

"Break that coal into smaller pieces," Mama would yell. Our back porch
was made of cement. My sister and I would drop the coal onto the porch
until it shattered.

Dick Gregory stated he walked to Mister Ben's grocery store and
stuck his pot into the soda machine to scoop out ice, and by evening the
ice would melt so he could wash. We had to heat big pots of water and
pour it into a big gray tub.

While bathing us, Mama would wash our hair and grease it with Royal Crown Grease. I was tender headed. I cried because the hair on my head was so nappy and brittle. I would listen to Mama speak softly as she greased my hair and it would give me thoughts of setting my goals as high as the sky.

Making the best of what she could do for fourteen children was a struggle at the time. Mama worked every day for rich white people who would always send hand-me-down clothes home. Every day I would look in the bags just to see what I could wear. Being ashamed was something Mama said we should never try to be. We were reminded that there were people worse off than we were.

Dick Gregory talked about being hungry and poor trying to survive from day to day. There were so many children in our family and there was not enough money for buying things we really needed. I always thought since we had to take baths in an old gray tub and had only cold running water, I would never tell anyone. I often wondered why the Owens family, our next door neighbors, could have the best of everything and my family suffered.

Mama had to be both Mama and Daddy to fourteen children. Whenever Father's Day came, I used to pretend that Daddy was always there, but as the years passed I had to face reality and realize that I was only dreaming for something that would never be.

There are times my sons ask questions about their grandfather. I begin by telling them he was a very proud man who had enough love for all fourteen children and although there were moments of sadness in our lives, we all pulled together and survived, because we had a strong, courageous mother. Even when times were hard, Mama never gave up.

Questions

1. How does this essay differ in tone from the story that inspired it?

2. Does the "Annie Mae" essay give you pleasure despite the harsh circumstances it records? If so, why?

3. Do you sense a rhythm in the writer's thinking that gives shape to the essay? Or do you (like one student) find it "choppy"? If you were to suggest changes in a revision, what would they be?

4. Where does Greene use vivid details to "catch the kaleidoscope of experience"? (Where, for example, does she report the sensation of heaviness, a brand name, someone's actual words?) In a revision, would you welcome more dialogue? A brief story?

5. In Chapter 1 a student remembers the loss of her father. How does the narrative point of view differ between "Annie" and "Laugh, Sherry!"?

For an African-American father's concern about his daughter's future, see "Explaining Race to a Child," by Leonard Pitts, Jr., in Additional Readings.

Consider the Themes

* Where does the writer present nonverbal details about Annie Mae's body build, voice, and touch?
* How many generations of the family are referred to in this essay?
* Do you know of situations where a living father is "dead" to the family?

STUDENT ESSAY 2

Goodman's essay explores a question, and Greene's a person. The following essay mulls over an abstraction.

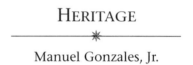

HERITAGE

Manuel Gonzales, Jr.

When I look into the mirror, I see black hair. Thick, curly, coarse black hair. Dark brown eyes. Light brown skin. My name tells people I speak Spanish; but until a year ago, when people asked, I'd say, "Sólo un poquito." Just a little.

Born in Fort Worth, Texas, I moved with my parents to Plano, Texas, an upper-middle class suburb of Dallas, when I was five. Throughout elementary school, middle school, and high school, I was one of a handful of Mexican American students in my grade. I remember one of them: Carl Martínez. His mother taught seventh grade Spanish in Plano. I also remember he didn't start speaking Spanish until his second year of college. As for me, the only Spanish words I could call my own, words I could understand, words I grew up with, were *mijo, mija* (My son, my daughter); *¡Ay, qué chulo!* (Oh, how cute!); *¡Ven p'acá!* (Come here!); *Te quiero* (I love you).

We ate *capirotada* (1) during Lent, we broke *cascarones* (2) for Easter, ate *tamales* (3) over Christmas, and for New Year's Day, *buñuelos* (4), sprinkled generously with sugar and cinnamon—the handful of traditions I not only claim, but clutch tightly, unwilling to loosen my grip, afraid that these last vestiges of the Mexican American culture would float away. I know how to make *tortillas* and *pico de gallo* (5) and *picante* (6), how to cook beans and rice and *fideo* (7), but only because I chose to learn. When I turned eighteen, before I left for college, I made sure my mother taught me how to cook.

I burn under the summer sun and my skin peels afterward. My circle of friends ranges from Texas Anglos to South Asian Indians to Brazilians to African Americans but, until my last year of college, too few Mexican Americans.

What am I?

Wrong question. Not *What am I?* but *Who am I?* My name is Juan Manuel Gonzales, Jr. My friends call me Manuel (sometimes pronounced Manwell, sometimes Manual, and it goes downhill from there).

As a writer, my stories deal with my heritage, my life, my experiences, but with very few Mexican Americans. I write in English. I am learning to write in Spanish and Portuguese, but it is slow going and difficult. A writer, to be true to himself and his stories and his characters, should write about what he knows, and I know about life in Plano and in Austin, and I know about the lives of my friends, and they are who I write about. If I were to move to Mexico, I would write about Coayacán or Guadalajara and the people who live there. In Brazil I would write about Bahia and Salvador and Río. In brief, I will write about what I know.

My heritage? I inherited my beliefs from the world I know and the friends who people that world. Some might argue that I have lost my heritage, that I have allowed it to fall by the wayside or that my parents should have passed more of their culture on to me. One mustn't throw the burden of an entire culture on the shoulders of two people and expect them to translate everything. No, not when my parents—migrant laborers—slept five to a room, and were ridiculed in school because they didn't speak English well; not when they dropped out of school to support their parents plus ten brothers and sisters. Culture? Hunger comprised much of their culture. Hunger for food, hunger for a change, and hunger for a chance, an opportunity to leave the one-bedroom, wood-framed house that tilted when the wind blew.

The opportunity also to end a day and look at your hands and see not hands rough and sore from picking cotton for seventy-five cents per hundred pounds, but hands that worked to move the family into a brick house, hands that worked to put children through college, hands that worked towards a future.

Yes, my name is Juan Manuel Gonzales, Jr. I am my parents' son, and I am proud of it. Proud of what I have inherited from my family and proud of what I shall leave for my children.

That is my heritage.

Notes

1. *capirotada:* A traditional Lenten Mexican bread pudding consisting of bread, cheese, cinnamon, and raisins. There is no set recipe since onions and sherry are added by some households.

2. *cascarones:* Dyed eggshells filled with confetti, usually made for Easter. They symbolize good luck when broken over someone's head.

3. *tamales:* A traditional Christmas food consisting of ground meat (beef and pork, mixed) rolled into a cornmeal dough, wrapped in corn husks,

and steamed. Some are made from fried pinto beans. Almonds and raisins may be added to the meat mixture.

4. *buñuelos:* Traditionally made during New Year's, they are fried wheat flour tortillas sprinkled with cinnamon and sugar.

5. *pico de gallo:* A Mexican sauce of onions, tomatoes, cilantro, fresh jalapeños, and lemon juice.

6. *picante:* A Mexican sauce of tomatoes, tomato juice, onions, fresh jalapeños, cilantro, cumin, and garlic. The recent English borrowing is *salsa.*

7. *fideo:* A Mexican dish made with vermicelli, salt, pepper, cumin, onions, tomatoes, and tomato juice.

Questions

1. Does this essay give you a sense of exploring the concept of "heritage" with the writer? Were your early expectations borne out?

2. Where does the essay take an argumentative direction?

3. Does Gonzales define his heritage in a way that seems paradoxical? That is, does he try to reconcile apparently illogical notions?

4. Do the appended definitions help you to understand and appreciate the author's conflict?

5. The word "heritage" is rich in positive connotations. "What am I?" largely defines "Who am I?" But when can a person's "What" start to chafe a person's unique "Who"? And when can one group's so-called heritage start to infringe on that of another?

Gonzales's concern for skin color invites comparison to two essays in the Additional Readings: Zora Neale Hurston's "How It Feels to Be Colored Me" and Leonard Pitts, Jr.'s, "Explaining Race to a Child." For the story of one person's struggle with the Nazis and their "master race," read Salomea Kape's story "Designer Genes" in the Additional Readings.

To compare an informal essay with its five-paragraph theme version, see Stephanie Owens McCall's "Pleasant Hill" in the Additional Readings, and Freda Green and Renee Michau's rewrite.

Consider the Themes

* How do details of personal appearance contribute to the essay?
* Whose hands are referred to in the paragraph beginning "The opportunity"?
* In a complication unimaginable to Columbus, Manuel, a descendant of aboriginal people and Europeans, tries to adapt to the United States and its mainly English-speaking natives. Can you imagine a conversation between Manuel and Andrés—in "Light Dawning"—of Chapter 1?

STRETCH:
WRITE AN INFORMAL ESSAY

Explore a subject, a question, a problem, or a hypothesis.

The informal essay will probably be meditative—that is, exploratory, reflective—but it should not be a meditation as defined in the previous chapter. Rather than following a three-phase sequence—composition of place, internal colloquy, and resolution—it should seek its own shape.

Ellen Goodman's essay, for example, begins with letters that have been saved and now moved with her household. She then contrasts present and past customs, praises letter-writing over telephoning, and circles back to the unpacked letters.

In "Annie Mae," Dorothy J. Greene begins with something she has read and then compares and contrasts it to her own experience. She mentions her father's death, recalls her mother's struggle to raise a family, and comes back to her father in the final positive context of her own children and Annie Mae.

Manuel Gonzales, Jr., starts with his appearance. He then explores the paradox of an English speaker with a Spanish surname. He shifts to Mexican-American foods, then to his light skin and non–Mexican-American friends. Having established himself as a cultural anomaly, he asks who he is and tries to answer the question. Defending himself and his parents, he proudly defines his heritage not as an ethnic culture but as a family sacrifice.

You will probably do yourself a favor by writing about your own concrete experience rather than an abstract topic like "creationism versus evolution" that can swallow up a writer.

Even if you prefer a less personal topic, still give your essay a personal flavor by its unique style, reflection, and easy, seeming-to-grow structure. Give it an air of improvisation, as in jazz, and avoid the point-one, point-two, point-three approach. Sound a bit like a person talking spontaneously. Reported one student: "To me the paper was very reflective, as if it served as a mirror for my thoughts."

If necessary, wean yourself from the five-paragraph theme. Find some other, more natural, enjoyable principle of organization. Do not supply a list of upcoming points in the introduction. If your essay does want to develop mainly by a series of points, introduce each one subtly rather than by a formula like "The second reason is. . . ." (For example, begin a new phase with a description or anecdote that leads to a statement of the new point.) And let your treatment of each point expand beyond the limits of a single paragraph. Do not end with "In conclusion. . . ."

Be sure to keep the emphasis on the movement of the mind rather than of chronology—a story is a "stretch" discussed in Chapter 1. If your subject depends mainly upon a cause-and-effect series of events for its interest—a narration with suspense, complication, and climax—save it for a later assignment. You could certainly tell one or more anecdotes, however, to enliven your essay. Perhaps devote one paragraph to such a brief story and let the reader enjoy connecting it with your train of thought.

Sensory details will help you catch the "kaleidoscope of experience." This is not a gray report. A boring essay is cold pizza. Do not aim to transmit information in the most efficient way, a purpose discussed in the next section of *Stretch;* you want to write an "essay" in the original French sense of the verb *essayer,* "to try." Both the writer and reader should relish a challenge.

Does your introduction catch the reader's interest? Be sure to avoid a stiff lead-in such as the following:

A good teacher is one that you have respect for. Respect may mean different things to different people, so I'm going to explain my version of a teacher that I consider "good."

Perhaps instead ask a question—"What does it mean to be a good teacher?"—and start exploring the possibilities. Or describe a teacher in action and then let your definition grow. In his essay on the custom of wearing clothes (see Additional Readings), Montaigne declares his frustration about having to get past cultural barriers to see things freshly, then challenges a traditional assumption:

Wherever I want to turn, I have to force some barrier of custom, so carefully has it blocked all our approaches. I was wondering in this shivery season whether the fashion of going stark naked in these lately discovered nations is forced on them by the warm temperature of the air, as we say of the Indians and Moors, or whether it is the original way of mankind.

Notice that his exploration enjoys a timely edge by arising from the current season and the "lately discovered" Indians. For more on beginnings and endings, read the sidebar in Chapter 1, "Titles, Starts, and Stops."

Time in a library can translate to power in an essay. You don't have to ransack the place, like Montaigne, but you can do some background reading to explore the topic. Even perusing an anthology of quotations can stimulate thought. Information from outside your own experience gives elasticity to a personal essay by complementing its subjectivity:

When I left Long Beach, California, the population was approximately 422,000. When I arrived in the town of Blue River, Oregon, I found the population wasn't quite 2,000 people.

Brice R. Becker

As for your audience, why not write your essay with readers of the school newspaper in mind? Or a newsletter or other print venue? Possible topics: "High School Honeys"; "That Old-Time Religion Meets College"; "Manners Meet College"; "Disaster Dates"; "Letters from Home"; "Hip Hop." Interview people to get ideas, examples, and quotations (using names only with permission). Be sure to write an informal essay with your personal viewpoint and flair rather than an objective analysis.

You might even compose your essay with a literal *audience* in mind—hearers—a group to whom you could read it aloud, at a banquet, for instance, or over the airwaves like one of the brief personal essays read on National Public Radio. Or write your essay in the framework of a letter: By addressing a particular reader or group of readers, you will sharpen your sense of an audience. (For a partial model, see Paul Rice's poem "Dear Christopher," which closes this chapter.)

Four Starting Points

Instead of the usual ten topics, here are four promising frameworks to help you begin and develop an informal essay:

1. A Subject. Start with a topic that engages your interest. Examples from student papers:

> "Boots, Spurs, & Pickup Trucks: Country Music"
>
> "Barnyard Baseball versus Little League"
>
> "On the Subject of Beer"
>
> "Rural Walking"
>
> "The Eighteen-Year Itch" (divorce as emancipation)
>
> "Dancing"
>
> "Working at X Job"
>
> "Running Track"

You could write about something inspired by readings in *Stretch*. Possibilities in this chapter: Street Children, Cultural Clash, Skin Tones, Family Routines, Food and Family, My Heritage, What I Am versus Who I Am. In other parts of the book: various kinds of "walls" in life after reflecting on the poem "Mending Wall" by Robert Frost (see Additional Readings); or "masks" (see Chapter 2); or immigration (see Chapter 6).

Or explore something of interest on campus—food, letters, encounters between ethnic or racial groups, clothes, and cliques. Instead of an objective report, aim for a personal essay that engages the reader partly through your personality and way of seeing things. But why not do some interviews to broaden your perspective?

Like Dorothy Greene, you could do a character sketch. You can declare an early judgment about the person and then support it, as Chaucer does when he calls the Knight a true, perfect, and gentle fellow and then offers evidence. Or you could skip any overall judgment and instead furnish details that add up to a portrait, as Chaucer does when he tells how the Miller pushes his thumb on the scale and rams his head into the door—see "The Miller" in Additional Readings. (See the drawing in Figure 3.2.)

However you do this profile, avoid the person-in-a-package technique of announcing several traits and then expanding on each. Instead, keep the reader a little off-guard and work more by association—as in the meditation form discussed in Chapter 2. Perhaps launch into an anecdote, shift to

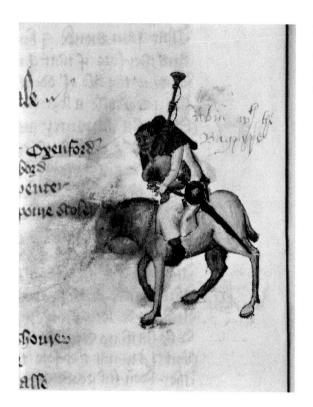

Fig. 3.2 ∗ CHAUCER'S MILLER WITH BAGPIPE

The Huntington Library, Art Collections, and Botanical Gardens, San Marion, California/Super Stock.

description, quote some memorable words, state a quality of the person and then expand on it. Stress not only the subject's personality but your own.

Or you could explore your memories of a place, as Robert Peterson did in Chapter 1. For more help with a locale, read Melissa Bjorklund's "Catholic School" in the Additional Readings.

You might use Zora Neale Hurston's essay as a model. Read "How It Feels to Be Colored Me" in the Additional Readings, then write your own "How It Feels to Be ———." Like Hurston, mark off sections of your essay with Roman numerals but do not announce the main "hows" as a pre-summary. This technique of artfully varying a model is a venerable practice in learning to write well.

For a comic exploration of a subject, read Dave Barry's "Bald Truth about Hair" in the Additional Readings.

2. A Problem. Explore something or someone that causes you some distress. Perhaps, like Ellen Goodman, take up a subject that arose from a change in your routine and provoked thought. The tone can be solemn, amused, ambivalent, ironic, anguished—or range among various emotions. Examples of student topics:

"Single Parenting"

"Beginning College" or "Going Back to College"

"Dormitory Life" or "Food on Campus"

"Trying to Survive X College Course"

"Having to Move to a New State"

"Slobs"

"Being———" (different from other people in some way)

3. A Question. Pose a question and then set out in search of the answer or answers. Examples:

"Should We Love Our Tourists?"

"What Is a Good Teacher?"

"How Did Being an Overweight Child Affect Me?"

"Why Do I Keep Making This Mistake?"

"Do I Want to Go into X as a Career?"

"Are Things Changing with My Friends (or Family)?"

4. A Hypothesis. If you're feeling brash, you might slap down an unorthodox proposition and test it out. Montaigne does this in "On the Custom of Wearing Clothes" (see Additional Readings). Entertain the reader with your ingenuity. You can take a stand as early as your title. Examples:

"All College Classes Should Begin with Calisthenics"

"X Is the Solution for Z Problem"

"Nobody Should Go to School for 17 Straight Years"

"The Dad Corps: Unwed Fathers Should Be Put to Work in Orphanages"

"Dance Should Be a Part of Religious Ceremonies"

"Housework Has No Sex"

Can you be "outrageous" without being offensive?

To find some techniques for generating ideas, review "Explore," and also take a look at the sidebar on clustering in Chapter 5.

REVISE TO MAKE THAT REACH

Read your draft to a friend or another student. What gives him or her the most pleasure? What would he or she like to see expanded? Clarified? Colorized?

Does your title arouse interest and hint at your topic or approach? Have you captured attention and interest with your introduction?

Do your paragraphs give the sense of thought-in-motion within themselves and between each other? At the same time, you don't want the reader to feel lost, so provide "directions," whenever helpful, in the form of transitions between paragraphs and sentences within paragraphs that express their main purpose or idea.

When you revise any draft of your personal essay, stress detail: Sesame Street numbers, the game of marbles played with rocks, Royal Crown grease, buñuelos. In Stephanie McCall's essay (see Additional Readings), what type of animal lives in the rafters? Your essay should be a cornucopia of sensory appeal, variety, abundance, surprise, drama, individuality. You might ask questions, wonder, analyze, remember, compare, qualify assertions, quote, allude, evaluate, describe, recount, philosophize, and even address the reader ("Tell me how can you wrap a lifetime of phone calls in a rubber band . . ."). Have you mined your subject for examples of nonverbal communication that blend the sensory with the significant?

As with a meditation (Chapter 2), welcome any dissonance that might arise between your ideas because it may help you to "essay" your subject more authentically and fully. Can you suggest the "multiple overtones" that Howard C. Brashear speaks of at the beginning of this chapter? This is not scientific writing with its ideal of a single, impersonal, one-to-one relationship between language and the world. A mixture of tones, unstated implications—both of these qualities can enrich prose exploration just as it can poetry or fiction.

Can you clarify the features of your mask or persona? (See Chapter 2.) According to one authority, the distinguishing trait of the personal essay is the sense it gives of the author's *presence* (Harvey). Try to accentuate the reader's impression that your essay was written by someone with individual experience, a unique perspective, and a distinct personality.

Where could you charge your wording with more impact through figurative language? Metaphors, for example: "Private history wrapped neatly"; "I feel a big glow of sunshine." (See the note on the poem at the end of this chapter.)

Are there any related sentences that should be combined into one paragraph? Any sentences that stray from the topic? That bog down the pace of reading? Should you develop any short paragraphs further? Should you split up any long paragraphs to give the reader a break? Make sure the length of your paragraphs and sentences varies to reflect the exact shape of your ongoing thought and to keep the reader alert. (Goodman uses a two-word sentence to help define a personal letter: "It waits." How does such grammatical brevity emphasize this benefit of a letter?)

Check for run-ons: Have you slapped down a comma and followed it with the subject of a new sentence? If so, change the comma to a period or make some other change. Read your paper aloud to hear where punctuation may help or distract.

Are all your sentences really sentences? Look at each one to make sure it can stand alone and shouldn't be linked to the previous sentence. But you may want a fragment if it works better than a sentence. Examples: "As fine and as ephemeral as a good meal" (Goodman); "No shopping malls, no movie theaters, not even a big grocery store" (McCall, in Additional Readings).

To get the most of your time, spend a little more of it to correct spelling errors. Run your paper through a spelling-check program on the computer, then search for misspelling it won't catch because of confusions such as *their-there* and *lead-led.* Check all possessives to make sure that nouns have them ("Mr. Ben's grocery store") and pronouns do not. Make sure that all contractions use apostrophes ("It's letters that let us take turns"). Eliminate all apostrophes mistakenly used before a plural *-s* ("grocery store's").

EXTRA CHALLENGE

You can try one of these bonus exercises by yourself or with another student:

1. Write a letter and send it. While writing, mull over its strengths and limitations in comparison to a phone call. Record these thoughts while you compose the letter or afterward.

2. As an experiment, recast the final draft of your informal essay to make it more formal—that is, more assertive in tone, more overt and logical in its organization, less personal. Do you appreciate the strengths of each version more fully by contrast? Do you favor one of them? Or recast your original as a stream of consciousness.

3. What are your "whats"? List a dozen or so of your affiliations, your roles, and any other easily definable groups to which you belong. (Begin each item with "I am" or "I am a.") Explore the extent to which such membership defines your "who?"

4. Write an essay called "How It Feels to Be Annie Mae" in which you imagine yourself as Dorothy Greene's mother.

5. Explore a place, person, event, or idea with the double-viewpoint format used by Bjorklund in the Additional Readings.

POEM: ADDRESSEE DECEASED

The descendant of a Creek Indian writes a letter to Christopher Columbus. It has five verse-paragraphs; does the sequence have an exploratory manner?

Notice the writer's precise vocabulary—one of the skills of poetry writing that carries over to artful prose. (*Fé y oro* were the dual motives of the conquistadors: conversion to the Christian faith and gold in Spanish pockets.) Also observe the nonverbal characteristics that Rice ascribes to his grandmother.

For a note on the attitude projected by the writer, see the sidebar on masks in Chapter 2.

DEAR CHRISTOPHER
listening
centuries beneath this Southern sand
I hear the dark hurt of hunted souls

reaching to the great white bloom of sail,
new sound of chain over gunwale,
light-skinned voices
cutting with tongues of gold
sharper than any stone,
and the will to put fire to dwelling,
fire to temple;
the will; always the will,
     fé y oro

listening
for my ancestor's voice,
I see her raptor face
her black hair;
I hear her keening,
nights on bloody paths,
burnt scrub oak and pine,
broken villages,
running wounds,
far from any shaman's heaven.

I see her flint eyes;
I have turned them up
with my racial memory's plow,
arrowheads of deep hatred
where rains have drowned
the dance
and the corn is gone to rot,
and the fires no longer shake
their weapons in the night.

for her, and every morning,
my heart raises new stone blades
against new Spanish sails—
hotels, restaurants,
condos on the beach.

old Creek women
take the earth's own shape,
but this has not made them quiet.
their eyes have become my arrows;
their distant voices
power the thunder in my words.

    Sincerely,

    Paul Rice

    Paul Rice

TIPS FOR PROSE

The boundary between poetry and prose is not completely surveyed, marked, and agreed upon. You might read a selection of prose, for example, and find it more poetic than an example of rhymed verse that fails to arouse aesthetic pleasure.

One resource of both prose and poetry is the metaphor. In "Dear Christopher" Rice uses numerous metaphors for compressed vividness. "Flint eyes," for example, has multiple power because it suggests the hardness of flint, its narrow shape, its sharpness, and its association with Native Americans.

Without looking back at the poem, try to write in the missing word in each of the following metaphorical phrases:

reaching to the great white _____ of sail

I hear . . . light-skinned _____ -s

turned them up with my racial memory's _____

rains have _____ -ed the dance

the fires no longer shake their _____ -s

new stone blades against new Spanish _____ -s

Now take another look at "Dear Christopher" to see if you can appreciate these metaphors more fully. Can you "translate" each one into literal, non-figurative language (e.g., "reaching to the great white sail," "I hear the voices of light-skinned people")? What is lost?

In your own prose, an occasional and original metaphor can please your reader as well as communicate the exact shape of your idea.

Works Cited

Brashear, Howard C. "Aesthetic Form in Familiar Essays." *College Composition and Communication* 22 (1971): 147–55. (The author has changed the spelling of his name from "Brasher" since the article was published.)

Goodman, Ellen. "Gentle Communication." *Boston Globe.* 3rd ed. 1 August 1985: 15.

Harvey, Gordon. "Presence in the Essay." *College English* 56 (October 1994): 642–54.

Rice, Paul. "Dear Christopher." In *Dear Christopher: Letters to Christopher Columbus by Contemporary Native Americans,* ed. Darryl Wilson and Barry Joyce, 62–63. Native American Studies. University of California-Riverside, 1992.

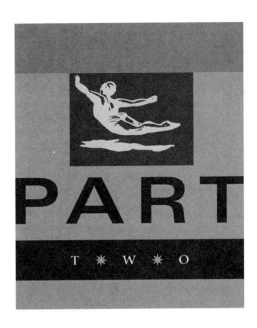

Explain

B end and twist in another direction, if you will, for this calisthenic textbook now leads you from *exploring* to *explaining*.

In such writing, often called expository, you clearly and fully set forth information. In contrast to exploratory writing, you aim to clarify the known rather than inquire about the unknown, so you tend to deal with the mapped over the unpredictable, the definite over the tentative, the objective over the personal. In these two chapters of *Stretch*, "Instructions" and "Other Exposition," you will emphasize a subject and deemphasize yourself—your process of thinking, your personality, your experience. Imagine the format of a memorandum: You will keep the emphasis on the SUBJECT instead of the FROM, going so far as to avoid the pronoun "I" unless it seems helpful.

How does expository writing differ from persuasive, an aim discussed in the next main part of this book? Your purview is the agreed-upon rather than the disputable, the dispassionate over the emotional. While persuasive writing tries to overcome resistance so as to modify beliefs or motivate action, expository writing simply conveys information to a reader who is deemed receptive. A review of a movie will judge its value as art or entertainment and may try to steer the reader into the theater; an objective description of the movie will simply furnish information about the actors, director, length, language, subject, plot, date, and so on.

The distinction is a blurry one, however. For one thing, you can convey information without intending to persuade, yet cause a change in a person's attitude or actions. An e-mail note to Carlos mentioning that "Tina will be there" might send him either to the party or to a movie.

For another thing, you can convey information to persuade someone without overtly making a judgment or recommendation, trusting instead that your selection of details will imply a point. Your own resumé is an example: It will provide objective, informative, and selective details about the kind of job you are seeking and about what education and employment you have had; but because it tries to snare an interview, its intent is persuasive.

Explanation and persuasion often work together like music and lyrics. In evaluating an argument, thoughtful people value the liberal use of expository techniques such as example, definition, narration, description, analysis into parts or steps, comparison-contrast, testimony, cause-and-effect reasoning, and numerical data. So any practice you can get with explanation will also give you a boost with persuasion.

You have probably noticed how difficult it can be to convey information accurately. The house of communication, no matter how well sealed, often admits a draft. Writing, however, can work well to get across complicated ideas because of the precision it gains from the writer's unhurried thought, revision, and research. Writing has special power to "fix, to define, to delimit" (Brashear 154).

WRITING VERSUS AUDIO-VISUAL MEDIA

When used to explain, the versatile written word, unlike material presented by magnetic tape and a VCR, can be assimilated at the reader's own pace. He or she can easily skim or slow down, skip a part or review it, even scan the material easily in search of a particular word or idea. And because writing does not fade away like speech, it can be studied, carried around, sent here and there by mail or computer, and stored as a record.

If printed on paper, the material can be read without machinery, photocopied, and even written upon or highlighted for analysis or emphasis. Unlike speech, writing can offer silence—an endangered creature in today's jungle of clacking printers, blaring car alarms, and beeping wristwatches.

For explaining, audiovisual media do sometimes have advantages over print. They can present the real processes, events, objects, places, animals, or people as lifelike, colorful images complete with motion and sound. This sensory information complements the verbal information provided by the human subjects or by the narrator (whether in a voice-over or on camera).

Examples of teaching videos: *How to Survive in a Step Family; Make Money Making Music; Handbuilding: The Art of the Potter; The Aztecs; Globalization in Theory and Practice;* and the filmed interview with the poet Simon J. Ortiz cited by Margaret Fritz in the Additional Readings.

In one job-training video, a pizza-maker reaches into the green-pepper bin twice—wasting time—whereupon the frame is frozen and a red X appears over the image. A print version, even with photographs, would be less cautionary.

Thanks to computer software, audiovisuals can also use animation that teaches while entertaining.

Audiovisuals can also work better than print in a group setting. They reach an audience efficiently because attendance (if not attention) is guaranteed, and they reinforce cohesion among the members. Students interviewing for jobs with the Walt Disney World College Program, for example, watch a video together on Disney World, on the role of its college program, and on the "Disney Look."

The strengths of audiovisual media for exposition, however, can become too much of a good thing. When overused, the images, motion, and sound can actually distract from the intended information. In an extreme case, a viewer-listener may have to absorb images (perhaps in a series of quick edits) along with the voice of a narrator, sounds captured by the videotape, and background music.

The inherent weakness of audiovisual material is its inability to convey dense verbal information. For this purpose, videotape is a skinny sumo wrestler.

To convey information systematically and completely, you will use writing not only in school, as in essay exams or lab reports, but on the job, in community service, and in your personal and family life. You might

* record the results of a physical exam
* write a report for the boss (perhaps with other employees)
* write up the minutes of a PTA meeting
* compose instructions for using a machine or following a procedure
* write a letter or memo to explain a new policy, convey news, or ask for an adjustment when a product or service is unsatisfactory
* draft a news release or a contract
* create a newsletter or brochure, perhaps with the help of desktop publishing software
* produce an audiovisual program, using the written word to get funding for the project, to establish its approach, and to compose its narration or dialogue

Here are three hints to keep in mind when you write an explanation. These guidelines can also be adapted profitably to public speaking.

CONNECT WITH YOUR READER

In all writing, you need to anticipate the reader's responses to avoid uncertainty and misinterpretation. Unlike a speaker, you can't monitor the nonverbal reactions of an audience or entertain verbal ones. Nobody will raise a hand to ask for clarification, nobody will scratch a head or furrow a brow. Take into account your reader's level of knowledge, purpose for reading, and degree of interest.

How much background should you furnish? What terms should you define that might be unfamiliar to your reader? Will he or she know that in radio jargon the word "cart" means a cartridge? That in football jargon it means a wheeled vehicle full of equipment? That "UNR" means University of Nevada at Reno? That "family dynamics" means the psychological interrelationships among family members?

Do you need to motivate your reader to devote time and attention to what you have to say?

Also consider that the reader, like an actor interpreting a script, will imagine a "voice" to your writing based on the verbal content. What kind will the reader expect to hear? One that reflects your own personality or one that sounds impersonal? What kind of voice do you want to project? What kind of "mask" do you want to wear in order to accentuate one attitude? (See sidebar on masks in Chapter 2.)

Although your teacher may be the only one reading your explanation, keep in mind an imaginary group that challenges you to shape your material according to its needs. You might keep in mind any educated adult, but even better, imagine a smaller group—for example, college students with an interest in the subject, or high schoolers with no particular interest. You might specify this narrowed readership on your title page: "Intended audience, X." The information will help your instructor evaluate how well your explanation has adapted to the reader. In other words, make *composition* serve *rhetoric:* All the parts and features of your writing—vocabulary, grammar, paragraphing, organization, development, and voice—should further your goal of imparting full and clear information to a particular audience.

HIGHLIGHT YOUR PLAN

Announce your subject in the title. An example in the next chapter is "Scripting for Video." While your title may be artful, it must primarily be clear: not "Tall Paul" but "Paul: A Case Study of a Step-Parent." Or "Student Internships in Business and Professions."

In contrast to the story, informal essay, or the meditation, you must also make your purpose clear in the first paragraph. For example:

> New college graduates often find it hard to get a job in their career field. They may have a lot of book learning but no experience in the area. As a college student you may want to try getting an internship. It lets you work for an organization while going to college, get credit hours (rather than pay), and learn about the field firsthand. *This report will give you an introduction to internships.*◆

Notice that this example offers some helpful motivation-to-read. Be careful, though, not to turn your explanation into an argument. Think about accomplishing a *purpose* rather than supporting a *thesis,* which is an opinion that invites controversy. Although you might have a personal slant, avoid argumentative techniques like appealing to logic and emotion, building a case with various kinds of evidence, and refuting objections. (For that "stretch," see Chapters 6 and 7.) Instead, focus on the systematic and detailed presentation of information.

Near the beginning you may even want to announce the areas to be covered, a technique called a pre-summary or essay map:

> This study will define work internships, explain their advantages, explain how to apply for them, and report one student's experience with one. ◆

Such an overview of your purpose, scope, and organization will give the reader a framework for making sense of the details to come.

When aiming to explain, consider announcing the subject or point of a paragraph and locating this information at or near the beginning. This technique does in miniature what the purpose statement does for the whole explanatory paper. Such a brief summary of a paragraph is traditionally called a "topic sentence." It provides a framework for the details to come:

> *Rastafarians make up only around thirteen percent of [Jamaica's] population but their influence on Jamaican music is out of all proportion.* Bob Marley is only the most famous of an enormous number of Rasta musicians. In the late 1960s and 70s, virtually every reggae artist seemed to have adopted or emerged from the religion. ◆
>
> *Salter 522*

In this case the second sentence provides an example of such influence and the third sentence makes a generalization about a certain kind of Jamaican music. Both sentences support and clarify the first one.

TWO LIGHT-HOUSES

Your title and first paragraph will help your reader navigate your entire explanation. How? Think of the reader as sailing along the coast at night. There are rocks and shoals in the area. He or she can determine the boat's location on a chart by a reference to two landmarks.

Suppose there is one lighthouse to the north and one to the east. Using a compass (sometimes built into a pair of binoculars), the sailor measures the magnetic bearing (i.e., the direction) from the observer to the first lighthouse. Then, on the chart, he or she draws a line in that direction from the lighthouse symbol out to sea. The sailor then does the same with the other lighthouse and its symbol. The point at which the two lines cross marks the position of the boat.

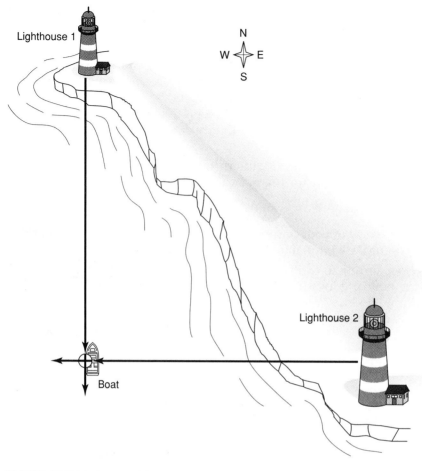

NAVIGATING BY LIGHTHOUSE
(Courtesy Thomas G. Hollinger.)

Here is what the chart might look like if the boat, facing northward, is headed directly north toward Lighthouse 1 (at a bearing of 180 degrees) and perpendicular to Lighthouse 2 (at a bearing of 90 degrees).

Just as a sailor can determine the boat's changing position, the reader can continually get his or her bearings by reference to your two lighthouses—the title and introduction, which state the purpose, the scope, and perhaps the method of your explanation.

In many cases one or more sentences add up to the central point of a paragraph:

Are birds stupid? Most definitely not. They have some quite remarkable learning abilities. My friend Juan Delius, an ethologist with a strong interest in both neurophysiology and experimental psychology, has spent much of his life studying the ability of pigeons to learn complex discriminations and solve problems. One of his discoveries is. . . . ◆

Robinson, in Additional Readings, p. 287

The central point could be distilled from these three sentences as "Birds are not stupid because they have some quite remarkable learning abilities."

Often a topic sentence will appear partway into a paragraph:

Many birds do many things with minimal learning. They seem to be hardwired to fly, build nests and so on. *Complex learning has been recognized, however, in a wide variety of circumstances ranging through singing, parent recognition, chick recognition, mate recognition and species recognition.* Some bird species learn song dialects but not the basic patterns of the songs, their basic "tunes." . . . ◆

Robinson 288

This topic sentence follows a concession that grants important limitations on bird intelligence.

Although often called "units of thought," paragraphs should not be confused with "production units," things made on an assembly line such as ceramic capacitors or even whole fryers. Paragraphs do not conform to one pattern. In fact, often there is no sentence or kernel from which a paragraph springs. All the sentences may add up to an unexpressed central subject or point.

Here is an example from a historical study of the family in Latin America. Discussing the nineteenth century, it follows a commentary on the unusual number of households headed by females during the seventeenth and eighteenth centuries, probably a social arrangement that reflects manufacturing done in the home. Notice how in the last sentence the paragraph shifts from interpretation of the *past* to conjecture about the *present:*

The prevalence of this form of household in nineteenth-century Latin America suggests much greater autonomy [independence] for women of all classes than had been perceived previously. It indicates that in this century the domestic unit was determined more by the productive organization of the household than by consumption, sexual ties, or affective needs. The reproductive unit (a natural mother with her children) was generally retained, but stable couple units were notable by their absence, particularly among the lower classes in urban areas. It is interesting to speculate whether the modern post-1960s phenomenon of female-headed households seen now in the U.S. and areas in the Third World, as well as very prominently in Latin America and the Caribbean, bears any analytical relationship to this earlier, distinctive household pattern. ◆

Stoner 310

This paragraph has no topic sentence to forecast the material on nineteenth and twentieth century households. In fact, logically, the "post-1960s" sentence could make up a separate paragraph.

If you avoid leaning too heavily on the "topic sentence" plan for your explanation, you will preserve the light touch of organic development, of naturally progressing thought, that keeps even impersonal writing from sounding robotic. (See the sidebar "A Paragraph Is a Committee Decision.") And as a reader, expect paragraphs to use unpredictable strategies within and between themselves. Paragraphs resemble the game of bridge, with its strategy and partnership, more than bingo.

Make sure that each paragraph follows logically from the next so that if the order were scrambled a reader could rearrange them by following transitions and key words. Here are two paragraphs from an excerpt in the next chapter that illustrate tight continuity. Italics have been added:

> Don't assume that a script that does not look like the examples shown here is somehow defective. There are many different methods to scripting. *Some* writers like to include every technical detail, including which camera will take the shot. . . . On occasion, the *script* will also list various running times, either the times of inserted tapes or an overall chronological listing of when each event in the program is supposed to happen.
>
> *But other scripts* contain few technical instructions, and their authors may simply choose to write everything out in plain English. Instead of "LS fire screen zoom to CU," they might write, "wide shot of the fire, then zoom in closer." ◆
>
> Hausman and Palombo 175–76

Notice how this paragraph begins with a transition from the previous one. It uses the contrast signals "but" and "other" (the latter echoing the word "Some"), and it repeats a key word, "script."

Often a transitional sentence will precede a topic sentence or blend with it. The paragraph below follows a paragraph on a Native American, Ira Hayes, who fought heroically in World War II but led a thwarted life afterward.

> *If Ira Hayes's life came to symbolize to whites what had happened to Indian veterans after the war, a group known as the Navajo code-talkers became the symbol of the great contribution Indians had made during the war.* Early in 1942 the Marine Corps recruited an all-Indian platoon. When basic training ended in July of that year, the men were assigned to units overseas. In battle the Navajos acquitted themselves with much glory and later attracted widespread coverage in the national press. During the war their mission had been kept secret.

Trained in communications, they had adopted the Navajo language as a code which helped in large part to foil the Japanese attempts to break the advance of American marines in the Pacific. In 1945, when it was revealed that the Navajo language had done so much to help the United States win the war against Japan, the "code-talkers" instantly became national heroes and part of American folklore. In the postwar years nearly every motion picture made about the fighting in the Pacific contained scenes of usually anonymous Indians speaking their native languages into field radios and leaving the enemy hopelessly confused and ready to be soundly defeated. ◆

Holm 156–57; footnotes omitted

The first sentence signals a contrast from the idea of the previous paragraph and forecasts the idea of the new paragraph.

For whatever reasons you break for a paragraph, and however overtly you announce its subject or point, be sure that it takes up tightly related material. The word for this feature is *unity*. For example, the paragraph above on Latin American families does have a central concern (although not expressed in one place): female-headed households in the last century and in the present. Each paragraph should cover, not confuse.

In an explanation of rain forests, for example, why do a few animals peep among the leaves in a paragraph on flora? Probably the writer should move the creatures to a paragraph or series of paragraphs on fauna. As you write, be on the lookout for paragraphs that scramble two ideas together instead of separating them and discussing just one. A reader expects writing to do most of this brainwork.

If a topic sentence at the beginning helps you to find the paragraph's purpose and enlighten the reader, use it. But otherwise you should trust your composing to find its own best shape.

If appropriate, use visual emphasis techniques for extra clarity. Headings, for example, help to distinguish a topic from its amplification, to make the logical visible. The more technical the treatment of a subject, and the longer, the more helpful are headings.

An example of the use of visual-emphasis techniques occurs in a manual of drugs called the *Physicians' Desk Reference*. Each entry must be utterly clear because of the potential effects of the drugs on users. So as each entry unfolds, it may employ the following major headings in boldfaced capital letters: **DESCRIPTION, PHARMACOLOGY, INDICATIONS, CONTRAINDICATIONS, WARNINGS, PRECAUTIONS, ADVERSE REACTIONS, DRUG ABUSE AND DEPENDENCE, DOSAGE AND ADMINISTRATION,** and **HOW SUPPLIED.** Each entry also uses italics for subheadings. (For an example of italics used to help separate the different provisions of a law, see "Indian Removal Act" in Additional Readings.)

A PARAGRAPH IS A COMMITTEE DECISION

The paragraph indentation indicates a separation. For what purposes? Here are several common ones:

First, to announce a *logical shift*. Like a turn signal, it helps your reader to expect a change in direction. The shift may be from background information to the first step of a process; from one type to another; from defining by contrast to defining by example or anecdote; and so on. A paragraph is an opportunity to develop some aspect separately and fully.

Second, to control *emphasis*. A short paragraph can place more importance on an idea than a long one. It says, "This is important enough for its own paragraph."

Third, as a way to give the reader *a break for the eyes,* like a speaker who quits talking for a moment to let the audience rest its ears.

A note about paragraphs in the column format. You should know, especially with the advent of desktop publishing, that the length of a paragraph also depends on its width. Since a hundred words in the page-width paragraph favored in school may run for twice as many inches in a column-width paragraph, you will need to provide more frequent paragraph indentations in, say, a newsletter.

So the timing of a paragraph indentation is a committee decision made by Logic, Emphasis, and Eye. Sometimes all three will agree, sometimes two, and sometimes one will prevail over the others.

For an example of such a decision, notice the contrast between video scripts quoted above ("Don't assume that a script . . ."). Instead of its two paragraphs, the "committee" could have decided to use either one or three. In a single, long, seamless paragraph it could have stated the point about a variety of scripts, defined the first type, and then defined the other. Or in a three-paragraph version—which would have emphasized logical distinctions and rested the eye—the first paragraph could have stated the point, the second paragraph could have defined one type, and the third paragraph could have defined the other type. The plan actually adopted by Hausman and Palombo represents a compromise between the strengths of these alternative possibilities.

COMPLETE THE DETAILS

Provide sufficient detail. Develop all material fully enough to meet the needs of your reader. Put yourself in the learner's place to avoid assuming too much. For example, suppose you are the manager of a retail store and there has been a spate of counterfeit $20 bills in your city. In your memo to cashiers, you want to explain what to do if a customer tenders such a fake—but should you first explain how to recognize one?

A complete explanation will keep the reader from telephoning for clarification, arriving at a formal party in a Little Bo Peep costume, delivering 35,000 Old San Diego bricks to the wrong lot, or wondering why, in a paper on cotton and the American Civil War, no distinction is made between the original long-staple variety (able to grow only on the coast) and the later short-staple variety (able to grow almost anywhere in Dixie).

Furthermore, if you want the reader to take some action, don't leave him or her wondering what to do, but spell it out: "Please report to the Human Resources Director at 8:00 a.m. on Wednesday, May 21."

Be sure that each paragraph amplifies its subject adequately. An occasional short paragraph can be used to emphasize a point, but a series of them can make the reader work too hard to combine splintered thoughts. At the same time, beware of overlong paragraphs that miss an opportunity to signal a logical shift or just give the reader a break from reading.

What are some of the ways you can expand on a subject? Here are a number of candidates. Notice how they can overlap, so two or more techniques can work simultaneously. Remember that most of these techniques can help you organize an entire explanation as well as develop sections of it. (For more help, see the sidebar on cubing, p. 14.)

Analyze into Parts. Like a military leader, divide and conquer. Subdivide a topic into major aspects to deal with each separately. For example, the home page of "The Edge-Man Cards and Collectibles" divides the business into four areas: Cards, Autographs & Memorabilia, Buying, and Other. (See the advertisement in Part III.) To analyze a subject into components, study it patiently and receptively—much as you would an undifferentiated hologram until it turns into a picture. You do this not with the eye, however, but with the verbal powers of the brain.

Analyze into Steps. Divide a process into its phases. Examples: making rye bread (Chapter 4), the encounter between Cortéz and the Aztecs (Chapter 5), the preparations and stages of marking the Jewish holiday Yom Kippur.

Define. State the class that something belongs to, then point out its difference from other members. *Pico de gallo* belongs to a class of food—Mexican sauce—and has the distinguishing ingredients of onions, tomatoes, cilantro, fresh jalapeños, and lemon juice. Tell something's composition or function: An axon is the core of a nerve fiber that carries impulses away from the nerve cell. Divide it: The three kinds of stretching are ballistic, slow, and static. Tell its purpose: "The **two-column script** format is used for most nondramatic video programs" (Hausman and Palombo, in Chapter 4).

Compare. Point out similarity. Mexican families in the last century seem comparable to the female-headed households that are widespread in the United States as well as in Latin American and Caribbean countries (Stoner, above). Woody Guthrie's "talking" style resembles rap singing because it deemphasizes melody. The treatment of the natives by Europeans forecasts the treatment of Jews and other minorities by the Nazis.

Draw an Analogy. In detail, compare one subject to another from an unexpected category: verbal concepts likened to a political map; families likened to dance troupes.

Contrast. Point out difference. Ligaments attach bones to bones, whereas tendons attach muscle to bone. Unlike the strings of a piano, those of a guitar can be plucked. Mexican families in the last century were organized according to what the members produced more than to what they consumed, to their sexual ties, or to their emotional needs.

Classify into Groups. Introduce some order among phenomena by putting them into categories. This technique relies on both comparison and contrast. All video scripts fall into three groups: the two-column, the film style, and the storyboard.

Cite an Example. Shift from the more abstract to the more concrete by naming a particular example of a class. An example of a ligament: the annular ligament of the elbow joint. Of Mexican food: *pico de gallo*. Of Rasta musicians: Bob Marley.

Connect Cause and Effect. Bodily flexibility must be maintained or it will fade. Personal letters allow time for thought. War hastens social change.

Furnish Testimony. "Then with bare head/He [i.e., Hannibal] met the frenzy of the storm, the falling sky"—Silius Italicus, one of many classical authorities quoted by Montaigne in the additional readings.

Present a Fact or Detail. "One Schwann cell myelinates only one axon" (below). Jamaica is an island that lies just south of the eastern part of Cuba. "In proportion to body weight, the bird brain is 5 to 20 times larger than the reptile brain" (Robinson, in Additional Readings).

Tell an Anecdote. One example of a brief story is the incident recalled by a Harley rider who stopped at a store (see Chapter 6). Another: "Someone or other was asking one of our beggars . . ." (Montaigne, in Additional Readings).

Give a Description. "A soft, white buckskin skirt, secured about the loins, descended nearly to the ankles" (Battey, in Chapter 4). "Anything that might have offered protection for the soldiers, such as trees and rocks, had been blown away" (Occhipinti, in Chapter 5).

Use Numbers. In your explanation be able to incorporate numbers, whether gleaned from library research or personal observation. They add the power of quantified measurement. They can convey everything from the size of an object like the tribal mask shown in Chapter 2 (41.6 centimeters high and 30.5 centimeters wide), to the extent of a social phenomenon like the number of one-parent family groups headed by a male in the United States (1,562,000).

Partly because computers make it more feasible to collect, store, and interpret data, and partly because governmental agencies make such information available, statistical analysis has become expected whenever possible. So as a writer and reader you should be able to wield basic mathematics and probably know something about statistics. You should at least know four terms:

1. The *mean,* or mathematical average. For example, the ages of all college students added up and divided by the number of students will establish a mean. The result will be closer to that of the younger students because there are more freshmen and sophomores than juniors and seniors.

2. The *median,* or middle number. Figuratively speaking, line up all college students in a row from youngest to oldest, then find the age of the student who stands at the halfway point.

3. The *mode,* or most popular number. Among college students, it's the age that turns up most often—say, 19.6 years.

4. A *correlation,* or co-appearance of two variables over many occurrences. If one thing occurs, the other also does to a significant degree (or does not to a significant degree). For example, a statistical correlation might be found between (a) dropping out of college and (b) working in a job for more than twenty hours a week while going to school.

Notice that correlation does not mean cause. Granted, it may signal causality at work somewhere, but it does not usually reveal a sole, direct cause. Dropping out of school may indeed reflect an excessive number of hours spent on an outside job, hours that subtract from study and sleep; but dropping out may also reflect a lack of academic interest—the same attitude that led many of the students to spend so much time at a job in the first place. So the two kinds of behavior may be effects of the same cause (lack of interest). Indeed, two things may have a high correlation but occupy different strands of a "causal web" (Albiniak).

Remember that statistics can be misleading—as when the state of California presumes a mother is unwed if she keeps her maiden name instead of taking her husband's. (See Ann Bancroft's article in Additional Readings.)

Provide Visuals. In explanation you will often use illustrations to supplement your verbal content. Visuals are expected in many kinds of writing—from advertisements to news stories to textbooks—and advances in computer graphics often make them possible to create.

In some cases, the words and graphics are inseparable, as with the movie poster in Chapter 1. An example from the realm of explanation is a CD-ROM study aid called *Microscopic Anatomy.* It presents photographs taken with the aid of an electron microscope alongside text such as the following:

Here is a cross section of a myelinated nerve axon. The myelin can be seen at the periphery of the electron photograph. Myelin is a lipid-rich substance that is formed by layers of Schwann cell membrane that have wrapped around the axons and had the cytoplasm extruded. One Schwann cell myelinates only one axon. **Microtubules** are the hollow circles in the axon, although they look solid at this low magnification. The **neurofilaments** are the intermediate filaments present. There are also several **mito-chondria.** ◆

Hollinger

The text, furthermore, allows the reader to interact with the illustration. The highlighted terms appear in colors that match arrows pointing to areas on the slide; the student can position a little magnifying glass over one of these arrows, click the "mouse," and enlarge the area.

These methods of development will help you fill out the details of your paragraphs. A paragraph should seem like a complete whole, in the context of neighboring paragraphs, rather than a splinter or fragment. In academic writing especially, if you see a brief paragraph, look skeptically at it; make sure that it works better than a more detailed one. Consider regarding it as a miniature rough draft that invites fuller amplification.

Despite the value of providing details and incorporating numbers, writing itself should not come in concentrated form like mathematics. Like all scientific communication, math condenses its steps to the minimum number, a goal known as "elegance." Beware of making your details impenetrable. How loosely or densely should you pack them? As a writer you must furnish as many steps as are necessary for the receiver to assimilate the information. For example, if explaining a myelinated nerve axon, you might need to define myelin: "A lipid-rich substance that is formed by layers of Schwann cell membrane."

The less understanding the reader carries in the brain, the more you must furnish to the eye. So be able to fill out your explanation rather than condense it. Slow your pace. Give plenty of specifics and examples. Build in repetition. And the more technical or practical your writing, the shorter the paragraphs and sentences should tend to be.

To get raw information, hit the library or the World Wide Web. "I agree that research can spice up a paper," wrote a student, "but no one wants to do it." Substance rather than spice, research not only helps you explain something more fully but also helps you get more interested in a topic and understand it better. As another student testified: "It really is interesting to find out a little more on your subject." Another wrote that research "gives you more angles to come at the paper from." Another: "It gives the paper more background and therefore makes it more interesting."

Although writing is not a tight mathematical formula, it is a promise to be more tidy than the spoken word. When you revise your explanation, watch out for the looseness, repetition, and imprecision that characterizes informal speech. Prime candidates for tightening: organization, paragraph unity, and sentence length and structure.

To reach your goal of conveying information, make sure to avoid any hint of Navajo code-talk by connecting with your reader, highlighting your plan, and completing the details.

Works Cited

Albiniak, Bernard A., Jr. Interview. Coastal Carolina University, January 1997.

Brashear, Howard C. "Aesthetic Form in Familiar Essays." *College Composition and Communication* 22 (1971): 147–55.

Hausman, Carl, with Philip J. Palombo. *Modern Video Production: Tools, Techniques, Applications.* New York: HarperCollins, 1993.

Hollinger, Thomas, Ph.D. *Microscopic Anatomy.* Software design by Richard Rathe, MD, and Tim Garren, BS. Gainesville: Gold Standard Multimedia/University of Florida, 1995.

Holm, Tom. "Fighting a White Man's War: The Extent and Legacy of American Indian Participation in World War II." *The Plains Indians of the Twentieth Century,* ed. Peter Iverson, 149–68. Norman: Oklahoma University Press, 1985.

Salter, Gregory. "The Loudest Island in the World: Jamaica, Home of the Reggae Beat." *In World Music: The Rough Guide,* eds. Simon Broughton, Mark Ellingham, David Muddyman, and Richard Trillo, 521–38. London: Rough Guides, 1994.

Stoner, K. Lynn. *Latinas of the Americas: A Source Book.* Vol. 363, Garland Reference Library of Social Science. New York: Garland, 1989.

"Valium Tablets." *Physicians' Desk Reference.* 48th ed. Montvale, NJ: Medical Economics Data Production Company, 1994: 1969.

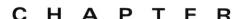

C H A P T E R

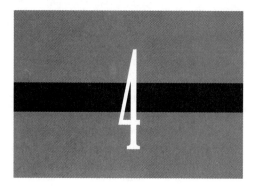

4

Teaching a Skill

Presently the dancers came from behind the screen; their faces, arms, and the upper part of their bodies were painted white; a soft, white buckskin skirt, secured about the loins, descended nearly to the ankles, while the breechcloth,—blue on this occasion,—hanging to the ground, outside the skirt, both in front and behind, completed the dress. They faced the medicine . . . [a bundle of sacred and powerful objects]—jumping up and down in true time with the beating of the drums, while a bone whistle in their mouths, through which the breath escaped as they jumped about, and the singing of the women, completed the music. The dancers continued to face the medicine with arms stretched upwards and towards it,—their eyes as it were riveted to it. They were apparently oblivious to all surroundings, except the music and what was before them.

Battey 175

This skill, a medicine dance of the Kiowa tribe, illustrates the way members of the human race have always taught each other without the written word—without so much as the dot of an *i,* the dash of a Hebrew vowel, or the *sukun* over an Arabic letter.

North American Indians, for example, passed on such skills as weaving baskets or blankets, making baby carriers from bark and root-stitching, embellishing dresses with beads or elk teeth, cooking with hot stones dropped into a hole lined with hide to boil water, making cakes of chokecherries pounded in a rawhide mortar, carving masks and totems, curing the sick by detecting witches, fashioning nose and ear ornaments out of shell, constructing a lodge with birch bark and willow poles tied together with ash splints and spruce roots, singing in a five-tone scale. They practiced scapulimancy by holding the shoulder blade of an animal over a fire and "reading" the darkened patterns. They recited stories to help the long winter pass. Fathers taught sons to shoot with a bow and arrow (see Figure 4.1).

Today oral instructions are still used for simple tasks. They may be supplemented by written ones, however, as when someone gives a handson explanation to clarify the manual. And writing is now indispensable for explaining complex skills to people not in the presence of the teacher. Speaking itself may be based on a written script, as with instructional videotapes like *Christy Lane's Funky Freestyle Dancing* or *Making A's in College.*

The more technical the instructions you write for this chapter, the greater "stretch" you will enjoy. Technical writing deals with concrete phenomena such as descriptions, procedures, processes, and standards. It uses specialized jargon, quantified information (numbers and measurements),

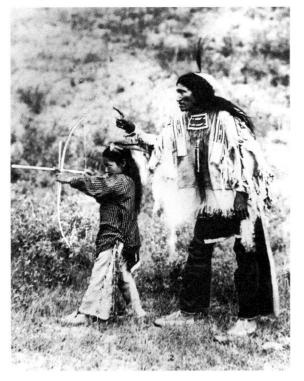

Fig. 4.1 ✳ **"KICKING BEAR," A SIOUX, TEACHING HIS SON TO SHOOT**

Lieb Image Archives, York, PA.

techniques of visual emphasis such as headings, and graphic aids such as tables and illustrations. It is rigorously objective in presentation, so that there are few clues to the writer's opinions or personality.

Your instructions will enable the reader to learn some practical skill. You can structure your explanation in a number of ways. Here are two:

Step by Step. You can view the skill as a process you want to teach and analyze it into its phases from beginning to end.

Examples:

* How to put together a bicycle from wheels to handgrips.
* How to form a legal corporation from first to last.
* How to install a piece of computer software in the right order.
* How to prepare for an athletic meet, day by day.
* How to write a sales letter from top to bottom (by getting attention, kindling interest, evoking desire, and asking for action).

Each stage of the process depends on the previous one(s) and must be finished before the next begins. This method of explanation is probably the most common type of instructions, but it is not the only method.

Pie to Pieces. Another way to teach a skill is to divide it into its logical parts or properties, rather than as a chronological structure.

Examples:

* The essentials of choreography: "There is no rule that says which comes first—theme, intention, motivation, or even a specific movement phrase" (Blom and Chaplin 8).
* The duties to be performed on a job (not treated sequentially).
* The principles a female executive should follow when buying a wardrobe.
* Ways to care for a cat (i.e., to meet its needs for health, safety, and affection).
* The traits needed by an employee at Burger Queen (such as friendliness, cleanliness, and efficiency).

Such subdivided aspects can occur in varying order or even simultaneously. The qualities of friendliness, cleanliness, and efficiency, for example, can be exhibited by an employee at any time and in any combination. (In contrast, a person assembling a toy baby-carriage must put each wheel on the axle *before* putting on the unremovable capnuts—as one inexperienced Santa Claus will testify.)

Instructions can combine these two methods. For example, someone teaching how to write a direct-mail appeal might divide sales writing into its major principles before outlining the steps of a sales letter. Or while discussing the need for cleanliness at Burger Queen, a writer might outline the steps of handling food with attention to hygiene.

The question-and-answer format is sometimes used to explain a skill. It can work by either the "steps" or "pie" method, or by a combination. It approximates the way skills used to be taught orally and personally because the questioner is a stand-in for the reader; the method seems to involve him or her in a slightly dramatic interplay. For an example, see Becky Fullwood's "Tips on How to Be a Cashier" (Additional Readings).

WARM UP FIRST

The boss has OK'd your proposal to produce a videotaped set of instructions on how to do your job. Make a preliminary list of five or ten actions that you want to film. You might want to specify which ones are close-ups. (For this warm-up exercise, use any job from your experience.)

PUBLISHED INSTRUCTIONS

Have you ever wondered how audio and video are coordinated for a news broadcast or other televised production? Someone had to teach this skill to the writers and videographers. The following explanation is adapted from "Scripting for Video," Chapter 13 of *Modern Video Production: Tools, Techniques, Applications* by Carl Hausman with Philip J. Palombo.

At the beginning of the chapter, Hausman and Palombo try to motivate the reader by stating that "putting words on paper is one of the most important facets of video production." This excerpt comes from the first section of the chapter, called "Script Formats." It covers three types of script: the two-column, the film-style, and the storyboard.

The authors, using the pie-to-pieces technique, divide a model two-column script into its components to help the reader compose one like it.

Notice how the instructions make use of boldface type for emphasis and numerous methods of development for amplification.

THE TWO-COLUMN SCRIPT FORMAT

❋

Carl Hausman with Philip J. Palombo

This paragraph defines the script first by its use ("non-dramatic") and then by its specialized columns. "Talent" has been defined as on-air performers.

An example will carry much of the information: In other words, for more on "how to," here's one.

The **two-column script** format is used for most non-dramatic video programs. The left-hand column contains technical instructions, primarily camera shots and movements, along with descriptions of the motion of talent. The right-hand column contains audio, such as dialogue and description of music or other sounds.

A page from a two-column script used in a news presentation is shown in the Figure.

Video	Audio
CU ANCHOR TED:	City fire fighters call it a miracle . . . they report no injuries in a fire that consumed a ten-story office building this afternoon
LS TILDEN BUILDING	TED (VO): The Tilden building, a landmark on the corner of Main and Delaware, erupted in flames shortly after two o'clock.
LS WORKERS EVACUATING	But all four hundred workers inside were able to safely evacuate . . . thanks, according to Fire Chief Tom O'Brien, to the fact that smoke detectors and sprinklers operated perfectly and gave the occupants of the building plenty of warning.
VTR O'BRIEN	O'BRIEN (SOT): It took about 20 minutes for what was a small garbage fire in the basement to start climbing up inside the walls. Nobody would have seen the flames until it was too late. But the smoke detectors went off right away, giving everyone plenty of time to clear the building. When the fire finally spread, it was like an explosion. If people had been in that building when the flames erupted, they never would have gotten out. No way.
CU ANCHOR TED:	O'Brien says the cause of the fire has not yet been determined, but arson has not been ruled out.

Just as "Stretch" provides Hausman and Palombo's explanation as a model, they provide a sample of a two-column script.

Fig. ∗ **A TWO-COLUMN NEWS PRESENTATION SCRIPT**

The pronoun "you" connects reader to information. SOT is defined in detail.

Some abbreviations in the script in the figure may be familiar to you: **CU** is close-up, and **LS** is long shot. The abbreviation **VO** means voice-over. VO is used to show whenever anyone is speaking over an image other than his or her on-camera picture. **SOT** means **sound on tape,** a term which indicates that the actual audio on the videotape is what will go over the air. Using the abbreviation *SOT* is often helpful to the director because it lets him or her know that the audio from the videotape is what the viewer is supposed to hear. In one scene from the illustration, for example, the viewer is watching pictures of the fire, but hears—*in the voice-over*—the anchor talking. The next scene shows an interview with the fire fighter and includes the audio from that interview too, meaning it is an SOT segment.

VO and SOT are common abbreviations, especially in news scripts. Abbreviations often used in all types of video scripts include those listed in the Table.

A subject of an earlier explanation, camera movement, is woven in to this later one, the two-column script, so that each gains clarity by its tie-in with the other.

Camera movements, which were first discussed in Chapter 2, are sometimes indicated on the left-hand side of the two-column script. But often, they are not because camera movements are typically left to the discretion of the director. Generally, camera movements are spelled out: zoom dolly, pedestal, truck, or tilt, are examples. Occasionally, the transitions are spelled out too: fade, cut, dissolve.

External sources of audio and video are also frequently abbreviated, as shown in the Table. None of the abbreviations in the Table apply specifically to news. Any type of video presentation can use these abbreviations and the spelled-out instructions. . . . [The authors refer to a second figure showing part of the script for an industrial training tape that uses many of the terms and abbreviations shown in the Table.]

The authors acknowledge the limitation of their examples, stress the variety of techniques, and explain one more type.

Don't assume that a script that does not look like the examples shown here is somehow defective. There are many different methods to scripting.

Some writers like to include every technical detail, including which camera will take the shot. (In most cases that's not really necessary, because a director can call shots.) On occasion, the script will also list various running times, either the times of inserted tapes or an overall chronological listing of when each event in the program is supposed to happen.

But other scripts contain few technical instructions, and their authors may simply choose to write everything out in plain English. Instead of "LS fire screen zoom to CU," they might write, "wide shot of the fire, then zoom in closer."

The "plain English" script is contrasted to the technical script.

Simple, plain-English scripts have decided advantages because they don't require a director, editor, or other crewperson to figure out an abbreviation that may be idiosyncratic to your style of writing or your department's script formatting guidelines.

The abbreviations used to indicate technical components of the script can be bewildering, which is why we have introduced them at gradual stages in the explanation of scripting.

* Table *

Common Video Script Abbreviations

Abbreviations	Explanation
XLS	extreme long shot
LS	long shot
MS	medium shot
CU	close up
XCU	extreme close-up
2S	two shot (a shot that includes two people, usually side-by-side)
OC	on camera . . .
OS	over-the-shoulder shot
SOT	sound on tape (a videotape played back with picture and sound)
VTR	videotape recorder or videotape recording
SFX	sound effects
VO	voice-over

Questions

1. Is the explanation clear to you? If not on the first reading, on the second?
2. What level of knowledge do the writers assume in the reader?
3. The sample script in the figure has five segments. Can you explain what the viewer would see and hear in each? (Use one sentence per segment.)
4. In which segment of the figure are there no traces of Ted's voice or hairdo?
5. Does this explanation use the "plain English" it recommends for script instructions?

For another such model used to teach a skill, see Figure 4.2, a business letter, published in 1607, showing how to ask a friend for a favor.

Consider the Themes

* What sort of news would you say that television is the best medium to convey?
* Audiovisual communication based on written scripts: Can you estimate how much time you spend during the week receiving it from

Emmanuel.

AFter my very harty commendations vnto you: I pray for your good health and pro-fperitie,& c. Thefe are moft heartilie to defire fo much your friendfhip and good will,to doe me this pleafure:as to receiue for me out of the Gabriel when fhe cómeth to S. Lucar, 6. tuns of Lead containing 150. peeces, being marked as in the * margent: & to doe fo much as make prefent fale of it, the beft you can as the time feructh. And when you haue made fale and re-ceiued monies for it, that you would bee fo good as to ride vnto Sheres and buy for me 8. Buts of very good Sacke, the beft that poffible can bee gotten, though they coft a Ducket or two the more in a But:& to lade them away as foone as is poffible abord the Gabriell, mark-ing thé with the former marke in the margent. And the reft of the monies that you fhall haue left,I pray you to paffe it with all fpeede hither to Siuill vnto me. Herein (if without feeming ouer bold)I may craue your paines to pleafure me:I doe affure you that you fhall finde me to the vttermoft of my power,both gratefull and mindfull to pleafure you againe in the like,and much greater if I can bee able. Little newes I heare woorth the writing. Thus taking my leaue I commit you to Almightic God. From Siuill the 27.day of Ianuarie.1589.

Your affured to my
power, R. A.

Fig. 4.2 ✳ MODEL LETTER, 1607

From *The Merchants Avizo,* London. The indentation of a paragraph has not always been a convention of writing. Where would you insert paragraph breaks in this letter?

television programs, advertisements, movies, videotape programs, even Internet resources?

✳ During World War II the United States used scripts as propaganda in radio programs (even soap operas), movies shown to the public or to the military, and news shown in movie theaters. When would you call such writing unethical in selection and slant?

STUDENT EXPLANATION 1
✳

Shifting from the audiovisual to the edible, here is a type of instruction that may be more familiar to you. Recipes usually list ingredients and then ex-plain the process, so they integrate both logical and chronological analyses.

MAKING RYE BREAD

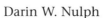

Darin W. Nulph

The Egyptians, more than 10,000 years ago, first started eating some type of prepared leavened or rising breads. Since then, people have included baked flour and yeast products as part of their diet. Being a veteran of bread making, I can claim that it is really not as hard as many people may think. In fact, it can be quite fun, and there is nothing like eating your own homemade breads.

There are two types of yeast breads, batter yeast and kneaded yeast. Batter yeast breads can be made into a very thick batter in the mixer. They are then poured into the baking pan and allowed to rise. You do not knead the batter for yeast bread. After baking, batter yeast breads have a yeasty smell and have a coarse and open-grained texture.

Kneaded yeast bread can also be made into dough in the mixer. But the dough is then kneaded in the mixer or by hand. If you knead by hand, here is a helpful hint. Place the dough in the mixing bowl and punch your fist into the center of the dough to release excess air. Then fold the outer edges into the center. Turn the dough over and let it rise. The kneaded yeast breads are then kneaded and allowed to rise, usually several times. The kneaded yeast breads usually have a fine, even-grained texture due to the gases being evenly distributed through the kneading of the dough.

An example of kneaded yeast bread is rye bread. Below is a recipe for rye bread:

> 1 package active dry yeast
> 1 cup warm water
> 1 tbsp. butter or margarine
> 1 tbsp. caraway seeds
> 1/4 cup cornmeal
> 1 tbsp. molasses
> 1 tsp. salt
> 1 3/4 cup flour (divided)
> 1/4 cup rye flour

The first thing that you must do is grease a large glass bowl and set it aside. Second, dissolve the yeast in warm water in a mixing bowl. Now add the butter, caraway seeds, molasses, salt, and one cup of the all purpose flour. Blend this sufficiently. At this point, add the rye flour, and mix this well. Now add the remaining all purpose flour and mix. At last when the dough is mixed, remove it from the bowl and form it into a ball. Then roll it in the greased bowl until it is well greased.

Afterward, cover the bowl with a cloth and let the dough rise for 90 minutes. Dough rises best between 80 and 90 F in a draft-free area. It is best to use a large, well-greased, glass mixing bowl because it will retain warmth better than a metal mixing bowl. You want the dough to stay slightly warm. If it gets cold, it becomes much harder to knead and form. It is also important to keep the dough in a draft free environment, because if the dough catches a draft, it dries on the exterior and becomes gritty and hard. This will make it harder to knead and form.

When 90 minutes is up, take the dough out of the bowl and rest it on a lightly floured board for 10 minutes. This process will remove any excess water before baking. Meanwhile, preheat your oven to 375 F. Also grease a cookie sheet and dust it with cornmeal. Now you are ready to form the dough into a loaf and place it on the cookie sheet. Slash the top of the dough with a knife a few times for decoration. Cover the loaf and let it rise another 50 minutes. Then bake in the oven for 40–50 minutes.

Many people frown upon making their own bread, often using the excuse of it being too hard and time-consuming. But the only time-consuming work involved is waiting for the dough to rise several times. The actual mixing and baking time is not a time-consuming process as people are led to believe. While waiting for the dough to rise, you can always pick up a good book to read and before you know it, you will have some delicious homemade bread to eat.

Questions

1. Can you make out the main parts of these instructions? Try labeling them in the margin. Can you then distinguish between main sections and their subdivisions?

2. What advantage(s) might this written version of this piece have over a videotape version? (For an instructional video on making bread with a machine, see *Better Bread,* Regal Ware, Inc., Kewaskum, WI.)

3. Would any visual aids help you understand the process? (See Figure 4.3 for a visual explanation of tobacco-making.)

4. In your opinion, should Darin Nulph omit references to himself? Delete the pronoun "you"?

5. To what extent can a written text furnish a sort of recipe for its own "preparation" by the reader?

Nulph uses other methods of developing a subject besides process analysis (the steps of the recipe). Notice how they overlap and reinforce each other in Nulph's directions:

Classification: types of yeast bread (batter and kneaded).

Contrast: batter versus yeast.

Definition: two meanings of "time consuming."

Description: batter bread's smell and texture.

Example: rye bread (one type of kneaded bread).

Cause and effect: problems caused by cold or dry dough.

Logical analysis: the ingredients of rye bread.

Testimony: "Being a veteran. . . ."

Background detail: Egyptians 10,000 years ago.

Breadmaking itself offers an **analogy** to the kneading and unforced rising of thought in the meditation form (Chapter 2). And a loaf of bread baking in the oven is probably a **symbol**—a concrete object or event that suggests something else—in "Heat in the Attic" by Gary Walker and Diana Jo Wilson (Additional Readings).

Consider the Themes

* How has bread helped to create your family bonds? How many specific ways can you remember?

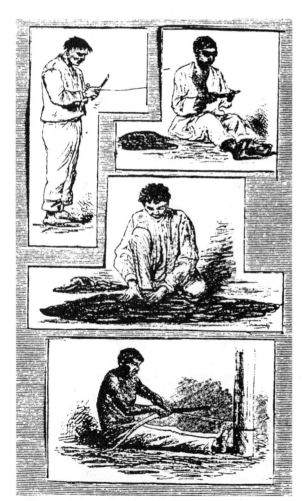

Fig. 4.3 * **PREPARING TOBACCO**
From Herbert H. Smith, "An American Home on the Amazons," 1879. Illustration by J. Wells Champney.

* "Paper is the bread of civilization"—Theodore Rosengarten, author of *Tombee: Portrait of a Cotton Planter* (1986). Does this maxim still hold true with all the nonprint resources available for communication?

STUDENT EXPLANATION 2

Like Darin Nulph, Kimberlie Chandler provides an introduction that offers background and motivation. She combines the techniques of logical analysis—dividing the job into its requirements for practices as well as game days—with step-by-step analysis.

PREPARING FOR A SOCASTEE HIGH SCHOOL FOOTBALL GAME

*

Kimberlie Chandler
For SHS Student Trainers

"There is no other person who can unify a health care program for the athlete with greater dispatch than the properly trained and accredited athletic trainer." –R. W. Redfern.

As a Socastee High School student trainer, you have many responsibilities. Your job is to help the head athletic trainer ensure that each athlete is able to perform to the best of his or her ability.

The responsibility of preparing the athletes and the trainers for sports events takes time. Time for after-school practices as well as time before, during, and following the games. Student trainers need this time to prepare equipment needed for practices and games.

The sport that is the most time-consuming and demanding is football. There are two times during the week when you must be present to carry out your duties during football season: on Monday and Tuesday you must go out to the practice field. Most of the time it isn't necessary to unload the cart until an emergency occurs. The only things that should be put out are the slush buckets, which are filled with ice, water, and two towels (Illustration 1).

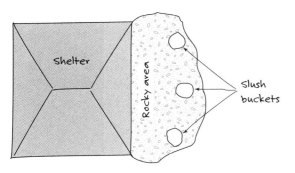

Illustration 1 * **PRACTICE FIELD SHELTER**

Shelter

Rocky area

Slush buckets

When practice is over, collect all the equipment—the cart, empty slush buckets, and used towels—and go back to the school building. Clean all equipment and put it where it belongs.

Game Day

On game day be in the training room at 5:00 P.M. The players will arrive for treatment at this time, and you must treat them as quickly as possible. After the players have received treatment, prepare the equipment.
Game equipment:

* trainer's kit
* splint bag
* tool box
* 8–10 towels bagged
* 2 coolers of water
* 2 coolers of Gatorade
* 1 cooler of ice

* 2 cup trays
* 4 sleeves of cups
* 2 water bottle trays with bottles
* 4 small bags of oranges cut
* 2 slush buckets
* pitcher
* pair of crutches

Again, remember to stock the trainer's kit and tool box.

When all of the equipment is ready, take out everything except the oranges and one cooler of Gatorade to the sidelines. The oranges and Gatorade are left in the hall of the school building for pre-game and halftime. To set up for pre-game, fill 50 cups with Gatorade and line them on a table for the players.

On the sideline, arrange the equipment according to Illustration 2.

Once the game has started, it is essential that you keep the water and Gatorade cups filled. The players must always have fluids readily available to prevent dehydration.

When there are about five minutes left in the second quarter, go back to the school building so that you can set up for halftime. Fill 50 cups with the Gatorade and set out the bags of oranges. Be sure that all players eat some fruit so that their bodies can replace lost fluids quickly.

After halftime, continue to watch the rest of the game. When the game is over, pack up all of the equipment and bring it inside. Once inside, clean all equipment and place it where it belongs. You will continue to perform these duties weekly throughout the season.

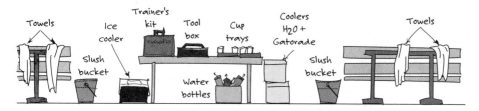

Illustration 2 * **SIDELINE OF PLAYING FIELD**

Questions

1. How does the writer try to connect her explanation to the reader in the introduction?
2. Can you label the main parts and subdivisions? Should Chandler have provided another heading that would parallel "Game Day"?
3. What detail about the perspective in Illustration 1 should Kimberlie add?

Consider the Themes

* The name "Socastee" comes from an Indian word. Can you list ten places that take their names from Native American languages?
* How important is music to the game of football? Do you find an incongruity between such a rough game and harmony at halftime? Is music important to any other American sport?
* Musical notation relies primarily on nonverbal symbols. Look at the instructions to the pianist in Figure 4.4: Can you translate them into words?

STRETCH:
TEACH A CONCRETE, PRACTICAL SKILL

Explain how to do some kind of human performance. Your instructions can work step by step or property by property ("pie-to-pieces"). Without having the person or people being instructed present, let the written word "speak" for you.

Here are a few contrasts with earlier assignments in *Stretch.* Instead of writing a story, meditation, or personal essay on playing in a band, give instructions on how to arrange a gig, set up for it, get through it, and get paid; or on the responsibilities of a good band member.

Provide a map rather than undertake an exploration. Your writing should be a means to an end rather than a pleasure in itself, so do not charm, entertain, or touch the reader. Deemphasize personal experience, variety, and surprise; present a fairly dry, systematic and complete exposition of a subject.

Fig. 4.4 * MUSICAL NOTATION
Courtesy William R. Hamilton.

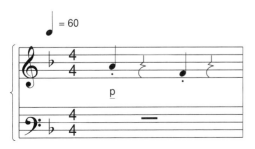

A few signposts may help you avoid the mistakes made by other pilgrims bound for the City of Instruction:

* Don't explain an impersonal process like internal combustion. Instead of telling how metals fuse, for instance, tell how to weld metals. And though a historical background might add interest, write mainly about the future: not "How Córtez Conquered Mexico" but "How to Travel Cheaply and Safely in Mexico."

* Don't be ironic. Although a how-to-do-it format can be used for humor (e.g., "How to Wreck a Date"), this assignment is to give you practice with straightforward explanation of the kind you will write in school and at work.

* Don't write a persuasive paper: No controversial point, emotional appeal, proof, rebuttal of opposing viewpoints. You are not trying to overcome resistance. In one paper on resurfacing hardwood floors, a former professional tended to warn the reader not to try the job himself or herself; instead, the writer should have directed his straightforward instructions to a new employee. Your instructions may, however, have a slight argumentative edge, as when you favor one method or product over another.

To help yourself remain impersonal, omit the word "I," as in a laboratory report, unless you judge that any personal references will lend special credibility, as in the breadmaking instructions, or interest. Instead of the personal "I will guide you through the steps of CPR," try a formula such as "These steps will guide you through the steps of CPR." (For an example of instructions that incline more to the subjective and interpretive than the technical, read Ronald V. Smith's informal essay "The Art of Watching Silent Films," in Additional Readings.)

Consider the following suggestions and use whatever helps. They adapt the techniques discussed in "Explain" to instructions.

Connect with Your Reader

Determine Who. As with all communication, try to compose your message with your reader's point of view in mind. Be able to adjust to his or her (1) level of knowledge and (2) degree of interest.

Envisioning your audience will help you know how much understanding of the subject you can take for granted. Are you addressing novices? People with a technical background? Your audience will determine how dense your instructions can be or how expanded—how long your sentences should be, how much ancillary explanation you should supply (such as definitions), and how much repetition you should build in. Envisioning your readers will help you anticipate questions and problems.

Name your intended reader beneath your title, as Kimberlie Chandler does. For example, one technical manual, called *Machinery's Handbook*, does spell out its audience: "A reference book for the mechanical engineer, designer, manufacturing engineer, draftsman, toolmaker, and machinist" (Green, title page).

Students sometimes fear taxing the reader's patience: "But this will be boring." Assume, however, that your reader already has some interest in the subject, so enrich his or her life by the new skill rather than the presentation itself.

Use "You." Address the reader directly using the pronoun "you." Although schools have often turned their nose up at this word as too chummy, it can "reach out and touch someone" in practical situations. Use the imperative form of the verb: "Dissolve the yeast" rather than "The yeast is dissolved."

Tell Why. Perhaps undertake a little motivation to reinforce the reader's interest. For example, in the chapter on scripting for video, the first paragraph begins by telling the importance of the skill:

Putting words on paper is one of the most important facets of video production. All the high-tech hardware in the world cannot compensate for clumsy expression on the part of the scriptwriter. . . .

Hausman and Palombo 175

A pamphlet called *The Disney Look,* which furnishes guidelines for clothing, accessories, hairstyles, and so on, to "cast members" of Disney World first tries to explain *why* a consistent look is important to the park's success. For motivation with higher stakes, here is an excerpt from the *Soldier's Handbook* of 1941:

Your rifle is a machine. It gives the best results when it is clean and properly lubricated. A dirty, poorly lubricated rifle may have stoppages which will make it useless in battle. Inspect your rifle daily and see that it is clean and properly lubricated. Neglect of your rifle may cost you your life on the battlefield. (39)

So to encourage attentive reading you may want to show how the subject meets some need. Think of the readers not as inert recipients of information but as collaborators; the more interested they are in the skill, the more attentive they will be. As one authority, Frank Smith, points out, reading "is not a passive activity—readers must make a substantial and active contribution if they are to make sense of print" (12).

Highlight Your Plan

Title Your Paper. The title is your first "lighthouse" (see the sidebar on p. 88); it should announce your subject precisely. "Preparing for a Socastee High School Football Game" offers more direction than "A Trainer."

Tell Purpose and Scope. Your introduction, the second lighthouse, should stand tall and have a lot of candlepower. Somewhere in the introduction, announce your purpose. Your phrasing will repeat or closely echo your title. Keep your reader as certain as possible from the beginning.

You might specify one or more behavioral objectives—that is, intended effects on what a person can do. Hausman and Palombo list three before launching into their explanation: "After completing Chapter 13, you will be able to: 1. Use standard script formats. 2. [etc.]" (175).

Also forecast the scope of your instructions. This step is a convention of technical writing. To guide the reader's expectations, tell how much your explanation will cover, and perhaps how much it won't. Be sure to narrow your scope enough to complete the task in adequate detail; for example, you might take up only one aspect of playing in a band, such as how to get the most out of a practice session.

You might also forecast the major subdivisions of your paper. This common use of an extra signal helps a reader keep the main phases of your paper in mind so that, in turn, each detail gains significance by its relationship to a framework.

Use Headings. Since you are not writing an essay, which unfolds more subtly, use organizational headings to reinforce your plan by highlighting the main sections of your paper. These examples of visual emphasis can appear over <u>underlines</u> or in CAPITAL LETTERS, **boldface,** *italics,* or color. One student used headings to divide his paper, called "How to Change the Oil in Your Car," into three main parts: Getting Set Up, Removing the Old Oil, and Replacing the Oil and Filter.

In technical writing, headings can replace transitional signals within the rest of the text: "*Perform a Title Search.* In the county courthouse, locate. . . ." To be safe, however, use headings to supplement other logical transitions, not replace them: "*Perform a Title Search.* After the contract has been reviewed, do a title search on the property. In the county courthouse, locate. . . ." In this approach, if the headings were omitted, the explanation would still have continuity between its parts.

Use a Vertical List. Whereas academic writing generally uses the paragraph, much practical writing uses lists presented vertically, often with heavy dots called "bullets":

* Free inspection
* 7 year or 70,000 mile protection plan on engine and powertrain

Be sure to insert a blank line before and after each vertical list.

Here is an example of such a list (with some of its items emphasized by italics) from "Fashion and the Woman Executive" in *Letitia Baldrige's New Complete Guide to Executive Manners:*

* *Buy with quality—not quantity—in mind.* Good fabrics are essential.

* *Accessories are all-important.* Shoes, handbag, jewelry, hosiery, scarf—everything a woman executive adds to her basic dress or suit is integral to the general impression she gives.

* She should know what colors look good on her and buy those, whenever possible. She should know which colors clash.

* She should move around and sit down in front of a full-length mirror whenever she tries on garments, so that she can see what happens to the skirt when she moves or sits.

* *She should follow fashion, but not blindly.* If the magazines are touting something only a young, pencil-slim model can wear, she should take along a frank friend, who will steer her away from something that looks really bad on her. If she doesn't have such a friend, she should ask a store fashion consultant to square with her and edit her selection with honesty. (Baldrige 217–18)

(For comic instructions on "the basics in hairstyle management," see Dave Barry's "Bald Truth about Hair" in Additional Readings.)

Use Other Emphasis Techniques. Use boldface or italics to emphasize important terms such as *SOT* (sound-on-tape). You might do the same to emphasize a warning, like an entry in the *Physicians' Desk Reference*. The explanation of Valium (trademark registered) Tablets uses boldfaced lower-case to look the reader in the eye: **"The prescriber should be aware of a risk of seizure in association with flumazenil treatment, particularly in long-term benzodiazepine users and in cyclic anti-depressant overdose"** (1969). (Misuse of this drug is pictured in Salomea Kape's "Designer Genes," in Additional Readings.)

Complete the Details

Cover Each Step or Part. Because you are so familiar with the skill, you may leave out something important because it's obvious to you. Beware of making the reader say "But what about. . . ?" Consider highlighting a step of gathering the necessary tools (like the ingredients for rye bread).

Define Terms. When you use a technical word, remember the analogy of language as a political map and make sure that your reader understands the location and shape of the "country" that the word stands for. A writer who uses the word "riff," for example, might define it as an improvised musical figure.

Use Methods of Development. At any point in your instructions would the reader appreciate another detail, some description, a contrast or comparison, an example, an analysis into parts, an explanation of cause or effect, a measurement?

Give Tips. From your experience, give advice or even warnings that will make the skill easier to perform, faster, safer, less expensive, and so on. Examples: "A salesperson needs to be able to stand for long periods of time"; "Cooperating with your buddy can make suiting-up for a game much easier and faster"; "Wash the fabric before sewing it."

Tell What NOT To Do. Include "Don'ts" to head off problems: "Don't hit the tennis ball so hard that you can't control the shot"; "Don't make this dish for company until you've tried cooking it one time"; "Don't try to mow over fallen apples—rake them up first."

Use Visuals. (See sidebar on Writing and Graphics.) To explain a skill fully, you may want to provide a sketch, like Chandler's picture of the football dugout. One student who described a tool used to decorate gingerbread figures furnished a picture of it. Your graphics need not be of professional quality, just clear enough to complement the written word. Or they can employ sophisticated computer techniques as shown in the sidebar.

WRITING AND GRAPHICS

Graphics do what writing alone cannot. They can present images (as in a photograph) or condense information (as in a graph). Illustrations are traditionally classified as either tables or figures:

Tables show the relationships between words and numbers by using the format of rows and columns. The table on video script abbreviations (p. 104) can also be called a "matrix," or a tablelike presentation in words alone.

Figures include visual examples such as the two-column script for news presentation on page 102. They include charts, graphs, diagrams, photographs, maps, and drawings.

The *Physicians' Desk Reference* supplements written explanations of drugs with photographs. One edition shows Valium as a round pill with a heart-shaped cutout that comes in three doses (color-coded by white, yellow, and blue). In the brochure called *The Disney Look*, drawings contrast acceptable and unacceptable hairstyles for men and women.

Your own visuals for this assignment need only be sophisticated enough to give the reader extra help. Or they can employ sophisticated computer graphics as seen in this example (Diagram 1):

For efficient use of an illustration (table or figure),

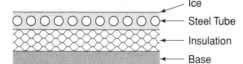

Ice
Steel Tube
Insulation
Base

Diagram 1 ✳ CROSS-SECTION OF INDOOR ICE SURFACE
Charlene Slugoski.

1. refer to it at the timeliest moment in your text—right when it will help out
2. supply it right after you mention it, or on the next page, or in an appendix

3. number it—for example, Figure 2

4. title it—for example, Figure 2. Cross section of indoor ice surface

5. give credit to any source—for example, author, name of book, city, publisher, date, page.

To follow the convention, like Hausman and Palombo, put the title above a table and below a figure.

To settle on a topic, consult an expert: yourself. Look at your own experience with jobs, athletics, hobbies, and unusual challenges. You could turn some aspect of your informal essay into instructions. One student who had explored the origins of her ice skating career in a story later explained how a four-layer ice surface is constructed for performances.

You might even write an exploratory essay first (e.g., about the job of a cashier). Narrow your scope for thoroughness but take on something that challenges you:

NOT "How to make a peanut butter sandwich"

BUT "How to plan a menu."

If you know another member of the class who also has some expertise in the subject, the two of you might collaborate, with the permission of your teacher.

Ten+ Topics

Here are some "how to" possibilities:

1. How to do something that you learned in a college course, such as a mathematical or scientific procedure, or a sports technique or computer process (e.g., scanning a graphic into a text, perhaps for use on the Internet).

2. How to do a job (or part of a job). This kind of explanation is called a job description; it can be kept on file for later workers. If you have experience in the military, you might draw on those duties for your paper.

3. How to perform a religious practice or ceremony (e.g., a Seder ceremony, or fasting for Ramadan and/or Lent).

4. How to do something you know from a hobby or outside interest (e.g., how to design a Web site using an HTML editor program).

5. How to do something familiar to you from your regional, ethnic, or racial heritage.

6. How to use the code of laws for your state. You may need to discuss annual supplements, CD-ROM versions, and commercial Internet aids.

7. How to do something that you learned because of an unusual experience.

8. How to do something on campus—apply for financial aid, get involved with an organization, live with a difficult roommate, work with a counselor.

9. How to get the most out of touring an area of a city, country, and so on, with which you are familiar.

10. How to deal with a challenge in family life.

To help you realize the wide array of "how to" topics available, here are some chosen by students:

* start a "fanzine" for other young people
* be a games supervisor at _____
* prep your dirt bike
* assemble your SCUBA equipment (a review for beginners)
* prepare your horse for riding (for children)
* relearn to walk after an injury
* replace tips and ferrules for Meucci billiard cues
* restring your guitar (for a beginner)
* barbecue correctly
* be a photographer at Dixie Stampede (for a job trainee)
* clean homes professionally
* prepare for opening day as a lifeguard
* shoot fouls
* swim the butterfly stroke
* tap dance (for beginners)
* care for a cat
* prepare for long-distance travel in a car
* drive a stick-shift car
* design a title slide with Microsoft Powerpoint
* interview for a job at Walt Disney World
* close XYZ doctors' office at the end of the day
* buy a house
* get a quick start in running track
* prepare a canvas for painting
* keep children safe when operating an afterschool program
* go through the divorce process

REVISE TO MAKE THAT REACH

With the help of your teacher or other students, ask: Does your explanation fan the reader's interest? Have a clear purpose? Suit the readers' level of knowledge? Follow a clear pattern? Cover a narrow-enough subject with adequate development? Anticipate problems?

A few hints:

* Review "Explain," Part II.
* Do a little research for more depth and detail. You can find technical material in the library of a technical college or elsewhere, and many libraries will have background information on your topic. You might talk with people familiar with the subject. If you need to acknowledge sources, there are several possibilities:

    1. Give a blanket acknowledgement at the beginning. Declare that the information comes from such and such. (Don't just rehash the pamphlet or whatever source.)

    2. Use parenthetical citations as you go (e.g., Jones 31); then document all these sources fully in a Works Cited page at the end of your paper.

    3. Append a list of Works *Consulted*—that is, material read and used to some extent but not actually quoted or cited in the text.

* Avoid overusing forms of the verb "be," whether to form the passive voice or to link words. Go through your paper and circle every *is* or *are* to see if you should replace any with an energetic verb. Two theoretical illustrations: Change "When the game is over" to "When the game ends"; change "It is important for the store to" to "The store should."

EXTRA CHALLENGE

Whether on your own or with one or more fellow students, limber up some more joints and ligaments by writing a variation on this chapter's "STR-R-ETCH" assignment:

1. Write an ironic (mocking) set of instructions. Examples:

    How to Prepare a Canvas Improperly

    How to Do the Worst Job as a Clerk at Wilson's Bakery-Deli

    How to Keep Smoking

    How to Sabotage a Family

    How to Just Get By in College

    How to Be a Bad Child

    How to Die of _____

    How to Be a Couch Potato

    A(n) X's Guide to Enjoying Z (e.g., The Four Star Hotel Dormitory)

2. Make a double-entry version of your instructions to contrast two perspectives. An excerpt from one paper:

To succeed at the job of waitstaff at X Country Club,
To work at X Country Club, you must first

Clothing must be considered very seriously.
Dress like a penguin.

Istana Hauber

3. Turn your instructions into an informal essay like Ronald V. Smith's on "The Art of Watching Silent Films" (Additional Readings). This set of instructions will be less technical, more subjective, more artistically pleasing, and less explanatory in intent.

   Examples:

   The Art of Dealing with a Difficult Roommate

   How to Quit Smoking

   How to Deal with a New Stepfamily

   How College Women Can Stay in Shape Safely

   How to Eat Healthy as a College Student

4. Convert part of the instructions you wrote into a two-column script for video. You will have to alter the prose to give the dialogue a lifelike quality. Keep the script simple. According to Hausman and Palombo, video is most effective as a communications tool "when it is used to engage attention, show compelling pictures, or motivate the viewer." Video has no special power, however, "for presenting dense textual information" (7).

   For a precedent, read the two versions of Brian Miller's "How to Choose a Kneeboard" in the Additional Readings. You might write instructions on how to do a communal dance and then try it out in class.

5. Rough out instructions for converting the essay by Zora Neale Hurston into a musical composition. (See question 5 following "How It Feels to Be Colored Me" in Additional Readings.) Perhaps lay plans to convert it to a musical play, an opera, a series of songs, or an instrumental piece with different movements. In a few paragraphs specify moods, orchestration, and styles.

POEM: WATCH FOR THE HOME VIDEO

In this brief excerpt, published in 1757, the writer tries to give poetic instructions for dealing with sheep diseases. Why does this method seem inappropriate?

FROM *THE FLEECE* (1757)

by John Dyer

Of grasses are unnumber'd kinds, and all
(Save where foul waters linger on the turf)
Salubrious. Early mark [*i.e.,* notice right away],
when tepid gleams
Oft mingle with the pearls of summer show'rs,
And swell too hastily the tender plains:
Then snatch away thy sheep: beware the rot;
And with detersive bay-salt rub their mouths;
Or urge them on a barren bank to feed,
In hunger's kind distress, on tedded hay;
Or to the marish [marsh] guide their easy steps,
If near thy tufted crofts the broad sea spreads.
Sagacious care foreacts: when strong disease
Breaks in, and stains the purple streams of
health,
Hard is the strife of art: the coughing pest
[pestilence]
From their green pasture sweeps whole flocks
away.

(17–18)

TIPS FOR PROSE

Can you translate this poem into simple instructions? Don't leave out any practical content. This effort will help you appreciate the straightforward nature of workaday prose.

Works Cited

Baldrige, Letitia. *Letitia Baldrige's New Complete Guide to Executive Manners.* New York: Rawson Associates, 1993.

Battey, Thomas C. *The Life and Adventures of a Quaker among the Indians.* Norman: University of Oklahoma Press, 1968. With an introduction by Alice Marriott. Originally published in 1875 by Lee and Shepard (Boston).

Blom, Lynne Anne, and L. Tarin Chaplin. *The Intimate Act of Choreography.* University Pittsburgh Printing, 1982.

The Disney Look. The Walt Disney Company, 1992.

Dyer, John. *The Fleece: A Poem.* London, 1757. Rpt. *The Poetry of Industry: Two Literary Reactions to the Industrial Revolution.* New York: Arno, 1972. Bracketed notes added.

Green, Robert E., ed. *Machinery's Handbook*. New York: Industrial Press, 1996. By Eric Oberg et al.

Hausman, Carl, with Philip J. Palombo. *Modern Video Production: Tools, Techniques, Applications*. New York: HarperCollins, 1993.

The Merchants Avizo. London, 1607.

Smith, Frank. *Understanding Reading: A Psycholinguistic Analysis of Reading and Learning to Read*. 2nd ed. New York: Holt, Rinehart and Winston, 1979.

Smith, J. Wells. "An American Home on the Amazons." *Scribner's Monthly* 18 (May-October 1879): 692–704. Illustration p. 695.

Soldier's Handbook. Washington, DC: United States Government Printing Office, 1941.

Work Consulted

Taylor, Colin. *Myths of the North American Indians*. New York: Barnes & Noble, 1995.

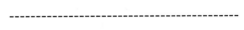

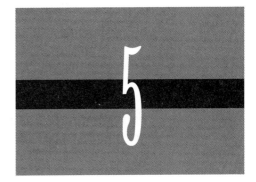

Other Exposition

Just as Chaucer's traveling Knight learned how to ride a horse early in his career, you will want to learn how to inform a reader with rhetorical tact, clarity, and completeness. This skill might take you places—if not to "Alisaundre, Ruce, and Turkye," to greater success in college, career, and other endeavors.

With this chapter you will extend your writing-range-of-motion by doing some kind of expository piece that differs from technical instructions. You will not teach a skill—that is, something intended directly to enable a particular behavior. Instead, you will inform the reader about a concept, person, animal, place, event, situation, relationship, problem, question, belief, requirement, even a process (but how-it-works rather than how-to-do-it).

To help you make this "stretch," here are some hypothetical contrasts with paper topics in Chapter 4, "Teaching a Skill." Instead of a subject like "Scripting for Video," you would pick "The Growing Use of Videotapes to Sell Goods and Services." Instead of "Making Rye Bread," you would write "A Comparison of Rye Flour to Whole-Grain Flours" (i.e., to whole wheat, barley, buckwheat, millet, oats, cracked wheat and bulgur, bran, and wheat germ). Instead of "Preparing for an X High School Football Game," you would write "Current Issues for Athletic Trainers."

As with all explanatory writing, you will connect with your audience, highlight your plan, and complete the details. The traditional methods of development will come into play for discovering ideas, organizing, and amplifying, and as with every writing assignment in this book, research will give it welcome depth. You might even generate new knowledge through your synthesis of other material or your interpretation—as long as you stay fairly detached and nonpartisan.

In college, exposition is persuasion. Why? Because a student who writes a clear and full explanation offers proof of understanding. At the start of an out-of-class paper or an essay question, show the professor that you know where you're headed. Here is an introduction that instills confidence:

The pilgrims on their way to Canterbury come from all walks of society. One character is a little on the hilariously raunchy side. In *The General Prologue,* Chaucer gives a very clear description of the Miller's appearance. Then in the link between *The Knight's Tale* and *The Miller's Tale,* the Miller's character is shown through his aggressive behavior toward the Host. Finally, his personality is expressed through the creation of his obscene tale.

Laura Cooke

Such a beginning announces both the purpose and organization of the paper. To the instructor it whispers assuringly, "This student has a clear focus on the way Chaucer characterizes the Miller, and the main parts of her paper will explain the different methods."

WARM UP FIRST

The memorandum is an everyday format for sending practical information. With the help of another student, write a memo to be posted in the employees' break room informing employees that they should give you their requests for summer vacation time. Basic information: They are entitled to one week off; they need to sign a sheet on your door and list their first, second, and third choices; the deadline is May 30. Add any details you think will clarify the situation. For a model of such workaday exposition, see the sidebar "Good News, Thelma!"

DIRECT-APPROACH MEMO

In practical matters, writers often use the direct approach to deliver routine information or good news. First they announce the main point (usually in a brief paragraph), and then they provide secondary details.

In this memo the writer, Ms. Gomez, announces her decision as early as the subject line—"APPROVAL"—so the reader doesn't have to wonder about the fate of her request. She repeats the news in her first sentence. Then she breaks for a new paragraph to emphasize the distinction between the main point and the subordinate details. The rest of the memo provides supporting information—including the exact day to begin and the exact work-hours.

TO: Thelma Anderson
FROM: Betty Gomez, Supervisor
DATE: May 11, 19—
SUBJECT: APPROVAL OF FLEXTIME

Your request for a change in work hours has been approved. On an experimental basis you may work at home on Wednesdays.

Please begin this flextime schedule on May 21. I will consider you on duty from 8:30 A.M.–12:30 P.M. and from 1:30 P.M.–5:00 P.M. You will be connected to us (and the customers) by telephone, computer, e-mail, and FAX. I will be sending out this news to other employees so they will understand the situation.

You have served Bay Area Supply well in the office and no doubt will continue to do so at home. From personal experience I know that it's hard to serve two masters—children and business—so I hope this experiment helps you. Let's meet in about six weeks and review the experiment.

To appreciate Gomez's straightforwardness, contrast this hypothetically poky beginning: "REQUEST FOR SCHEDULE CHANGE. I have received your request for a change in work hours. You have served Bay Area Supply well over the years. The businessplace is changing. . . ." The reader must drum her fingers while the writer gets to the point. When Thelma finally gets to the news, she may be too anxious to assimilate it accurately, so clarity is jeopardized.

PUBLISHED EXPLANATION

World Music: the Rough Guide (1994) classifies the world into thirteen musical regions, North America being one of them. Another is the Caribbean, the subject of Chapter 10. Among that chapter's subdivisions, which include "Cuba," "Haiti," and "Salsa," is one called "The Loudest Island in the World." What is this place? According to the subtitle, "Jamaica, Home of the Reggae Beat."

The editors' brief preface to this subdivision helps motivate people to read on by arousing their curiosity. For despite the great impact of Jamaican music upon the world, "its diverse strands are hardly known." The editors credit the writer, Gregory Salter (one of about seventy-five contributors to the book), and forecast the half-dozen roots "that underlie the great Caribbean powerhouse that is reggae music."

Here is a discussion of one of those roots, a religion known as Rastafari. Comments in the margin will help you follow the plan for the whole explanation, the strategy of its individual paragraphs, and the methods of development.

"RASTAFARI FOR I AND FOR I"

❋

Gregory Salter

The title and first paragraph clarify the subject and pique curiosity.

Rastafarians make up only around thirteen percent of the island's population but their influence on Jamaican music is out of all proportion. Bob Marley is only the most famous of an enormous number of Rasta musicians. In the late 1960s and 70s, virtually every reggae artist seemed to have adopted or emerged from the religion.

The first sentence seems to announce the point of the paragraph: "non-doctrinal." But the next sentence declares that "certain themes recur." Perhaps this is the topic sentence. The paragraph then focuses on an *example,* the belief that Jah is a living force on earth and the *effects* of this idea on language—a subject that leads to another theme, "Babylon." So in retrospect the reader might see the whole paragraph as advancing this point: Although "non-doctrinal," Rastafari does reveal certain themes.

Rastafari is non-doctrinal, in the sense that no one church is powerful enough to impose its version of religious purity and heresy, and that one person's version of it is as valid as another's, as long as he or she is possessed of the Spirit of Jah (God). Certain themes, however, do recur. Among them is the belief that Jah is a living force on earth, and not a mere otherworldly palliative. Jah enables otherwise disparate humanity to unite. To embody this in speech, Rastas refer to each other as "I." Thus I am I, you are I, and we are I and I. Such is the Rasta emphasis on the importance of the spoken word that many other words are similarly altered: "Unity" becomes "Inity", "brethren" becomes "Idren", and so on. Unity, or Inity, is essential if Rastas are to stand strong against the wicked forces of Babylon—the oppressive (or downpressive) system.

Again, the first sentence seems to announce the paragraph's topic. But Garvey points the way to Selassie. Details explain the effects of both figures on many Rastas.

Marcus Garvey, a forceful campaigner, in the 1920s and 30s for black unity, pan-Africanism, and a return to Africa, is of great importance to many Rastas, who revere him as a prophet, and even as the reincarnation of John the Baptist. In one of his pamphlets, he urges Africans of the New World to look to Africa for a Prince to emerge. This was taken by many to mean the then Emperor of Ethiopia, **Haile Selassie I.** His claimed descent from Solomon, and his battles in 1937 with the wicked forces of Rome (Mussolini), were taken as fulfilling the prophecies of the Book of Revelation, and Selassie was worshipped as Christ come again. Selassie was deposed in 1974, and died a few years later, although to Rastas "Selassie cyaan dead" and is living still. Rastas believe that they are awaiting repatriation to Africa—Zion—and regard themselves, and all New World black people, as living "slavery days" in bondage.

From time to time Rastas hold reasoning sessions. Larger and more protracted reasonings are called **nyabinghis.** Like their Revival Zion and Pucomaniac counterparts [discussed in earlier sections], nyabinghis feature Bible-reading, hymns, foot-stamping, and drumming. Rasta drumming, though, is much slower, with a beat more or less the speed of a human pulse. Other differences include the reasoning itself, in which matters religious, social, political and livital (about life) are discussed collectively, aided and abetted by copious consumption of *ganja*—Jamaican colly weed, the good herb, the *Irie*. Rastas adore ganja and lovingly cultivate it, cure it, smoke it, brew it (non-alcoholically), use it for medicines of all sorts, and, above all, talk about it. For this, Babylon brutalizes them no end, but to little avail. As Jah Lion sings, "When the Dread flash him locks, a colly seed drops."

There are some good recordings of traditional Rasta music, though, inevitably, they fail to capture the Dread atmosphere and significance of the real thing, which is recommended to anyone interested. Nyabinghis occur quite frequently in Jamaica, are generally well advertised and easy to find. By far the best Rasta sounds on record are the extraordinary "Grounation" sessions, performed by the late, great **Count Ossie and his Mystic Revealers of Rastafari.** Count Ossie was master Rasta "repeater" drummer from the Kingston ghetto. In the early 1960s, a number of very talented musicians came under his influence,

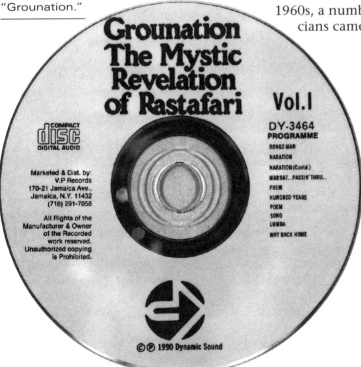

"GROUNATION" CD

By permission of the Mystic Revelation of Rastafari.

including most of the subsequently legendary Skatalites. Listen to "Grounation" (copies turn up on various obscure labels) and you will find astonishing Rasta drumming and chanting, bebop and cool jazz horn lines, and apocalyptic poems.

Questions

1. Can you write one word next to each of Salter's five paragraphs to indicate its subject?
2. If you were to read these paragraphs in a scrambled order, could you put them into the original sequence? Is Salter's order the most effective? If so, why?
3. Do the phrases "the wicked forces of Rome" and "the wicked forces of Babylon" seem to reflect Salter's personal attitude? Or is he wearing a mask of amused and affectionate tolerance?
4. Should Salter explain the meaning of "When the Dread flash him locks"? Should he point out that ganja is plain old marijuana?
5. Do you know of any popular musical style besides reggae that is influenced by religious music?

For an essay that accuses reggae of selling out to what Rastas might call Babylon, see Ruffin's "Do You Hear What I Hear?" in Additional Readings.

Consider the Themes

* When Columbus arrived on the island of what became known as Jamaica, it was populated by the Arawaks. Why does *World Music* not trace the Arawak influence on present-day Jamaican music?
* Do you belong to a group that derives any sense of "Inity" from its speech? From its rituals?

STUDENT EXPLANATION 1

In the following piece, a freshman wrote about her grandparents' experience during World War II. She did some research over the telephone with primary resources (firsthand records—in this case, interviews). She also consulted the library for secondary sources (interpretations of primary materials).

Notice how Laurie Ann Occhipinti uses the back-and-forth method of comparison-contrast. She switches between the battlefront and the home-front rather than discussing Mary in one part of the report and Anthony in the other. This pattern allows her to emphasize the differences between their experiences as well as the simultaneity.

ANTHONY'S WAR TIME, MARY'S HOME DESPAIR

Laurie Ann Occhipinti

World War II began on September 1, 1939 with the invasion of Poland by the Germans. The Allied powers were the United States, Great Britain, and the Commonwealth, the U.S.S.R., France, and China. The Central Powers were Germany, Italy, and Japan. Throughout the war, Japan was a world power that the United States was battling. World War II ended on September 2, 1945, six years after and almost to the exact day it began. The government of Japan surrendered to the United States on the battleship *Missouri* in Tokyo Bay.

At the time of the war, many American men were being drafted from their businesses and families from the age of eighteen and up; one of those men was Anthony John Occhipinti of Spring Valley, New York, who was drafted in 1944. Anthony was a twenty-four year old farmer with a wife and two children. His business was in poultry and it was quite time consuming. So, when Anthony was drafted into the war, the business fell into the hands of Mary, his wife, who still had the responsibility of looking after the two children, Jean and Angela, ages seven and five.

Mary knew hardly anything about how to run the poultry business and had a very difficult time managing it. Much of the time, Anthony's father would come over to help Mary feed and take care of the turkeys each day. When there was a shipment coming in, he would help Mary unload, uncrate, and keep track of the number of turkeys that came in, along with figuring out the cost of the shipment. When there was a shipment going out, he would again help Mary crate and load the turkeys, count how many crates went out in each shipment, and figure out the profits made. Meanwhile, Anthony's mother helped out by minding Jean and Angela and by preparing the meals. Since Mary would be out in the barns all day long, she had no one to watch after her two girls or feed them. So Anthony's mother volunteered herself to help out in the home.

When Anthony was drafted, along with countless other young men, he was sent to Fort Dix, New Jersey, for military training for a couple of months. Immediately afterwards, he was sent to the Pacific Islands of Japan. [The writer supplies a photocopied map.] While in the jungles, many of the soldiers became ill with malaria and acquired types of fungi on their bodies. Because these men would become so infected with these sicknesses, they would sometimes have to lose an arm or a leg; and then others just simply died.

While the men were battling the war, many things were happening to the factories and supplies around the United States. Because everyone had to gear up in a hurry, all of the United States' natural resources were taken and rationed for the military such as sugar and flour. Gasoline was also a major natural resource that was seriously rationed—three gallons of gas per week. All the factories were devoted to building weapons, tanks, vehicles, and planes.

Mary remembered how she and her children would always anxiously await the sight of the mail carrier in hopes of good news from their loved ones in the war. [See Figure 1.1 for a V-mail letter.] However, they would shudder at the sight of someone from Western Union or someone dressed in a military uniform. These people would always bring the news that someone became either a casualty of war or missing in action (M.I.A.).

Meanwhile, out in the jungles during the Japanese war, many casualties were incurred by our own men on their fellow soldiers! According to Anthony—"Many of our own were killed because you just couldn't see in the jungle who was who." [The writer supplies photocopied photographs.] All the men lost a significant amount of weight while in the jungles. "The temperatures would reach 110–115 degrees," said Anthony:

All that you could do was drink water all the time because it was just too hot. I remember when I came in, I weighed about one hundred and eighty five pounds. When I came out, I was one hundred and forty pounds. There were many bad situations. We were surrounded many times by the Japanese. I remember killing at least fifteen to twenty of the enemy. I didn't feel any remorse, it was either him or me.

Anthony was stationed the longest on the two islands of Saipan and Pelelieu. His memories were still quite vivid when he spoke of the virtually "blind" warfare that went on in the jungles of Saipan and how it was clearly every man for himself in the open, destroyed areas of Pelelieu. Because of the extensive bombing that occurred, anything that might have offered protection for the soldiers, such as trees and rocks, had been blown away. In order to get any precise shot of the enemy, the soldiers had to be out in the open since there was nothing to hide behind. This then made the soldiers very susceptible to getting shot themselves.

While stationed together, all of the men became quite close friends with each other. It was the only way to survive the horrid feelings the war brought about. However, many times friends were separated and killed by the enemy. These tragic incidents many times had long lasting effects. "I remember having two real close pals that I lost to the enemy during battle," said Anthony. "It was so long ago but I still remember them."

Lots of times the soldiers had to leave the war scene and return home for emergency reasons. In Anthony's case, he had been in Japan for fifteen months when he was summoned home to New York for emergency medical reasons because Mary was very ill. "I remember before I came home, I had acquired a fungus on my feet and none of the medical ointments could cure it. So on my way home, I did not change my socks for a week. When I finally took them off, the fungus was gone."

World War II was one of the most dramatic, drastic periods in the world's entire history. Millions of casualties occurred and many soldiers came back physically and mentally disturbed for life. Victory should be sweet, but not at such a cost!

Works Consulted

Morison, Samuel Eliot. *History of the United States Naval Operations in World War II*. 1st ed. 15 vols. Boston: Little, Brown, 1947–62.

"World War II." *Collier's Encyclopedia*, 1989.

New York Times, May 1942.

Questions

1. Does Occhipinti's explanation fulfill the promise made by the title? Why or why not? Is the title clear enough to you? Would you suggest another one?

2. Judging from the introduction, the writer (remember the **FROM:** heading of a memo) assumes that her audience (the **TO:**) has what level of knowledge about World War II (the **SUBJECT:**)? How might the **DATE:** of her paper influence its value and reception?

3. Label each paragraph except the first and last. If it discusses Anthony, label it *A;* if Mary, *M;* if both, *A,M.* Can you see how this back-and-forth pattern counteracts the narrative momentum that starts to build in each story—that is, the appeal of "What happens next?"—to juxtapose the two experiences instead?

4. Does the conclusion move you? Or does it distract you by shifting away from dispassionate explanation? For an experiment, replace the last sentence with one of your own, perhaps one that furnishes a summary.

5. Can you find the Mariana Islands on a map of the South Pacific Ocean and locate Saipan among them?

STUDENT EXPLANATION 2

Here is another comparison between two experiences. In this case, however, it is two versions of the same meeting.

FIRST ENCOUNTERS: CORTÉZ VS. AZTECS

Kathy Coleman

It's graduation night. "I am so happy. Now that I'm a graduate, I can marry my boyfriend and we can all live under mom and dad's roof." "My daughter is finally graduating. This means that she'll be moving on to law or medical school and also out of my house." "This night means a lot to counselors like me. I took this girl under my wing and look where she is tonight." In this one event, three people said what it meant to them and yet none of the statements are alike. Did this ever happen in historic events? Of course it did. For example, when the Spanish first met the Aztecs, both groups of people had highly different meanings, interpretations, and impressions of the same event just like the graduate, mother, and counselor during graduation.

It was the search for gold, silver, and conquest that drove Cortéz and his army into Mexico. When he first arrived at the Island of Cozumel and the Cape of Yucatán, he wrote letters to Charles V of Spain describing how the natives looked, acted, worshiped, and ate. He described their features as "well-proportioned." He noticed that they had body-piercing in the ears, lips, and noses and that they put "large and ugly objects in them." Much of the food that the natives ate was not unknown to the Spanish with the exception of the "roasting of large peacocks," which were turkeys and unheard of in Europe. The types of houses that the natives lived in were not that unusual to Cortéz. He described their houses as well built. The religion was the most shocking to the conquistadors:

"They have another custom, horrible, and abominable, and deserving punishment. . . . [T]hey may take many boys and girls, and even grown men and women, and in the presence of those idols, they open their breasts . . . and take out the hearts and entrails . . . and burn the entrails and hearts before the idols."

MacNutt; qtd in Wheeler and Becker 8

At one point during their stay, Cortéz ordered his soldiers to break up the idols and roll them down the stairs and set up an image of Our Lady in their place.

During his stay, Cortéz thought that he was very ill provided for. Upon arriving in Tenochtitlán, he felt himself assaulted. The native envoys made sacrifices in front of Cortéz and they offered him blood. He grew angry and struck the envoy with his sword (Díaz del Castillo 63).

The natives' account of the same events are quite different. The Aztecs got word that strange people were heading toward their city, and they thought that these people were their gods and were to be worshipped. The natives brought gifts to the "gods" and sacrificed in front of them, which was the highest honor. When the "gods" became angry at them for their gifts, they all became confused and terrified. When they first saw the Europeans they described them as being "completely covered, so only their faces can be seen." Their skin was like it was made out of "lime" and their hair was yellow. The Europeans' food looked like straw to them, which was probably some kind of pasta. The natives had never seen the animals that the Europeans came with (Leon-Portilla 21):

"Their deer carry them on their backs wherever they wish to go . . . [and] are as tall as the roof of a house. Their dogs are enormous, with flat ears and long, dangling tongues."

Leon-Portilla 30

The most shocking to the natives was the Europeans' weapons. They had never seen a gun or cannon before, and when they heard the cannons they thought it was magic.

Both groups had very little understanding of the other. The Europeans' goal was conquest, but they also viewed the Aztecs as evil because they were not Christians. As a result, the gifts offered by the natives were taken as an insult since it was nothing that the Europeans could relate to. On the other hand, the natives at first thought Europeans were gods. Then confusion arose when the "gods" were not acting like gods.

So you see, different interpretations or meanings of events could sometimes lead to disaster as in the Aztecs' case. The next time you hear your friends talking about some event, try to think of what that event would mean to someone else.

Works Cited

Díaz del Castillo, Bernal. *The Conquest of New Spain.* Middlesex, England: Penguin, 1963.

Leon-Portilla, Miguel. *The Broken Spears.* Boston: Beacon, 1959.

MacNutt, Francis Augustus. *Fernando Cortés: His Five Letters of Relation to the Emperor Charles V.* Vol. 1. Cleveland: Arthur H. Clark, 1908. Quoted in Wheeler and Becker.

Wheeler, William Bruce, and Susan D. Becker. *Discovering the American Past: A Look at the Evidence.* 2 vols. Vol 1: *To 1877.* Boston: Houghton Mifflin, 1994.

Questions

1. Does Kathy Coleman arouse your interest by using a hypothetical present-day situation to introduce a historical event?

2. The body of this explanation has two main parts. Which sentence announces the second part?

3. Could Coleman have used Occhipinti's method of switching back and forth? If so, what would be the points of contrast between the two interpretations? Which method of comparison would be more effective for her purpose?

Consider the Themes

* Where does the misinterpretation of nonverbal behavior aggravate this bad encounter?

* In which cases did the language of one group have no word for the other's animals? What do you suppose were the enormous dogs?

STRETCH:
EXPLAIN A NARROW SUBJECT TO A PARTICULAR AUDIENCE

This "stretch" can be a traditional research paper—a clearly organized, fully developed, and fully documented study of something of general public concern, written to an educated audience in a strictly impersonal tone.

Or it can be a magazine article, feature story for a newspaper, pamphlet, part of a home page on the Internet, or a paper that challenges you to adopt your material to a narrow group of readers. In other words, it may differ from the traditional research paper in a number of ways:

Subject. The topic can be something of local interest or even something of little interest—at least until you connect it with your reader. Leaving the old term paper war-horses such as Abortion and Capital Punishment to chew grass in the pasture, try a subject that arises from your own concerns.

Audience. This exposition can have a sharper sense of audience. Under your title specify your intended readers: for example, To Readers of the College Newspaper, or To Anyone Interested in Chiropractic as a Career, or To People Unfamiliar with X War. Although academic writing usually has no audience other than the teacher, this paper will give you practice in adjusting to the needs, interests, and constraints of different readers, even if imaginary.

Style. Your paper may have a degree of flair, like Gregory Salter's piece on Rastafarians. Explanation has a broad range of tone, from the severely impersonal (as if there is no writer) to the individualistic. Just be sure to subordinate your personality to clarity of presentation.

Your exposition may also use headings, other techniques of visual emphasis, and illustrations. (For a photograph or drawing, at least rough it out or specify wherever it would go.)

Length. It may be shorter than the traditional research paper and may have fewer quotations, depending on your teacher's guidelines.

Here is a brief review of the techniques covered in "Explanation" that will tailor them to this assignment.

Connect with Your Reader

You might adapt the subject, introduction, organization, development, and style to a specified readership—to their degree of knowledge and interest, their needs, their expectations. This paper, like a memorandum, can have a clearly envisioned **TO:** rather than a TO WHOM IT MAY CONCERN. For example, the readers of *World Music: the Rough Guide* expect a discography of Rasta recordings (and get one).

Here is the introduction to an expository article called "Human Papilloma Virus." This virus is a sexually transmitted disease (STD), widespread on college campuses, that is known to cause genital warts and is suspected of causing cancer. Notice how the two-paragraph introduction establishes the importance of the subject and, in the final sentence, explicitly connects it to the interests of the intended audience:

Safe sex awareness campaigns usually hone in on the dire consequences of risky sexual behavior: AIDS, syphilis, herpes, unplanned pregnancy and others. But none focus on cancer as a consequence of sexual risk-taking, despite that the most commonly transmitted viral STD, human papillomavirus (HPV), may be responsible for countless cases of cervical and other cancers.

One study estimates the lifetime cumulative risk for acquiring HPV infection to be as great as 79%, meaning that eight in 10 people will be infected with the disease during their lifetimes [Crum C et al. Papillomavirus-related genital neoplasia: Present and future prevention. *Cancer Detection and Prevention.* 1990; 14 (4): 465–469]. Proper diagnosis, treatment and counseling are acutely important for clinicians in every setting. (Gerchufsky 21; his parentheses)

The audience is medical clinicians, who are in the position to treat or prevent the disease, rather than people who are at risk for it. Indeed, the article appears in a professional journal, *Advance for Nurse Practitioners.*

So your intended readers should affect the way you present the **SUBJECT.** Consider trying to kindle interest, as Coleman did in her introduction to the Spanish-Aztec encounter. Use your ingenuity to relate the subject—whether from history, mathematics, biology, psychology, or any academic course—to the reader's life. For example, a paper on some aspect of World War II could start by asking college students to imagine what they would be doing if they'd been living in the early 1940s and by citing possibilities.

Also connect the information with the reader's framework of knowledge. For example, "France is about twice the size of Texas." One student contrasted Islamic prayer to that of religions and denominations familiar to his intended readers.

Your explanation may have a slightly argumentative angle, like Kathy Coleman's, to get attention or otherwise add illumination. You could encourage an understanding of the topic, express your opinion about it (as Occhipinti does at the end of her report), or recommend a certain way of looking at it. Just be sure that your primary aim is explanatory.

You may even address the readers with the pronoun "you" if the word helps motivate them to read and otherwise connect them to the subject.

Highlight Your Plan

Narrow your scope to give a sense of thoroughness. Make the most of those two lighthouses of title and introduction. The latter can always start with a wide scope and then narrow down: from basketball, to female teams, to a single example.

Use headings if they will help distinguish major sections and will be welcomed by the reader. Make the subject of each paragraph clear enough that the reader can label each paragraph with a word or summarize it in a sentence.

For all or much of your framework, consider the following often-used methods:

Analysis into Parts. Divide the subject logically into two or more aspects and develop each fully.

Gregory Salter does this to some extent in his explanation of Rastafarians and their music because he tries to cover everything important, although in a brief way. "Logically" can range from the necessary to the probable. Not everything can be divided into tight logical compartments, but make sure that you have covered every aspect your reader will consider important. For example, any explanation of Rastas would probably include the subtopics of Bob Marley, Marcus Garvey, Jah's power to unite humanity, and nyabinghis.

Cause and Effect. Explain the cause(s) of a situation or event, or the effect(s) of one.

Your discussion will be more illuminating if you know a few basics about cause-and-effect reasoning. (1) Usually there are multiple causes rather than just one: A car wreck may result from a combination of alcohol, fatigue, and bad weather. (2) Causes range from the nearer to the farther: Alcohol and fatigue may be "proximate" causes (i.e., nearer to the event), whereas a "remote" cause (farther from the event) may have been the loss of a job or relationship.

Comparison and Contrast. There are at least two basic formats for comparing and contrasting. Suppose, for instance, that you want to contrast the Paleolithic era to the Neolithic. You can first explain the Paleolithic, perhaps covering a few features, and then you can explain the Neolithic while highlighting its differences to earlier points. This half-and-half method can sometimes work best, especially when there is some cross-referencing between the two parts.

To emphasize these differences, however, you might juxtapose the points of contrast (put them side by side) by using the back-and-forth method:

Introduce feature 1
    Explain relevance to the Paleolithic
        "   "   " " Neolithic
Introduce feature 2
    Explain relevance to the Paleolithic
        "   "   " " Neolithic
Etc.

You could even blend these methods to discuss each era mainly by itself but with an occasional cross-reference to the other.

Definition. Write an extended definition of a term, for example, by using various methods of development. Like an organist, press all the keys, pump the pedals, pull or push all the stops—flute, reed, and brass. Divide your subject into parts, explain causes and effects, describe it, give examples, furnish background, analyze it as a process, compare it, contrast it, use an analogy, and provide more details (including numbers). Consider telling what it is *not:* A coffee house is not a restaurant.

One commercial catalogue defines a thousand "themes" available as background music for industrial videotape productions, those created for businesses and other organizations. It does so by using an array of expository techniques. For example, the theme titled "Full Potential" is classified as "Industrial" in type and "Energetic" as subtype. Its style and instrumentation are analyzed:

The classic Network industrial featuring a triumphant brass melody, driving rhythm and orchestral punctuation. *Inst: French horns, brass, strings, electric guitar, piano, bass, drums and percussion.*

Network Music 499

Keep your plan in the foreground. It will help the reader follow your sequence and grasp the connection between one part and another as well as between each part and your main idea.

At the end, would the reader value a restatement of your main points to be reminded of them? To appreciate them from the perspective of the complete explanation?

Complete the Details

A reminder: You will gain credibility, force, and accuracy by incorporating research. Your teacher will furnish guidelines as to how much and what kind. Information might come from interviews, print material, videotapes, reference works on compact disk, or the Internet. In the library, look at books, newspapers, periodicals, pamphlets, government documents, and audiovisual material.

The borrowed material that you weave into your paper might be central or peripheral—that is, it might focus exactly on your subject or help to furnish a background for it. An explanation of corporate "downsizing" (maybe intended for students preparing to enter the workplace) would rely heavily on sources that discuss the practice; whereas a profile of a "downsized" worker who has returned to college would include fewer sources and use them for background.

Avoid rehashing one secondary source. How? Use more than one, perhaps including your textbook and lecture notes. And narrow your topic: Instead of writing on all seven pillars of Islam, choose just one of them, such as praying five times a day. Instead of trying to cover everything about computer viruses—who invents them and why, what kinds exist, and how to prevent them—consider focusing on how different kinds operate. The narrower scope invites you to use more specialized sources.

Artfully weave sources into your explanation (rather than sticking them on top like a postage stamp). Synthesize them—weave them together—whenever it would help to point out their different emphases.

For extra variety and authenticity, interview someone. You should reveal the person's name and expertise before you present his or her ideas. If you wish to document the interview at the end of your paper, there are various ways. An example:

Takamatsu, Mineko. Interview. Milwaukee. 8 October 19—.

You might also conduct a survey. Ask the same questions of each person. These can be "forced answer" (yes-no, age, favorite television program, etc.) or open-ended ("Why do you watch television?"). Stick to questions that respect privacy.

You will probably use longer sentences and paragraphs than in your technical instructions because the material is probably more complex and abstract.

In this assignment let explanation carry as much of the message as possible. Be easy on value words that express your opinion about the worth of something. As a case in point, you would omit the underlined word: "The Food Pyramid is a *great* alternative to the traditional diet, and is something more Americans should become accustomed to for a long, healthy life." You can, nevertheless, take up controversial material as long as you frame it neutrally, like a newspaper reporter: "Adherents believe that to receive the gift of tongues one should pray, believe, and act in faith." (Contrast this partisan version: "To receive the gift of speaking in tongues, pray, believe, and act in faith.")

For using illustrations, please see the sidebar, "Try a Drawing, Bar Chart, or Table."

TRY A DRAWING, BAR CHART, OR TABLE

Sometimes you can present explanatory details more effectively with the help of images and numerical tables. Here are three examples—a drawing, bar chart, and table. They come from different issues of *MMWR: Morbidity and Mortality Weekly Report*, published by the Epidemiology Program Office, Centers for Disease Control and Prevention, Public Health Service, U.S. Department of Health and Human Services, Atlanta, GA 30333.

Notice how the segmented pyramid offers a visual analogy to the types as well as the relative amounts of food eaten in a healthy diet. The drawings of food also complement and reinforce the text.

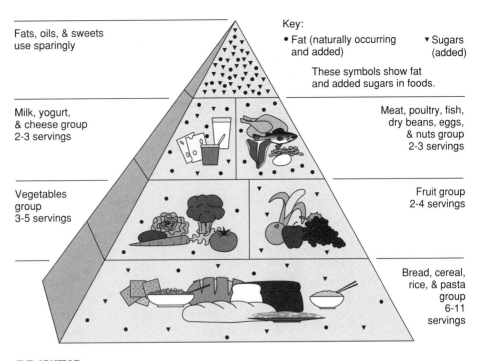

DRAWING

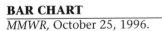

MMWR, June 14, 1996.

In this chart, the bars are doubled for comparison between blacks and whites. The vertical axis displays the unit of measurement (percentage), while the horizontal axis presents a series of responses (from "Excellent" to "Poor"). Notice how easily the visual contrasts strike the eye: (1) between blacks and whites at each point and (2) among the five different gradations.

Look at the center pair of bars: How would you put into words the information they convey?

BAR CHART
MMWR, October 25, 1996.

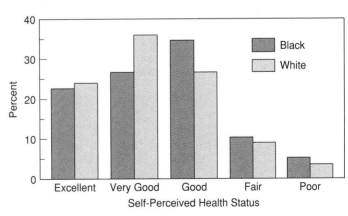

The table below looks complicated with all its headings, subheadings, numbers, and footnotes. (For this exercise, please ignore the plus-and-minus figures for "confidence interval.") But imagine how daunting its data would

Percentage of high school students who used cigarettes or smokeless tobacco, by sex, race/ethnicity, and grade—United States, Youth Risk Behavior Survey, 1995[*]

| Category | Cigarette use | | | | Current smokeless tobacco use[¶] | |
| | Current[†] | | Frequent[§] | | | |
	%	(95% CI[**])	%	(95% CI)	%	(95% CI)
Sex						
Female	34.3	(±3.1%)	15.9	(±3.0%)	2.4	(±1.3%)
Male	35.4	(±2.4%)	16.3	(±2.8%)	19.7	(±2.5%)
Race/Ethnicity[††]						
White, non-Hispanic	38.3	(±2.6%)	19.5	(±3.5%)	14.5	(±1.7%)
Female	39.8	(±3.2%)	20.8	(±3.8%)	2.5	(±1.1%)
Male	37.0	(±3.3%)	18.4	(±3.7%)	25.1	(±3.0%)
Black, non-Hispanic	19.2	(±3.0%)	4.5	(±1.8%)	2.2	(±1.0%)
Female	12.2	(±3.0%)	1.3	(±0.7%)	1.1	(±1.2%)
Male	27.8	(±5.6%)	8.5	(±3.4%)	3.5	(±1.4%)
Hispanic	34.0	(±5.2%)	10.0	(±3.3%)	4.4	(±1.8%)
Female	32.9	(±5.8%)	9.3	(±4.0%)	3.1	(±3.3%)
Male	34.9	(±8.2%)	10.7	(±4.2%)	5.8	(±2.4%)
Grade						
9	31.2	(±1.7%)	9.6	(±2.7%)	11.2	(±1.7%)
10	33.1	(±3.8%)	13.3	(±3.0%)	9.6	(±2.2%)
11	35.8	(±3.6%)	13.3	(±3.0%)	9.6	(±2.2%)
12	38.2	(±3.5%)	20.9	(±4.0%)	11.2	(±2.8%)
Total	34.8	(±2.2%)	16.1	(±2.6%)	11.4	(±1.7%)

[*]Sample sizes: 10,473 for current or frequent cigarette use and 10,772 for current smokeless tobacco use. Sample sizes differ because of missing data.
[†]Smoked cigarettes on ≥1 of the 30 days preceding the survey.
[§]Smoked cigarettes on ≥20 of the 30 days preceding the survey.
[¶]Used smokeless tobacco on ≥1 of the 30 days preceding the survey.
[**]Confidence interval.
[††]Numbers for other racial/ethnic groups were too small for meaningful analysis.
(*MMWR*, May 24, 1996)

be to a reader if presented in a graph or in a series of paragraphs! With practice you will be able to interpret such tables as well as to compose them.

To understand the table above on smoking, first study the title to grasp its three main parts: Measurement used (percentage), people studied (certain kinds of students), and categories (by sex, race/ethnicity, and grade). Then try to find these terms in the headings—vertical and horizontal. Each number in the grid falls at the intersection of a vertical column and a horizontal row; so to understand its significance, look at the heading to its left and the heading above it.

For example, the first number, 34.3, belongs (1) to the row-heading "Female" and (2) to the column-heading %. (This abbreviation means percentage of current cigarette use.) The number indicates that 34.3 percent of female high school students (in this survey) currently smoked cigarettes.

Now look at the number 16.1 in the "Total" row at the bottom. This number means that 16.1 percent of high school cigarette smokers (in this study) smoked frequently. Notice that the heading at the top, "Frequent," gives a footnote that defines the term.

What does the number 8.5 indicate in the center of the table? Can you put the meaning into words?

Ten + Topics

Here are some diverse possibilities for your exposition:

1. Introduce other students to a concept, historical figure, and so on, that you learned in another course this semester. Challenge yourself to make your presentation relevant to the readers' needs and otherwise interesting.

2. For the campus newspaper, write an explanatory piece on something that will have a ready-made appeal to students. Introduce a campus organization, a course, a sports opportunity, a nearby restaurant, a musical group. Look for a photograph possibility and, to add human interest, incorporate an interview.

   Or do a profile of someone on campus. For an example that was printed in the college newspaper, see "Trip around the World" by Shayla Gore (Additional Readings). One pair of students even interviewed a drag queen and wrote a thoughtful interpretation of the man's career and personality. A tip: If you profile someone from another country, furnish some background about the place—location, size, and population.

   To help you with the organization of a profile, read Chaucer's two sketches in the Additional Readings.

3. After doing some research on the subject so as to ask informed questions, interview a person who remembers living through World War II, or another war, as a soldier or civilian. You may want to record the interview on audiotape, transcribe portions, and edit the transcription. Write up the results with background information. Try to get your explanation published in a local newspaper along with a photograph.

   Or interview an immigrant after reading "The Immigration Myth" in Chapter 6. For example, two freshmen interviewed two other students who were husband and wife. Hong Dao had been caught trying to escape from Viet Nam in a boat and then had been forced to help dig a canal with her hands. Published in the student newspaper, this distressing profile emphasized the local connection in the title, got attention in the first sentence ("Have you dreamed of escaping from somewhere?"), told the couple's story with an emphasis on freedom and education, and furnished quotations, among them this concluding one: "People in the United States do not appreciate freedom. . . " (Tinter and Hall).

4. For an imaginary *Handbook of Religions,* explain one or more tenets, rituals, and so on, of a religion or denomination. Do so in an objective way rather than as an advocate. Use phrases such as "in the eyes of many" or "according to Islamic belief." Examples: the relationship of men and women according to the Baha'i faith; the mourning period for Orthodox Greeks; the origin of the Koran or Quran. Don't give away your own convictions (if any).

   Or define a secular ritual or practice that most Americans are probably unfamiliar with. For example, the Día de la Raza, or Day of the Race, a holiday that honors Columbus in the United States but in Mexico honors the origin of the mestizos, people of mixed European and native ancestry.

5. As an article for your town or campus newspaper, take a subject of public controversy and present the views of two sides without revealing your own position. One controversy: the safety of smoking marijuana. This experience should broaden your outlook.

   Or discuss the pros and cons of tracking by "ability groups" in schools, a practice that Jing Dai inveighs against in the next chapter.

6. Introduce students to a language other than English that may be heard on campus—for example, Spanish, Chinese, Japanese, Korean. Explain only one feature, or a few at the most. Don't try to teach a skill in this brief effort, only a concept.

   Or introduce the idea of body language by reporting on instances that you observe. Narrow your scope to a certain type (e.g., clothing), group (e.g., diners in the cafeteria), or place (e.g., the weight room). Incorporate theory and avoid controversy. Or report on some narrow aspect of body language in televised soap operas or in a music video. Or do a study of the ways that body language contributes to Salomea Kape's story "Designer Genes" (Additional Readings).

7. Inform other students about the use of videotape programs as a business and professional tool (e.g., for recruitment, or training, or sales, or public relations, or motivation). Research will probably help you decide on a focus.

   Or for other students do a report on one kind of persuasion: packaging techniques. These mix verbal and nonverbal resources (images, color, layout, shape, etc.). For example, look carefully at a number of cereal boxes and then explain how the front panels invite the customer to reach for the cereal. (To sharpen your sense of the verbal-nonverbal distinction, type out all the words on a white piece of paper and see what is lost.

   Or introduce other students to what advertising jargon calls the "creative" in various print advertisements—that is, to the interaction between image and words. Do a little research on ad techniques.

Or do a report on design and layout in a magazine. How does it use space, typography, text boxes, pull quotes, color, illustrations, introductions (larger print used at the beginning of an article to invite the eye), captions, columns, and headings? You might consult a book on the subject, perhaps one on desktop publishing.

For these last three topics, include the originals for the teacher's benefit.

8. Write a report for the Musical Notes section of your college newspaper. Listen to songs played by a radio station during a one-hour period (perhaps tape the hour so you can review it); reason inductively from these concrete instances to some general pattern and then write a report on the lyrics. Stay as objective as you can. Possibilities: Explain recurrent themes or subjects; classify the songs into groups according to some principle; or take one group and define it.

9. Explain something suggested by material in *Stretch,* whether in the chapters or in the Additional Readings.

You might define a certain kind of dysfunctional family; write a guide to typical family life in an ethnic or racial group that you know well; discuss some current research on homosexuality or bisexuality; give a historical background on letter-writing; supply a historical introduction to the Indian Removal Act (Additional Readings); explain something about the indigenous people of the Americas (e.g., the Arawak tribe), Rastafari, motorcycle riders, mestizos, immigration (see the argument in Chapter 6). Do a study of the "Singles Seeking" phenomenon in newspapers: How widespread is it? How successful is the method? What are the risks?

10. For an audience that you specify, compare or contrast X to Y. Possible topic: two spiritual views of humankind's relation to the earth. For example, compare Native American beliefs with orthodox Judeo-Christian tradition. (See Margaret Fritz's interpretation of Simon J. Ortiz's poetry in the Additional Readings.)

You might make a comparison based on something you studied in another course—for example, the Taiwanese view of Taiwan's political status versus the mainland Chinese view—and thus use writing to both teach and learn. (For a contrast between two views of native peoples, see the poem on artifacts in a Seattle museum, Chapter 2.)

You might compare the AIDS epidemic to the one in Latin America caused by Chagas disease, a parasitic illness that has infected millions.

REVISE TO MAKE THAT REACH

Re-read the guidelines for writing good explanations in the preface to Chapters 4 and 5.

Should you make your organization clearer? Do you use "turn signals" to help the reader follow your thought? For clarity should you beef up predictions and transitions? Could the reader easily insert headings to mark the main parts? Or, to the contrary, would your explanation seem unnecessarily

Certificate of Registrar

This is to Certify that pursuant to the Rationing Orders and Regulations administered by the OFFICE OF PRICE ADMINISTRATION, an agency of the United States Government,

(Name, Address, and Description of person to whom the book is issued:)

Park _____ Frances _____ Elizabeth ·
(Last name) ____ (First name) ____ (Middle name)

_____ R.F.D. 2 _____
(Street No. or P. O. Box No.) ____ (Street or R. F. D.)

Bergen _____ New York _____
(City or town) ____ (County) ____ (State)

····t not be detached except in the presence of the reta

5 ft. 3 in. 120 lbs. grey light 28 yrs. Sex { Male / Female ☒
(Height) (Weight) (Color of eyes) (Color of hair) (Age)

has been issued the attached War Ration Stamps this 5 day of May, 1942, upon the basis of an application signed by himself ☐, herself ☐, or on his or her behalf by his or her husband ☒, wife ☐, father ☐, mother ☐, exception ☐. (*Check one.*)

Harold W. Davis (Signature)
(Registrar)

Local Board No. 18-0-1 County Genesee State New York

his employee, or person authorised by him to make delivery.

WAR RATION STAMP	WAR RATION STAMP
22	20
WAR RATION STAMP	WAR RATION STAMP
19	17

The Stamps contained in this Book are valid only after the lawful holder of this Book has signed the certificate below, and are void if detached contrary to the Regulations. (A father, mother, or guardian may sign the name of a person under 18.) In case of questions, difficulties, or complaints, consult your local Ration Board.

Certificate of Book Holder

I, *the undersigned,* do hereby certify that I have observed all the conditions and regulations governing the issuance of this War Ration Book; that the "Description of Book Holder" contained herein is correct; that an application for issuance of this book has been duly made by me or on my behalf; and that the statements contained in said application are true to the best of my knowledge and belief.

Frances Elizabeth Park [Book Holder's Own Name]
(Signature of, or on behalf of, Book Holder)

Any person signing on behalf of Book Holder must sign his or her own name below

and indicate relationship to Book Holder Husband

C. B. Park
(Father, Mother, or Guardian)

☆ U. S. GOVERNMENT PRINTING OFFICE : 1942 16—29651-1 OPA Form No. R-302

UNITED STATES OF AMERICA

War Ration Book One

WARNING

1 Punishments ranging as high as *Ten Years' Imprisonment or $10,000 Fine, or Both,* may be imposed under United States Statutes for violations thereof arising out of infractions of Rationing Orders and Regulations.

2 This book must not be transferred. It must be held and used only by or on behalf of the person to whom it has been issued, and anyone presenting it thereby represents to the Office of Price Administration, an agency of the United States Government, that it is being so held and so used. For any misuse of this book it may be taken from the holder by the Office of Price Administration.

3 In the event either of the departure from the United States of the person to whom this book is issued, or his or her death, the book must be surrendered in accordance with the Regulations.

4 Any person finding a lost book must deliver it promptly to the nearest Ration Board.

OFFICE OF PRICE ADMINISTRATION

№ 848353 -315

Fig. 5.1 ✳ WORLD WAR II RATION BOOKLET WITH STAMPS REMAINING
Courtesy Mrs. Frances Park.

mechanical to the intended readers? Is it the Tin Woodman in writing? Should you at least oil its joints?

Are any of the paragraphs in your explanation skimpy? Too formidable? Should various strands of thought be separated into different paragraphs?

Do your sentences show a variety of length and structure?

Here are further pointers:

Be More Direct—Or Less So. Should you proceed more directly into your explanation? Readers in the sciences and social sciences even expect an article to begin with a summary of its methods and conclusions. Here is an example from the professional journal *Families in Society*. The title: "What about Dad? Fathers of Children Born to School-Age Mothers."

ABSTRACT: Information regarding fathers of children born to school-age mothers is minimal. In this study, the authors describe paternal age, relationship and contact with the mother of the child, help provided by fathers, and the natural history of paternal drug use and other illegal behaviors of 170 fathers through three and one-half years postpartum [after birth]. Results indicated that fathers tended to be older than their partners and have intermittent patterns of contact and changing relationships with mothers over time. Many fathers engaged in illegal activities, including selling drugs. Potential predictors of ongoing contact between fathers, their partners, and their children are explored.

Larson et al. 279

Sometimes, however, explanation works with a touch of exploration. The writer avoids laying out everything up front and instead piques the reader's curiosity and satisfies it gradually.

One example is the article "Empire of Uniformity" from a popular magazine called *Discovery*. Between the title and the body text, in colorful type, appears an eye-catching bridge (called an "introduction" in textual design):

With its vast area and long history of settlement, China ought to have hundreds of distinct languages and cultures. In fact, all the evidence indicates that it once did. So what happened to them all?

Diamond 79

You might experiment with a variation on the No Surprises formula. You could engage your intended reader (and teacher) by a lead-in such as the following that although clear, promises a touch of indirection and even exploration:

The Aztec Empire arose in the mid 1300s in Central America. A highly organized society with a strong central government, it comprised somewhere between ten and twenty-five million people. After flourishing for over two hundred years, it fell apart. What were the causes of its downfall?

The more you spell out your purpose and plan, the more certainty your reader feels; the more you artfully postpone, as in storytelling, the more curiosity you evoke. In this paper, stress certainty. But always ask yourself, "How much do I want to reveal, how much to conceal?" And as a reader, like a volleyball player, stay on your toes, since the ball won't always come right to you.

Don't Beat on *Be*. Tighter grammar can help transmit information efficiently. For an energetic style, avoid overusing the verb "be" in its various forms (*is, are, was, were,* etc.). This verb, although indispensable, tends to make an explanation stodgy, static, and wordy. Contrast these two versions of a paragraph:

Maintaining proper soil compaction *is* just one of the skills a superintendent needs to do his job successfully. Soil compaction *is* just one small aspect of golf course maintenance. Very often the work of the superintendent *is* over-looked while praise for the condition of the course goes to the Head Golf Professional. It *is* important for you, as a golfer, to *be* knowledgeable of the "Whys?" and "Hows?" of golf course maintenance.

The revision:

Maintaining proper soil compaction *is* just one of the skills a superinten-dent needs to do his job successfully. Soil compaction encompasses one small aspect of golf course maintenance. Praise for the condition of the course very often goes to the Head Golf Professional and overlooks the hard work of the superintendent. It *is* important for you, as a golfer, to know the "Whys?" and "Hows?" of golf course management.

Circle every form of the verb "be" in your paper to check for anemia. Do you use the passive voice too much? Its subject doesn't do anything but in-stead receives the action: "The work is overlooked." If so, replace it with the active voice: "Praise . . . overlooks the work." Do you overuse *be* as a link-ing verb—that is, one that connects a noun with another noun or with an adjective? Examples of this function come from the paragraphs above: "Compaction is one skill" and "It is important. . . ." If so, replace the *be*-for-mula with a verb that names an action: "As a golfer, you should *know*. . . ."

EXTRA CHALLENGE

Lengthen the fibers in your writing muscles with one more exercise.

1. Recast your familiar essay from Chapter 3 as an explanatory piece. Turn as much of the original content as you can into rather impersonally conveyed information. This experience will give you a sharper sense of how any subject can be developed in innumerable ways.

2. Recast your explanatory paper in another format. One possibility: a dialogue. For instance, one student wrote a very brief introduction to ancient Western schools of philosophy that defined each school and compared it to others. He then recast the paper as a little drama be-tween personalities. Here is an excerpt:

Epicurean: . . . So everyone should feel that their minds have been "re-leased from worry and fear," and another point—
Cynic: "Released from worry and fear," would you please stop your mumbo-jumbo sob story for just one minute? We, as Cynics, believe that we are supreme individualists. . . .

A. L. Rohm

Another possibility: In an eye-catching metamorphosis, keep the same con-tent as your explanatory paper but recast it in a desktop-publishing format. Try some or all of these techniques of document design:

* columns (two or three)
* a visual "introduction" between title and text
* a "pull text"—that is, a brief quotation selected from the text, enlarged or boldfaced, and positioned where it will catch attention, sharpen the point, and add visual variety
* a text box
* frames or rules
* color
* illustrations, decorative or informative

Any practice with these nonverbal resources will give you an alternative to the traditional academic format. For example, the newspaper feature on Hong Dao and Boc Tran used two columns; these were broken up about halfway down by a pull text within a rectangle of lines and space:

"People in the United States do not appreciate freedom..."—Hong Dao.

3. Interview an imaginary person such as the motorcyclist in "Why Write?" or Chaucer's Miller (Additional Readings).
   Or Read Tracy Graham's "Flirting Nonverbally" (Additional Readings) and then write a mock-anthropological report on patrons of a coffee house (or whatever) as if investigating an exotic tribe.
   Or imitate the mushroom poem in the next section of this chapter, using some other item or substance.
4. Draft a law. As your model, use the Indian Removal Act (Additional Readings) and/or use laws published in your state's code of laws (found in the reference section of the library). The law may be ironic in tone.
   Or draft a contract such as a prenuptial agreement.
5. As business manager of a band called the Food Pyramid, write an informative letter to Le Club Dance confirming arrangements for an upcoming gig. Type the letter in a business format (perhaps following the example in the next chapter). Create your own letterhead with color and a logo.

POEM: TRY OUR TWO-ITEM SALAD BAR

The Aztecs viewed the mushroom as a sacred plant. Two varieties are defined in the following poem (which was preserved by a Spanish monk and translated into prose centuries later). How do these prose mushrooms seem more poetic than Dyer's sheep at the end of Chapter 4?

TWO MUSHROOMS

1

It is round, large, like a severed head.

2
It grows on the plains, in the grass. The head is
small and round, the stem long and slender. It is
bitter and burns; it burns the throat. It makes
one besotted; it deranges one, troubles one. It is
a remedy for fever, for gout. Only two or three
can be eaten. It saddens, depresses, troubles one;
it makes one flee, frightens one, makes one hide.
He who eats many of them sees many things
which make him afraid, or make him laugh. He
flees, hangs himself, hurls himself from a cliff,
cries out, takes fright. One eats it in honey.
I eat mushrooms; I take mushrooms.
Of one who is haughty, presumptuous, vain, of
him it is said: "He mushrooms himself."

(Rothenberg and Quasha 301)

TIPS FOR PROSE

Notice how fully these two poems draw upon various methods of developing a subject.

They define both mushrooms by implied comparison to each other. They also define them by a blend of description, detail, analysis, and cause and effect. They tell where, who, why, and how: "One eats it in honey" (a strangely matter-of-fact detail to bring closure to the bad drug trip).

As with some artful types of prose, all this explanation, with its complexity and variety played off against its brevity, has an aesthetic appeal. That is, the poem offers enjoyment as an end in itself, for its workmanship, not only as a means to understanding *Basidiomycetes*.

Notice that these Aztec poems, like the explanation of Valium in the *Physicians' Desk Reference,* explain each subject by physical description (what it looks like), operations (what it does), and contrastive features (what it's not like).

Works Cited

Diamond, Jared. "Empire of Uniformity." *Discover* 17.3 (March 1996): 79–85.

Gerchufsky, Michael. "Human Papilloma Virus." *Advance for Nurse Practitioners* 4.5 (May 1996): 20–26.

Larson, Nancy C., Jon M. Hussey, Mary Rogers Gillmore, and Lewayne D. Gilchrist. "What about Dad? Fathers of Children Born to School-Age Mothers." *Families in Society: The Journal of Contemporary Human Services* 77.5 (May 1996): 279–89.

Network Music. Vols. 1–120. San Diego: Network Music, 1993.

Rothenberg, Jerome, and George Quasha, eds. *America a Prophecy: A New Reading of American Poetry from Pre-Columbian Times to the Present.* New York: Vintage–Random House, 1973. The translators, Arthur J. O. Anderson and Charles E. Dibble, worked from texts compiled by a monk shortly after the Spanish conquest.

Salter, Gregory. "The Loudest Island in the World: Jamaica, Home of the Reggae Beat." In *World Music: the Rough Guide,* ed. Simon Broughton, Mark Ellingham, David Muddyman, and Richard Trillo, 521–38. London: Rough Guides, 1994.

Tinter, Elissa, and Jan Hall. "Vietnamese Find Freedom, Education in Myrtle Beach." *The Chanticleer* (Coastal Carolina University), 14 November 1995.

U. S. Department of Health and Human Services. *MMWR* 45.20 (May 24, 1996).

_____*MMWR* 45.RR-9 (June 14, 1996).

_____*MMWR* 45.42 (October 25, 1996).

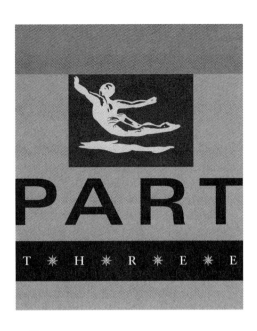

Persuade

"**D**o you believe in UFOs?"

"Well . . . not really."
"I do."
"Mm-m."
"Want to know why?"
"I guess."
"My uncle in Brooklyn—one day he went around the corner to buy a cigar—and he never came back!" ◆

This actual conversation shows how people tend to view life—and to measure reasonableness—from clashing perspectives. When you try to persuade, you must overcome resistance caused by other ways of looking at the subject.

Perhaps you intend to influence habitual attitudes or actions mainly by presenting information, like *An Employer's Guide to Islamic Religious Practices,* distributed by a Muslims' rights group in an effort to combat discrimination. Perhaps you want to motivate or reinforce some interest in your rather uncontroversial material. Or perhaps you want to put a persuasive spin on material that is pretty convincing by itself. But often you must overcome more serious resistance by building an argument—by marshalling evidence to support an opinion.

Resistance may arise from experience or expertise, from conscious or unconscious drives, from pride, from fear, from entrenched attitudes, from vested interests—in other words, from concerns for any practical, private benefit at risk, especially to that most sensitive part of the body, the wallet. In such cases, aiming to convince requires even more tact.

Whereas explanation tries to increase knowledge, persuasion has the touchier job of changing attitudes or motivating action. Such an effort can draw on any of the methods of development discussed in the previous section of *Stretch,* not so as to inform but to influence. Persuasion converts information to evidence.

Attempts to persuade can be ethical or unethical, impassioned or low-key, rational as geometry or irrational as astrology with its supposed planetary influence on human beings. Depending on one's point of view, an argument can withstand an earthquake of objection or collapse at a gust of reason. Attempts to persuade can alleviate prejudices or inflame them. Persuasion can help a family put a little dance in its act, unify one part of a community—perhaps at the expense of another—and cause people to give blood or shed it.

Despite the rhetorical, logical, and ethical challenges it presents, persuasion can give you more control over your own life. It can save you from playing the role of passive observer. It can also help you contribute to the welfare of the larger group by offering the benefit of your unique viewpoint. Look for opportunities for persuasion at school, at home, on the job, in the community. If like many people you avoid trying to sway others, this assignment will be a specially beneficial "stretch" because it will expand your versatility.

The effectiveness of even the best persuasion has its limits. No matter how heartfelt and eloquent, efforts to persuade may fail to produce "conviction in the soul of the listener" (adapting Plato's words). There was a general outcry against the Indian Removal Act of 1830 (see Additional Readings), a call that was joined by Christian missionaries as well as a senator from New Jersey, Theodore Frelinghuysen, who spoke for six hours in defense of the Cherokee tribe. Addressing the president of the Senate, he declared:

> I believe, Sir, it is not now seriously denied that the Indians are men, endowed with kindred faculties and powers with ourselves; that they have a place in human sympathy, and are justly entitled to a share in the common bounties of a benignant Providence. And, with that conceded, I ask in what code of the law of nations, or by what process of abstract deductions, their rights have been extinguished? . . . How can Georgia . . . desire or attempt, and how can we quietly permit her, to invade and disturb the property, rights, and liberty of the Indians? . . . How can we tamely suffer these States to make laws, not only not founded in justice and humanity "for preventing wrongs being done to the Indians" but for the avowed purpose of inflicting the gross and wanton injustice of breaking up their government, of abrogating their long-cherished customs, and of annihilating their existence as a distinct people? ◆

Jahoda 44–45

Frelinghuysen's effort at persuasion was partly nonverbal—his delivery, which is lost to history. It was partly verbal—his text with its ringing premise that Indians are people, with its rhetorical questions about their human rights. And it was completely unsuccessful—the racist and cruel bill passing in Congress by a vote of 102–97.

Although plenty of bad things happen despite persuasion, few good things happen without it. In order to counteract inertia (the force of habit that continues to do things in the same way) someone must catch an eye or ear, define a need, offer a solution, pat a shoulder, touch a heart, make a deal, find a means, and probably tap a keyboard.

Persuasion often combines writing with speaking. A writer may warm people up about a document by talking with them before or after they read it. Writers who collaborate, moreover, usually talk about their uncertainties, possibilities, strategy, and progress.

And writing often gains persuasive power from graphics. Photographs, drawings, maps, charts, and graphs can help make a case along with the alphabet. An example is the movie poster in Chapter 1: Its image of the praying woman helps to catch attention, carry meaning, and arouse interest. Of course, advertisements strive for just the right blend of word and image. For an example of an advertisement displayed on the Internet, see Figure III.1.

Even the design of a printed text can have a nonverbal persuasive appeal. A business letter will make a better impression on heavy paper, under an attractive letterhead, and in a conventional format. The annual report of a large corporation, will use glossy paper, lavish color, attractive layout, handsome typography, abundant graphs and charts, and artistic photography to help make an impression of substance.

Of course, *Stretch* will emphasize persuasion undertaken by written symbols, with all their amazing ability to communicate with relative precision, complexity, and density. But be on the lookout for ways to combine writing with nonverbal stimuli to help gain attention, whip up interest, enhance clarity, arouse feeling, even gain credibility with an impressive presentation.

Here are a few principles that will guide you. They arise from the memorandum format, simple but illuminating, already discussed in Chapter 5. You will notice that these three elements are interdependent, so a change in one brings a change in the others.

DATE:

Consider the "Day"

What's in the air on the calendar date or, more broadly, at the current time? Socially, politically, economically, what issues might influence the discourse? What buzzwords (those temporarily in vogue) might you want to use or avoid?

Can you refer to some recent event to lead into your argument or otherwise bring out its topical importance?

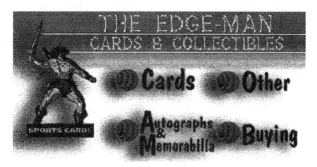

To receive information about our *"HOTTEST"* specials,
be sure to sign our guestbook.

Links to our hottest items below:

[NEW RELEASES: BOXES/LINEUPS !!]
[Mirages: In Stock/ Latest Pricing]
[ALLIANCES!!!!!!!!!!!!!: New/Better CURRENT PRICING]
[ICE AGE OUT OF PRINT!!: INFO + CURRENT PRICING]
[RARE SET FIND:92 PROLINE "EMBOSSED", PRICING AND INFO]

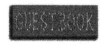

10835 Sanden Drive * Dallas,Texas 75238
214-349-9690 * fax 214-349-5083
E-Mail: edge@airmail.net * Website: http://www.edgeman.com

000013629

"Last updated on Oct 6, 1996.
All prices quoted subject to change,
according to our current needs."

Fig. III.1 * HOME PAGE OF "THE EDGE-MAN CARDS AND COLLECTIBLES"

Used by permission.

What urgency is there in the communication? What is timely or pressing about the subject? Is your own timing for your letter, report, or memo tactful? Is the date important as a legal record?

Envision a Campaign?

Should you think of your document as just one part of a series that may involve further writing, audiovisual presentations, formal speaking, and informal speaking (with elbow squeezing and other techniques of nonverbal persuasion)?

TO:
* ■

In persuasion, as in explanation, your reader not only receives your message but shapes it. So you should consider the following guidelines:

Narrow Your Audience

Don't try to convince everybody. Get a sense of one particular group you can address, even if it is "educated adults with X attitude toward the subject." Use the pronoun "you" if such direct address gives the topic a helpful nudge from the theoretical toward the personally relevant.

Adapt Purpose to Reader

Given the nature of your audience, how much persuasion do you need to employ? Should you try to convert your readers? Modify their beliefs? Conciliate them by offering a compromise? Plant an eggplant of doubt among their pansies?

Some audiences will not be convinced; there is no "give," no rhetorical latitude for persuasion. They may have substantial reasons, they may not: What people lack in proof they furnish in certainty. So you might want to target readers who may have some "give." Don't deliver an oration to the deaf.

Work Either More or Less Directly

You can announce the main point as early as the title or declare it in the final sentence. As always, composition serves rhetoric: The organization and development of your paper depends on your sense of the reader's attitude and degree of understanding. Here is a brief definition of the two approaches:

Direct. You have probably used the clear-from-the-top approach in the academic papers you've written. The writer makes a claim near the beginning and then supports it.

If your thesis is simply unfamiliar, or provocative, or a little unsettling but not threatening, you can probably work directly. Straightforward, easy to follow for the reader, and reliable for the writer, this technique is indispensable not only in college but in the workplace and in public life generally. This "deductive" method will be discussed in Chapter 6, Direct Persuasion.

Indirect. The direct method, however, has only so much flexibility. When a writer should tiptoe, it clumps. The more your idea challenges the audience's emotional condition, cultural assumptions, temperament, and vested interests (such as gold on the Cherokees' land in Georgia), the more indirectly you might work. The indirect approach invites someone to accept a gradually evolving proposition. It avoids making an early thesis statement that can put a reader on the defensive—just as a rap on the shell causes a turtle to retract his head. You can reveal part of the thesis near the beginning but withhold the rest until later. Or reveal it toward the end. Or imply it and never overtly express it.

As a writer (as well as a reader, speaker, and listener) you should be familiar with the indirect, "inductive" sequence of persuasion discussed in Chapter 7.

The problem-solution format, which is very common in persuasion, can work directly or indirectly. The writer tries to establish that a problem exists and then urges a solution; the latter can appear as early as the title or as late as the final sentence. Similarly, the proposal format establishes a need and makes a recommendation that can be expressed early or late.

However you proceed, try to do the following to adapt to the reader.

Find Common Ground

Discover a value you share with the reader. It can reduce the emotional distance between you and provide grounds to support your point.

In 1997 the lieutenant governor of South Carolina urged that the Confederate battle flag be removed from atop the State Capitol to the lawn in front. He knew that foes of the plan revered the banner and considered it an emblem of their heritage, so he took pains to establish the honor in which he held both his Confederate ancestors and the flag. He thus tried to reduce any static electricity arising from him as a person.

Moreover, he was able to turn this same value of honoring one's heritage into evidence against flying the flag atop the Capitol. For, he argued, the controversy surrounding it actually distracted from the attempt to honor the generation of soldiers who fought and died: "The flag now flies in a position without reference or reverence to these same men" (Peeler 4–A).

Fill a Need

Especially when you propose an action, try to show how your idea will answer some need or needs. Will it help the reader become more prosperous? Capable? Safe? Attractive? Successful? Powerful? Admirable? Self-respecting? Stimulated?

Can you actually get your reader to *want* to do something? Then you can draw on his or her own motivation to carry the point.

For a few words of Socrates on the need to find different means of persuasion for different people, see the excerpt from Plato's dialogue *Phaedrus* (in Additional Readings).

Support Your Thesis

Do more than make an assertion and hope the reader will go along with it. When you state something controversial, like the arguments in the next two chapters, you depart from commonly accepted ideas, take a risk, go out on a limb.

Do you recall the swimmers described in "Explore," who climbed a tree, grasped a trapeze bar, and swooped down toward the Waccamaw River and then far above it? Those who try to persuade must relinquish the conventional ground and swing by themselves into the air. To keep from merely plummeting like a rock, they must secure their thesis to its support—just as the trapeze bar is attached to the cypress bough by a cable.

A judicious reader will expect you to provide evidence in a logical framework. You can read an example (see Additional Readings) where Michael H. Robinson argues that birds are surprisingly intelligent. He depends on two main areas of proof: (1) Absolute brain size is not a measure of braininess, and (2) birds have some remarkable learning abilities. Each of these premises is supported in turn by explanation drawn from theory and experiment—from such specific evidence as running kiwi birds and pecking pigeons. Robinson's thesis (to expand the analogy of the tree-swing) is attached to solid logic, which is itself deeply rooted in evidence.

What about research? Will your readers expect it? If so, what kind? How quantified? In a magazine article they may appreciate a reference but will not expect full documentation. Will they expect illustrations? Your teacher will probably furnish guidelines on this aspect of the assignment.

You will probably cite sources as you go. Try to point out relationships among them. Does one reinforce another? Touch on a particular aspect of another? Contradict another? You should make your research varied and current (unless the subject is timeless).

The reader will expect you to deal with points advanced by the opposition. Ignore these at the peril of your credibility. Instead, take them up and try to show their flaws or limitations.

So to persuade most effectively keep in mind the reader, just as Senator Frelinghuysen did when he looked into the eye of the president.

FROM:

Your own credibility makes a powerful resource for persuasion. In fact, Aristotle averred that it makes up a triad with the other appeals of logic and emotion. You build your credibility as you write: Do you seem well disposed to your audience? Knowledgeable? Logical? Emotionally in control? Experienced?

Your own experience could indeed be persuasive, so you might include a firsthand anecdote or example. But save a long story for Chapter 1 because this "stretch" should derive power from a logical, rather than chronological, relationship among its parts. And let the informal essay, discussed in Chapter 3, emphasize the writer's personality and thoughts-in-progress; instead, emphasize the connection between reader and thesis—between **TO:** and **SUBJECT.** Do not write a flippant or primarily entertaining paper.

Here are a few guidelines about the writer as an element of persuasion:

Know Thyself

Anyone who would undertake persuasion might profitably look at himself or herself as well, as the product of a certain era, culture (including language with its prescribed ways of looking at the world), personality, experience, vested interests, even sociobiological drives—biologically inherited social tendencies that have enabled *homo sapiens* to survive in a hostile world. (If such things exist, they would be "hard wired," to use Robinson's metaphor for some bird behavior.)

Scrutinize your motivation. Often people have more than one reason for doing something, one more admirable than another. Do you want to look good? Be sure to keep this secondary aim from calling attention to itself. Do you want to poke somebody in the ribs? Be honest with yourself and ask if you should temper your message in order to persuade rather than punish. Do you really want to express intense feelings more than change minds? Then don't put on a fireworks show, especially in writing, a medium that sets up an expectation of restraint and precision. Keep—actually, create—the reader's trust in your level-headedness. Use your steam to propel a constructive argument rather than ventilate an overheated boiler.

Perhaps write an exploratory essay on why you believe a certain way, or jot down a few influences and ponder their value and limitations. One major question in philosophy and psychology is how to distinguish between the seen and the seer. ("The vision of the maker informs the eye," declares the poet in "Reflections on a Visit to the Burke Museum," Chapter 2.)

People use more calories to protect their habitual way of thinking than to broaden it. A lesson from Columbus: So determined was he to believe that Cuba was Asia that he threatened to cut off the tongue of anyone who said otherwise (Todorov 21–22).

Should you enrich your understanding by doing more research? Perhaps you should even collaborate with one or more people to benefit from their viewpoints, experience, expertise, and credibility. Even the Lone Ranger had help from Tonto.

Determine a Persona

Like this famous cowboy, you should don a mask. (See the sidebar in Chapter 2). It will not conceal your identity, but it may conceal your hostility when anger will jeopardize your goal. Wrath puts the reader on the defensive, so after sending a nasty letter you may have trouble getting your room re-wallpapered for free in the pattern you originally specified; or after squirting a colleague with ink you may spend years cleaning the shirt.

Project an attitude that you judge will make your reader most receptive. Your "mask" can be detached, prophetic, sarcastic, impassioned, cajoling, whatever seems most effective, considering your purpose and readers.

Are you the sole proprietor of the truth? You might stay a bit humble; at least avoid appearing righteous and "mushrooming yourself," in the words of the Aztec poem in Chapter 5.

Notice that an impersonal, official mask can disguise a dearth of ethics, as in the Indian Removal Act with its mechanical series of "and be it further enacteds" (Additional Readings). Conversely, highly charged feelings can betray a dearth of substance; a restrained mask can encourage you to present evidence rather than express emotion. To arouse feelings, though, try to give your paper the stirring power of music with your ideas, word choice, figurative language, and grammar.

Avoid Logical Fallacies

Human beings, by language, culture, and temperament, value a sense of order. To achieve it we are ever ready to impose patterns on life, as when we connect a few stars that despite their widely varying distances from earth seem to make a two-dimensional picture of a familiar object or figure.

When you argue, you propose connections. They may be between cause and effect, whole and part, general and specific, subject and properties. Make sure that you support the pattern you envision by providing as much support as is necessary or feasible.

Be especially careful not to oversimplify causality. Be more convincing than the chain letter in the Additional Readings (see Anonymous). Humans tend to impose cause-and-effect relationships where they may not exist: Striking the cow made the milk go sour in the kitchen; going outside in the cold causes colds; human sacrifice will appease the gods; censoring lyrics will protect women and children. Your job is to make the connection as probable as you can.

Usually there are multiple causes of an event. For example, *fé y oro*— faith and gold—were the double motivations of the conquistadors, who wanted to take Christianity to the Indians and take wealth away from them. (See Paul Rice's poem in Chapter 3.)

And there are always remote causes—often powerful social, economic, and psychological forces—that might be acknowledged. For example, the Treaty of Versailles, which ended World War I, required that Germany pay immense reparations to the Allies; German resentment over this provision helped Hitler rise to power—which in turn provided an immediate cause of World War II.

Here are a few notes on some major fallacies to avoid:

Either-Or. Presenting only two options when there are more commits the either-or fallacy. "They have taken prayer out of the schools" is a statement implying only two choices: official prayers or none. It ignores the options of individual or privately communal prayers.

American culture may reinforce a dualistic way of looking at the world with its paired verbal symbols: religious-secular, heaven-hell, black-white (racial categories), right-wrong.

Argumentum ad Hominem. Criticizing the person instead of the position is argumentum *ad hominem.* People easily succumb to this temptation when they cannot hold their own with an argument that draws on principles and evidence, or when they are just too upset to argue. "As a Democrat, you should support gay marriages," or "As a Republican, you should oppose gay marriages." One student, exasperated at a critic's review of an opera, asked, "Can he do any better?"

Red Herring. Diverting the argument to an irrelevant point is creating a red herring. Like the argument against the person, this fallacy opens a new front rather than combating a challenge on another. If the opera critic charges that the scenery was inadequate, a strictly logical rebuttal is "We disagree for these reasons," not just "Well, we didn't have enough money for elaborate scenery."

Bandwagon. Everybody's doing it, therefore *you* should is the bandwagon approach: "Hey, this is a dorm—have a beer!"

Hasty Generalization. A statement about many particulars that is not adequately supported is a hasty generalization. "The Patel families always stick together in the motel business." To be safer, qualify the assertion; that is, limit it: "From my experience, the Patel families . . .," or "The Patel families typically stick together. . . ." Even better: Also give examples, testimony from a Patel, or other evidence for your view. Hasty generalization characterizes off-the-cuff speech more than careful writing.

Post Hoc Ergo Propter Hoc. Since X came after Z, it must have been *caused* by Z. This is a *post hoc ergo propter hoc* stance. The causal relationship may indeed have been thus, but supply evidence. An example is found in the chain letter in Additional Readings: "Dallan Fairchild received the letter and not believing, he threw the letter away. Nine days later, he died." Maybe his failure to continue the chain killed him, maybe not, but let's hear evidence to link effect to supposed cause.

Non Sequitur. A non sequitur is a generic fallacy that overlaps with others. "It doesn't follow." The writer sees a connection, hopes the reader will, and doesn't bother to weave strands of evidence into a cable to connect them: "After all, where would American music be without African influences?" After what "all"? Don't quit prematurely, but instead furnish examples—syncopation, the blue note, the call-and-response pattern, the gospel choir, and so on.

A non sequitur to one audience is a "sequitur" to another. Will the distribution of condoms increase sexual activity among the unmarried? The debate over this question characterizes public health policy making almost everywhere in the United States. Can the true relationship be determined objectively?

Argumentum ad Populum. *Argumentum ad populum* is an appeal to unexamined and automatic emotional responses, especially those widely shared by the populace. "This socialistic liberal program—" Whoa! Do more than invoke the out-of-favor term "liberal" and appeal to the natural resistance to taxes: Offer a critique of the program itself.

As with all these fallacies, argument to the people can have drastic implications; in World War II, German, Italian, and Japanese leaders aroused tribal instincts that brought death and destruction to them and to many others.

Begging the Question. Slipping in an assertion in hopes the reader will go along with it without demanding support is known as begging the question: "This healthful product," "This tax-and-spend measure," "Such a ridiculous proposal. . . ." Logically, this fallacy is the equivalent of "Excuse me, could you spare a buck?"

Beware of these fallacies and any other unacceptable shortcuts in logic. Like driving through a corner gas station to avoid an intersection, they skirt the painstaking requirements of building an argument with logic and evidence.

SUBJECT:

Limit Your Ambition

As with explanation, be sure to limit your subject to something manageable, given your allowance of words. Consider announcing that you will take on only part of the question—for example, whether the movie was true to the book, not whether it was worthwhile on its own terms.

Be ready to narrow your subject by limiting your argument's claim: Instead of declaring that "single-parent families put extra burdens on children," perhaps reduce the probability to "may put" or narrow the scope to "single-parent families headed by teenage mothers."

Given the nature of your audience, consider making a strategic concession. This is an admission, a point granted to the audience, an acknowledgment that their way of looking at a situation has some value. (Sometimes people are relieved just to know that their concerns have been heard.) For example, you might acknowledge that free condoms will encourage some young people to have sex. This concession renders the audience more receptive, portrays you as more balanced, and narrows your focus to what may be more defensible territory: That most determined teens will find a way, with or without protection.

You can also narrow your argument by agreeing that someone's plan may be *desirable* but declaring that it is not *feasible:* A swimming pool proposed for a certain elementary school may be an attractive idea but not a practical one in view of local tax conditions.

Anticipate Custom

Any topic you address will encounter the natural conservatism that characterizes human beings—not only your readers but yourself. This attitude will be a factor in any subject you take on. Just as most students expect to have the same chair in the same classroom day after day, all people count upon pretty much the same world tomorrow as the one that they woke up to yesterday.

Also, be aware that a subject will be viewed differently by people of different cultures or subcultures. People see the world through the language and other assumptions of their group. "Wherever I want to turn," writes Montaigne in the beginning of his essay on clothes, "I have to force some barrier of custom, so carefully has it blocked our approaches" (see Additional Readings).

In one culture, dance may be central to religious ceremonies; in another, antithetical. Even directness itself in communication depends on a culture for its value: Admired in the United States, it is eschewed in Japan. The more you and your reader share basic assumptions about a subject or strategy, the more likelihood for persuasion. But an argument that tries to cross the border from one culture to another may be charged a heavy toll in understanding or acceptance, and it may even be halted by armed guards.

Keep all these guidelines in mind as you use some art to persuade. **DATE:**, **TO:**, **FROM:**, and **SUBJECT:** are constituents you can borrow from the memorandum to help you develop any kind of persuasion, from the simplest to the most complex. As Socrates declares about rhetoric, "The method which proceeds without analysis is like the groping of a blind man" (Plato 274).

Works Cited

Gerchufsky, Michael. "Human Papilloma Virus." *Advance for Nurse Practitioners* 4.5 (May 1996): 20–26.

Jahoda, Gloria. *The Trail of Tears*. New York: Holt, 1975. Ellipses are Jahoda's.

Peeler, Bob. "Heritage Act Serves the State Best." The *Horry Independent* [Conway, SC], 9 Jan. 1997: 4-A, 8-A.

Plato. *Phaedrus*. From *The Dialogues of Plato,* Trans. B. Jowett. Introduction by Raphael Demos. 2 vols. New York: Random, 1937. 1: 233-82.

Todorov, Tzvetan. *The Conquest of America: The Question of the Other.* Translated from the French by Richard Howard. First published in France in 1982. New York: Harper/Collins, 1992. Harper Perennial.

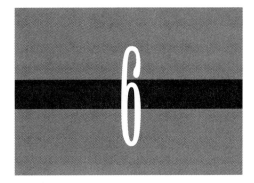

Direct Persuasion

"**E**at, buy and grow organic food."

This commandment appears on a T-shirt, and below it appears the rationale "Good health from the good earth." Like this screen-printed shirt, a writer often makes a claim or recommendation and then offers evidence to support it. For a World War II poster that jumps directly to its point, see Figure 6.1. For a bumper sticker, see Figure 6.2.

Just as the clearest *explanation* announces its purpose at the beginning, the most direct *persuasion* announces its thesis. A thesis is an opinion. It is a proposition advanced by the writer and not automatically accepted by readers. It may concern such questions as the value of something, a course of action, or an interpretation, whether of an event or a literary work. The writer must support this opinion to gain assent or at least reduce resistance.

Persuasion, even more than explanation, needs to adapt its strategy to the reader's (or listener's) point of view. Generally, the more receptive the reader, the more directly you can go. Practice in writing direct

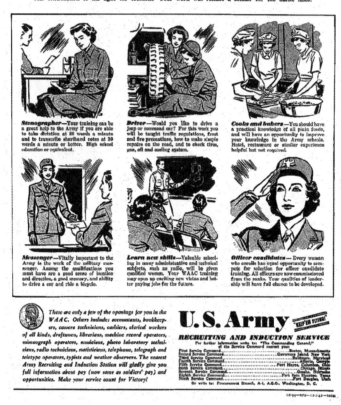

Fig. 6.1 ∗ **POSTER FOR WOMEN'S ARMY AUXILIARY CORPS (WORLD WAR II)**

This poster addresses the viewer directly and tries to put her to work immediately. Contrast the more gradual approach used by the poster in Chapter 7.

persuasion will help tone up your writing ability (as well as your reading and listening skills) because in many cases the more straightforward the approach, the clearer and better received the message.

Suppose you are concerned about the growing number of single mothers in the United States. You believe that this phenomenon negatively affects the child, the mother, the community, and the country, and you want to write about it in hopes of changing people's behavior. How would you develop your argument directly?

You might try a preliminary thesis like this one: "Children need dads, not just fathers." In other words, it's one thing to conceive a child in min-

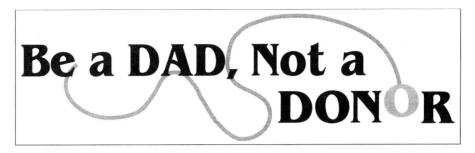

Fig. 6.2 ✳ BUMPER STICKER THESIS
© R. Wells and P. Olsen, 1996.

utes, but it's another to raise it for decades. What are some kinds of help a dad gives in raising a child? You could turn up some ideas with an exploratory paper, a list, one or more interviews, library research, any of or all these discovery techniques.

Examples: A dad brings home at least a few strips of the bacon, helps with child care, offers a different perspective from a mother's, helps keep the house in shape, and gives attention and love. (See Figure 6.4 for a family with Dad at the handlebars.)

But before you can write, you need something else. Not another job to fill out the dad's job description, but a sense of your audience. Lacking an intended reader, your argument sounds too generic. You need to address a particular group that has its own values, needs and interests.

Should you focus on adults? Teenagers? Since having a child is a joint responsibility, maybe you should address both sexes. Perhaps you might be able to write a better paper if you focus on young males who are at risk for premature fathering, though. Besides, addressing only teen boys allows you to make a corollary point that responsibility belongs to both partners. This stand is not a typical one, since people usually expect girls alone to take the responsibility for pregnancy. Now you are ready to state a tentative thesis that reflects your intended audience: "Don't just *father* a child, *Dad* it."

How can you back up this exhortation? You could tell how a real dad helps the child, the mother, and society. You could even argue that the satisfaction of being a dad is worth waiting for. You could try to discover such reasons by making a cluster drawing like the one in the sidebar on being a dad. From it you could choose the strongest reasons and then convert them to a preliminary outline such as this one:

Point 1: A dad helps the child

   a. by giving love

   b. by enforcing discipline

   c. by meeting material needs

Point 2: A dad helps himself

   a. by enjoying companionship and love

   b. by having pride in raising kids well

**CLUSTER
DRAWING
ON DADS**

You can generate ideas with lines and circles. Write down a general idea and draw a large circle around it. Then draw lines that radiate out from the large circle to subdivisions or associations, which you label and enclose with smaller circles. Then draw more lines from these circles to even smaller ones that enclose more specific details.

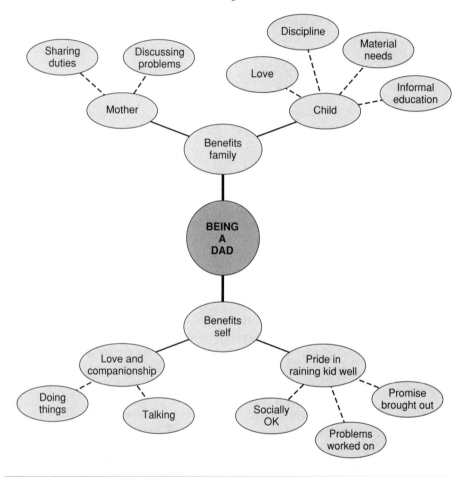

Will young men be persuaded by these arguments? Could you strengthen your support by adding the testimony of dads, or of non-dads who regret their choice? Should you touch on the potentially negative effects of dad-less children on the community?

How widespread is the problem of the fathered and forsaken? You could go to the library to search for those comprehensive little symbols called numbers. First of all you could negotiate your way around the *Statistical Abstract of the United States*. This compendium is published by the U.S. Department of Commerce and updated yearly. It includes hundreds of tables that analyze the population of the country according to many different measurements.

In the table of contents of one recent edition, for example, is the heading "Vital Statistics" and the subdivision "Births." This section of the book includes many tables on the subject, for example, "Births to Unmarried Women, by Race of Child and Age of Mother: 1970 to 1992." A person could also circle back to the table of contents to try a different heading, "Population." The subheading "Marital Status and Households" refers to a section with many more tables, for example "Female Family Householders with Spouse Present."

To help illuminate the causes, effects, nature, and ramifications of the problem you might consult the *Social Issues Resources Series*. This reference work reprints articles written on a number of controversial topics and collected in looseleaf volumes that are classified according to some thirty social concerns like "Sexuality." After finding the classification "Family," you might prospect through the articles to find gold, a connection between single-mother households and welfare:

Three factors—job discrimination against women, the time and money it takes to care for children, and the presence of only one adult—combine to make it nearly impossible for women to move off of welfare through work alone, without sufficient and stable supplemental income supports.

Tilly and Albelda, Art. 40

You can find even more information by consulting a newspaper index. One article informs you that the proportion of American children who grow up in fatherless homes has quadrupled since 1950, according to the Annie E. Casey Foundation. What are the effects of such a large demographic change?

The report said children who grow up without fathers are five times more likely to be poor, twice as likely to drop out of high school and much more likely to end up in foster care or juvenile justice facilities. Girls who are raised in single-parent families are three times more likely to become unwed teen mothers, and boys without fathers at home are much more likely to become incarcerated, unemployed, and uninvolved with their own children when they become fathers.

"Number of Fatherless" 3A

So with a little effort you have profited from a lot of work done by others: Your paper can establish the extent and the effects of a problem before it offers a solution.

WARM UP FIRST

The following letter was actually written to the advice columnist Ann Landers. Try answering it by using the direct approach. Begin with the words "I think," render a verdict, give at least one reason, and use fewer than seventy-five words.

Dear Ann Landers: I am now 27. Nine years ago, "Judy," the girl I was going with, became pregnant. I now know sex is strictly for adults and there are responsibilities and consequences that go along with it. But I was only 18 and very naive.

I went on to college. Judy began harassing my family, first with phone calls and then through bizarre behavior. She vandalized my girl-friend's apartment and trashed my car and my parents' car.

Nine days after I married my girlfriend, Judy filed for child support. The court has ordered me to pay 25 percent of my annual income. I am really burned up. I never wanted to have this child, so why should I have to support it?

I firmly believe that a woman has total control of her body. Judy de-cided ON HER OWN to have that child. I ordered her to get an abortion or put the child up for adoption. She refused. In my opinion, she should be totally responsible for taking care of that child.

I am not able to pay child support. I have an enormous amount of debt—college loans, car payments, credit card bills, rent and graduate school tuition. I am a newlywed and just getting by. My major asset is my car. The court has said I should sell it.

When my wife and I decide to have children, it will be a mutual de-cision, and I will be happy to provide for that child financially and emo-tionally. Judy is physically able to work but refuses to do so. I feel like an innocent bystander who is being taken for a ride. What do you think?

—A Dad Too Soon in N.J.

PUBLISHED ARGUMENT

It was Asia to Columbus; to the indigenous people it was home. Like the ar-rival of the European on the shores of the "New World," the arrival of im-migrants to the United States has always provoked resentment from many of those already established. These newcomers have incited anxiety that is fed by sometimes muddy streams: economic, political, religious, ethnic, linguistic, and racial.

The complexion of the United States—both its social composition and its skin color—depends upon this issue of immigration. Do immigrants help or harm the country? This controversy is ready-made for resolution by bias rather than by fact and logic. The following article takes up a number of "myths" that have grown around the subject of immigration and tries to refute them with evidence. The argument was published in May 1996 by *Reader's Digest,* which sells almost as many copies each month (27 million) as there are people in California. The magazine tends to prize individual ef-fort, conservative social values, and limited government.

According to an introductory note, Linda Chavez is president of the Center for Equal Opportunity; John J. Miller is a Bradley Fellow at The Heritage Foundation (a conservative research institute).

Comments in the margin will highlight the authors' use of (1) the direct approach and (2) persuasive techniques.

For a negative view of immigration, see the home page of FAIR, The Federation for Immigration Reform: http:www.fairus.org.

Their yearning to be free is good for all of us.

The Immigration Myth

※

Linda Chavez and John J. Miller

Americans like immigrants as individuals—the decent, hard-working Korean grocer on the corner, the Russian computer programmer who lives down the

The subtitle (which precedes the title) probably states the thesis of the article in one brief declarative sentence.

The authors earn good will by using the pronoun "we" and by giving credit to Americans.

Americans like immigrants as individuals—the decent, hard-working Korean grocer on the corner, the Russian computer programmer who lives down the street or the Filipino nurse who works at the local hospital. But as a nation we don't seem to think much of immigration in general.

A survey and an editorial help to establish the extent to which Americans hold the opposing viewpoint.

In a 1994 *Newsweek* survey, for example, half the public agreed that "immigrants are a burden because they take our jobs, housing and health care." Passions run high. "We are flooding areas of the country with millions of uneducated immigrants," complained one *Wall Street Journal* reader. They "take over, impose their culture and don't even try to assimilate."

The authors limit the scope of their argument to legal immigration. But they point out the current political threat to all immigration.

Everyone agrees that we must police our borders against illegal immigrants. But some, including Presidential candidate Pat Buchanan, want to declare a moratorium on *all* immigration. Sen. Alan Simpson (R., Wyo.) has sponsored a bill that would reduce the number of legally admitted non-refugee immigrants from 675,000 annually to 540,000.

The authors make several assertions that add up to a thesis; the last echoes the title and seems to forecast the plan of the article.

Yet in sharp contrast to the prevailing rhetoric that feeds on misinformation, the evidence shows that the problems attributed to immigration are false or greatly exaggerated. In reality, today's immigrants contribute positively, in much the same way our own ancestors did. We would only hurt ourselves by shutting the door in their faces. It's time to debunk the myths that are clouding our public debate and policy.

Indeed, the article will work by debunking each myth.

MYTH: Today's immigrants are less educated than in the past.

In fact, the educational level of immigrants has been increasing, not decreasing. About one-third of all new immigrants in 1960 had less than eight years of schooling. In the past decade, that proportion has dropped to one-quarter.

The percentage of immigrants with a college education and with advanced degrees has been increasing too. In the 1980s, for example, there were about 11,000 foreign-born engineers and scientists here. By 1992 that number had doubled.

An astonishing 40 percent of engineering doctorates at American universities in 1993 went to foreign-born professionals, who have become a vital force in the high-technology sectors critical to our future—telecommunications, biotechnology, chemicals and computers.

"How important are immigrants to my company?" asks T. J. Rodgers, president and CEO of Cypress Semiconductor, a manufacturer of high-performance computer chips in San Jose, Calif. "We would be out of business without them." In the research and development offices of the firm, pins on a world map represent employees' places of birth. Almost half lie outside American borders. Home countries include China, Ghana, India, Panama, the Philippines, Russia, Taiwan and Zimbabwe.

This is true of countless firms in America's computer industry. At giant Intel, maker of the Pentium processor used in millions of home computers, many of the people working on the Santa Clara–based company's top projects are immigrants. Take Indian-born Ryan Manepally. He co-developed the concept for a computer-to-computer video-conferencing product that would allow, for instance, doctors in different states to discuss X rays simultaneously. Intel CEO Andy Grove is from Hungary, and at least six of the company's 29 corporate vice presidents are also immigrants.

"Without immigrants, we would have to send work overseas," notes Anant Agrawal, Indian-born vice president of engineering at Sun Microsystems, Inc., a leading designer and manufacturer of workstations used for commercial and technical computing. "That certainly would not help the American economy."

MYTH: Immigrants steal jobs from Americans.

Behind this myth, notes economist Julian Simon, is a basic fallacy: that the number of jobs is finite, and the more that immigrants occupy, the fewer there are for others. Numerous studies dispute this myth. For instance, the Alexis de Tocqueville Institution in Arlington, Va., found that between 1960 and 1991, the ten states with the highest immigrant presence had a lower unemployment rate than the ten states with lowest immigrant presence. Blacks—often portrayed as economic victims of immigration—were found to earn more when they live in cities with large immigrant populations than they do in cities with small ones.

Immigrants, notes Simon in a recent Cato Institute report on immigration, "make new jobs by spending workers." What's more, less skilled immigrants take work Americans shun. IBP, Inc., near Garden City, Kan., operates the world's largest meatpacking plant. Workers at IBP are reasonably well paid—$7 to $10.35 per hour. Yet most of the workers on the "kill floor" there and at a nearby competitor, Monfort, are from Mexico or Southeast

Asia. Meatpacking is the most hazardous job in the United States. Workers make several cuts on a carcass every few seconds for eight hours a day, six days a week. The kill floors can get wet with water and blood, and even the most experienced worker can fall or get cut. "There are jobs that native-born Americans simply won't do," says Steve Orozco, a program specialist at Job Service Center, a state agency in Garden City. "Meatpacking is one of them."

The 40 workers at the Dalma Dress Manufacturing Company in New York City are all foreign-born. "Hardly any Americans apply for a job here," says Tonia Sylla from Liberia, an 11-year veteran. "Even when they do, they don't last long." Says Dalma's owner, Armand DiPalma, "Immigrants are the only labor pool we have."

Half of the 800,000 garment workers in the United States are immigrants, part of a $120-billion industry. If they were not doing the work, the jobs would probably move overseas.

"Every time you see a 'Made in the USA' label on a piece of clothing," says Bruce Herman of the Garment Industry Development Corporation, "chances are you can thank an immigrant."

Citing statistics, examples, and testimony, the argument tries to show that immigrants make positive contributions because they (1) help to support other workers and (2) accept work that others shun. The irony of the last quotation challenges any simplistic distinction between American and non-American.

MYTH: Immigrants are welfare moochers.

After a concession the author points out that most legal immigrants depend less on welfare than do the native-born, and that foreign-born males have a greater rate of employment than native-born.

Because immigrants admitted as refugees are guaranteed cash and medical assistance by federal law, the proportion of foreign-born on welfare is 6.6 percent, versus 4.9 percent of native-born. However, only 5.1 percent of nonrefugee working-age immigrants—the vast majority of legally admitted foreign-born—receive welfare benefits, compared with 5.3 percent of working-age native-born.

In reality, the work ethic of today's immigrants is just as strong as that of the Irish, Italians and Poles of yesteryear. According to the 1990 census, foreign-born males have a 77 percent labor-force participation rate, compared with 74 percent for native-born Americans. Hispanics have the highest rate of any group, 83 percent.

Chavez and Miller acknowledge that public money helps to support many immigrant but locate the root source of conflict in extravagant federal and state programs.

No doubt, too, many immigrants receive government benefits. However, the problem is not the immigrants but our overgenerous welfare state. California, for example, burdened as it is by federally mandated programs, is also laden with state-sponsored aid programs. The strain on the state's taxpayers boiled over in 1994 when Proposition 187, a ballot measure that denies benefits to illegal immigrants, passed by a huge margin.

A contrast between policies helps to show that fear of welfare mooching reflects overgenerosity of state aid.

Texas, on the other hand, spends less on welfare. It has taken in millions of immigrants in recent years without the public backlash. Gov. George W. Bush opposes laws modeled on Proposition 187, which have gone nowhere in the Texas legislature.

"Immigrants have the determination to succeed," declares Patricia Charlton, who arrived penniless from Jamaica in 1981 and started work at a McDonald's in Manhattan. She worked her way up, eventually being named a regional Manager of the Year. She's married, owns a house and has a child in private school.

"Often immigrant-owned businesses invest in inner cities where rents are cheap, becoming a revitalizing force there," says Stephen N. Solarsh, a New York City business and real-estate adviser to many immigrant-owned businesses. Korean immigrant Kim Suk Su, for example, currently owns property in some of the worst areas in Brooklyn, N.Y. Each was vacant when he bought it, but today most are back on the tax rolls.

> Examples, explanation, and testimony suggest that most immigrants are go-getters whose drive helps the community and nation.

Koreans Choi Duckchun and his wife, Hae Su, work seven days a week at their New York City delicatessen, paying a $15,800 monthly rent and a $10,000 monthly payroll, while trying to save enough to eventually send their three young children to college. It's a struggle, and crime is a problem. Nevertheless, their hard work pays off. "In Korea, money and politics determine everything," Choi says. "Here it's the land of opportunity."

There is one final irony in the charge that immigrants are welfare moochers. Most immigrants arrive in their prime working years, their late 20s. "The payroll taxes of these young immigrants," notes economist Simon, "help underwrite the Social Security checks of America's senior citizens."

MYTH: Immigrants don't want to assimilate.

> Immigrants learn English for practical reasons.

Language is the key issue for assimilation, and self-interest impels most foreign-born to learn ours quickly—unless government gets in the way.

"I didn't speak any English when I came here in 1984," says Miguel Angel Rivera, who lives in Baltimore. "I didn't need to because I was washing dishes and busing tables."

Then the Salvadoran decided to become a waiter. "I started working the floor and picked up English from the customers," he says.

Today Rivera is fluent. He also owns and operates Baltimore's Restaurante San Luis, which specializes in Chinese and Salvadoran cuisine. "I have no problem communicating with any of my customers," he says.

> One person's testimony is supplemented by the findings of a study.

Although many immigrants don't speak a word of English when they arrive here, most recognize that learning it is the key to their economic success. A study of Southeast Asian refugees in Houston found that fluent English speakers earned almost three times as much money as those who only spoke a few words.

> Assimilation, the authors argue, can be hindered by the government's policy rather than the immigrants' attitudes.

Progress might even be faster among the young were it not for bilingual education, which can reinforce the native tongue and delay the learning of English for years. Failed policies such as bilingual education and multicultural curricula are not being demanded by Mexican laborers or Chinese waiters. Instead they are being rammed down immigrants' throats by federal, state and local governments, at the behest of native-born political activists and bureaucrats.

Culturally, immigrants believe in the melting pot and want to join the mainstream. Ninety percent of Hispanics are "proud" or "very proud" of the United States, according to a recent Latino National Political Survey.

Greg Gourley teaches citizenship classes at several Seattle-area community colleges. To become citizens, immigrants must speak, read and write in English, and pass an exam about U.S. history and government. The test is not easy. "If they didn't want to be Americans, they wouldn't be here," Gourley says. "We've got a waiting list a mile long."

The authors return to the importance of this issue to national policy. They name various enlightened politicians and restate the idea that the country gains by its immigrants. The final quotation with its door-shutting metaphor and its emotional diction echo and reinforce the first part of the article.

So the argument has enlisted the values of the magazine and, presumably, of its readers—the ideals of personal responsibility, patriotism, and minimal government—as support for the pro-immigration view.

NOT EVERY POLITICIAN has jumped on the anti-immigration bandwagon. Many, including House Majority Leader Dick Armey (R., Texas), Sen. Joe Lieberman (D., Conn.) and Gov. George Pataki (R., N.Y.), see through the myths, and understand that the United States gains when legal immigrants arrive. As Sen. Spencer Abraham (R., Mich.) says, "We should not shut the door to people yearning to be free and to build a better life for themselves and their families."

Questions

1. Do you think that the direct approach is the best one, given the middle-America readership? Or should the authors have come on less strong in the beginning? Should they have furnished a noncommittal subtitle ("Is their opportunity good for all of us?"), then asked a question ("Does the evidence support the rhetoric?"), and then promised to look into immigration myths?

2. Does this pro-immigration argument persuade you? If not, what disagreements do you have? Reservations?

3. Do the authors present these four myths in the most effective order? Could the sequence of myths be rearranged without loss? Why might you agree that "assimilation" serves well as the final myth?

4. The paragraph beginning "Progress might even be faster" uses the phrase "failed policies." Do the authors beg the question (i.e., make an assertion without providing evidence)?

5. In that same paragraph, do the authors let their mask of reasonable earnestness slip by using an overemotional image? Replace the metaphor to tone it down and then compare the impact.

Consider the Themes

* Do you personally know any immigrants who have mastered cultural disruption through family cohesiveness?

* Would you consider the original Spanish, Portuguese, English, Dutch, and other colonizers of North and South America as "immigrants"? Why or why not? What about Africans, whose first recorded arrival in North America was in 1619?

STUDENT PERSUASION 1

One young immigrant, Jing Dai, condemns the grouping of students by ability as a failed practice (to borrow Chavez and Miller's term for bilingual education and multicultural curricula).

Revised a number of times, the argument was written at the University of California-Berkeley.

TRACKING HARMS STUDENTS IN ALL ABILITY GROUPS

*

Jing Dai

As young people attend public schools, their different abilities become increasingly apparent. As a result, tracking, ability grouping, is widely practiced in today's educational system. Robert Slavin, an educational psychologist at Johns Hopkins University, estimates that 88 to 90 percent of U.S. public schools practice tracking (Shell 62). Many people think that tracking could help slow learners learn things at the pace that they feel comfortable. Fast learners would not be held back by slow learners. These are the good intentions of the advocates of tracking. Yet does tracking work? The answer is no.

Tracking brings negative effects that are the opposite of its original intentions. It harms the intellectual development of students in all ability groups. According to the article, "Blowing Up the Tracks," in the *Washington Monthly*, "Over time, slow kids get slower, while those in the middle and in the so-called 'gifted and talented' top tracks fail to gain from isolation" (Kean 31). Because of these serious effects, I strongly recommend schools end tracking.

Instead of allowing students in high tracks to advance freely, tracking puts tremendous amounts of pressure on them. They feel that scoring well on tests is more important than learning the materials since scoring well on the placement examinations is the only way to keep themselves in high track classes. Ann Wheelock, the author of *Crossing the Tracks: How Untracking Can Save America's Schools*, says, "Kids in the top tracks stop taking risks. They think that if they make mistakes, they will get booted into a lower track, so they play it safe. This attitude is not conducive to creative thinking, or to learning" (qtd. in Shell 62).

Mike Rose also points out the value of errors in his book, *Lives on the Boundary: A Moving Account of the Struggles and Achievements of Educationally Underprepared*. He suggests that when students start making "grammatical errors," it is a "sign of growth." It means that students are trying out new sentence structures or expressing more complex ideas. Instead of denouncing these errors, teachers should encourage students to try out new things and not worry about making mistakes (Rose 188–189). Tracking, however, brings exactly the opposite result. When it takes slow learners out of fast learners' classes, it also gives the fast learners a strong message: keep up those high test scores, or you are out of the high track. They lose their curiosity and become test machines.

If tracking can harm the intellectual development of students in high tracks, it completely stops the development of many students in low tracks. Tracking usually causes them to receive "mediocre schooling" which includes disorganized curriculums and unfit teachers (Drake 123). In her study, Ann Wheelock tells of a little girl in the third grade who thought that students in high tracks will be "smarter," because "they've been taught more." (Wheelock 82). Mike Rose experienced this treatment when he was in Vocational Education. His English teacher was a football coach who was unfit as an English teacher. He did not teach the class and only asked the students to read the same play over and over again.

Those who teach low track classes often give up on their students by having low expectations. Jeanne Oakes, an authority on the issue of tracking, did a study on the expectations of teachers in different ability groups. The study shows that teachers who teach slow track students only expect their students to learn low level skill such as memorization. As a result, not many teachers want to teach slow track classes, and these classes are usually given to less experienced teachers (Shell 62). Luis J. Rodriguez, the author of *Always Running: La Vida Loca: Gang Days in L.A.*, endured this treatment when he was in school. On the first day of school, he had an inexperienced teacher who "did not know what to do with him" because he did not speak English. The worst thing is that she made him feel "unwanted" (Rodriguez 26). When Rodriguez was in Taft High School, he decided to take "photography, advanced art, and literature." His counselor, instead of encouraging him, told him that he was not "academically prepared for his choices" (Rodriguez 138). Once again, Rodriguez lost interest in his school work, but who can blame him? Like many other students in low tracks he was labeled as second class and incompetent.

Low expectations of teachers have serious effects on students in low tracks. The students usually have low self-esteem. Ann Wheelock asked several seventh graders in low tracks why they should not be in the same class with students in high tracks. Their answer was that "we would hold the smart kids back" (Wheelock 82). Students in low tracks do not think that they are "smart" or have the potential to be "smart." They are "unwanted" and hopelessly lost in the tracking practice which supposedly exists to help them. Basically, right now tracking only prepares them for "mindless" and nonexisting jobs which are low skilled blue collar jobs (Kean 31). Schools and teachers, instead of helping them develop intellectually, just try to keep them busy.

Tracking also locks up the low-track students and throws away the key. A few students overcome great difficulties—low expectations, inexperienced teachers, and disorganized curriculums. Their test scores finally show that they can go into high tracks, but these tracks are glass ceilings to them.

When I first came to the United States, I was put into ESL (English as Second Language) classes. It was reasonable since I could not speak any English. But two years later, when my placement test scores and my performance in classes clearly showed that I was ready to go to regular classes, the school held me back. I did not understand and felt this was unfair since colleges do not accept grades earned in ESL classes, which means I had no chance of going to a four-year university. The school only put me into a regular English class after my parents wrote a letter to the school officials. However, not every parent can write letters (most immigrant parents speak little English), so many of my friends stay in ESL classes until the day they graduate from high school. Some of them do not even have the confidence to go to community colleges. They tell me that they are too stupid to learn English.

Tracking is often misused in many schools. The article in *USA Today* shows that capable black and Hispanic students (determined by their 8th grade test scores) are more likely not taking college preparatory courses than white and Asian students. They are usually placed into low track classes ("Tracking . . . " 13). Black and Hispanic students are trapped in the stereotype that they are not as smart as white students. This is exactly what happened in Keppel High School when Rodriguez attended. "They [Anglo students] were in the journalism club that put out the school newspaper. They were in school government sessions making decisions about pep rallies, the annual Christmas party and the Prom. They made up the school teams, the cheerleading squads" (Rodriguez 173). Chicano students, who were 40 percent of the student body, did not join any of the school activities, and they were in low track classes. They did not receive the education that they needed. Many students who want to go to college do not know that they are not taking college preparatory courses because schools do not want parents and students to "complain and demand better placements" ("Tracking . . . " 13). Under the name of the good intentions of tracking, many students become victims.

Under the practice of tracking, slow learners do not get the special attention they need, and they are being mistreated. Fast learners lose interest in advancing themselves. Yet what is the purpose of staying in high tracks when they cannot develop intellectually like they are supposed to do? Support for or against tracking is not the ultimate issue here. Our goal is to help our children to be the best they can be. School should be fun and challenging for them, not a place that creates pressure and glass ceilings. For the future of the next generation, please join me to create a better learning environment for our children by taking tracking out of schools nationwide.

Works Cited

Drake, Daniel D., and Rosemarie Mucci. "Untracking Through the Use of Cooperative Learning." *Clearing House* 67 (1993): 123–26.

Kean, Patricia. "Blowing Up the Tracks: Stop Segregating Kids by Ability and Watch Kids Grow." *Washington Monthly* 25 (1993): 31–33.

Rodriguez, Luis J. *Always Running: La Vida Loca: Gang Days in L.A.* Willimantic, CT: Curbstone Press, 1994.

Rose, Mike. *Lives on the Boundary: A Moving Account of the Struggles and Achievements of America's Educationally Underprepared.* New York: Penguin Books, 1989.

Shell, Ellen Ruppel. "Off the Track." *Technology Review* 97 (1994): 62–64.

"Tracking Harms Many Students." *USA Today* 123 (1994): 13.

Wheelock, Ann. "More Students Learn More with Untrack." *Educational Leadership* 51 (1993): 82.

Questions

1. How well do the two "lighthouses" of title and introduction help readers get their bearings throughout the paper?

2. Does Jing Dai offer strong enough rebuttals to the orthodox view of tracking? In your opinion, how much weight does her own story carry as testimony?

3. Are her points clear? Try completing this sentence by listing them: "Tracking should be abandoned because . . ."

4. Which paragraphs begin with a miniature thesis to be supported? Which of these also provides a bridge from the previous paragraph?

5. How many bad effects does she allege come from putting students in the *lower* track (paragraphs 3–6)?

Suppose you were to extend the idea of tracking from an educational practice to a metaphor? What light could this figure of speech shed on the experience of Andrés-Andele ("Light Dawning," in Chapter 1)? On the disparity between the Jeter and Owens families in "Annie Mae" (Chapter 3)? On the efforts of Mr. and Mrs. Gonzales in "Heritage" (Chapter 3)? On the suffering of Ola in "Designer Genes" (Additional Readings)? On the Indian Removal Act (Additional Readings)?

Consider the Themes

* In the paragraph beginning "Mike Rose," the writer maintains that taking out the slow learners "gives the fast learners a strong message." Would you call that message a *nonverbal* one?

* When did the first Asians immigrate to the areas now called North, Central, and South America?

STUDENT PERSUASION 2
✳

The writer offers a defense of behavior that many regard as antisocial. This essay takes up a local concern that would interest the intended readers. For a photograph of one female Harley-Davidson enthusiast, see Figure 6.3.

Harley-Davidson Women:
Why We Look the Way We Do

✳

Amy C. Weaver

Intended Audience: readers of the Myrtle Beach, S.C., *Sun News*

Imagine being able to indulge your senses through a simple trip along a country road. Your eyes see everything crystal clear and unobstructed. Your nose catches the slightest odors, from the fresh smell of cut grass to the scent of honeysuckle along the road to smell of frying bacon. Your ears hear the steady rhythmic chug of the motor as you gracefully weave along the highway. You can feel the sharp freshness of the air as it rushes by and the heat of other vehicles as they pass. You can taste your independence as you succumb to the legendary Harley-Davidson experience.

Unfortunately, many women have never experienced what I have just described, although it is very real. Some women may not be scared of riding a motorcycle, but may be wary of the old-fashioned Harley-Davidson image. They are intimidated by the rough looking men and women straddling the loud bikes. If not intimidated, they simply may be snobbish, not realizing that they may be snubbing a well-respected member of the community.

As a lady rider I fully acknowledge the negative stereotypes of Harley riders, especially those who are women. However, not all fit this "bad girl" image that has survived through the generations, although it may appear to be true by our unkempt or daring physical appearance when on the bikes. Actually, there are practical reasons why we look the way we do when we ride—reasons which I hope will make sense to women everywhere and open the door to a wild ride for some.

Lady Harley-Davidson riders often look kind of grungy. They don't usually have the best hairstyle around. You may see one of us get off a Harley and say to yourself, "If my hair looked like that, I would have stayed home!" Well, her hair probably looked great before she rode sixty miles an hour into the wind. Many lady Harley riders seem to be either stuck in the seventies with that outdated feathered hairstyle or just plain homely with the old braided pony tail with bits and pieces sticking out here and there. The reason for such outdated hairstyles is simple—the feathered style is the only one possible with a wind-blown part in the middle of your bangs and no hair spray or curling irons available. For ladies with longer hair, the only sensible style is a braided pony tail or French braid; otherwise, they would never be able to untangle all the knots caused by the wind. This style doesn't look its best when you dismount from your iron horse with little strands of hair sticking up all over your head, but it's much easier to handle.

Riding a Harley is as destructive to make-up as it is to hair. When you get on a Harley, your foundation can be flawless, your eyes beautifully outlined and accented, your cheeks wonderfully defined. While you rumble from point A to point B, road grime gets embedded into your

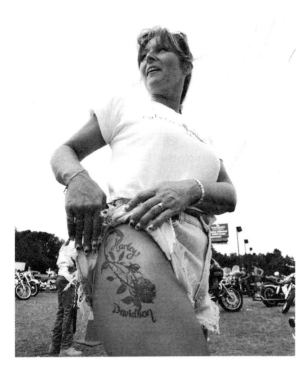

Fig. 6.3 ✳ MS. ANITA WEISS, A RACER, HAD HER FLOWERED TATOO DONE IN PURPLE AND TEAL TO MATCH HER CYCLE.

Myrtle Beach, S.C., Sun News.

pores. You no longer look fresh as a summer day. The wind blowing into your eyes makes them water, ruining your eye make-up. I admit that an easy solution to this problem is not to wear make-up, but some women feel more secure with make-up on than without it. Many feel "naked" without their cosmetics on. If Maybelline would just develop products which are invulnerable to road grime, female Harley-Davidson riders would be eternally grateful.

The typical Harley-Davidson wardrobe gets some heavy criticism from non-Harley women. I admit there is something shocking about a woman clothed mainly in a sheer lace body suit, but to each her own. I've seen many outfits worn in public which would have been much more appropriate for the bedroom. But such tasteless outfits don't represent the majority.

Every year the third week in May is marked by thunderous roars as hordes of Harley-Davidson riders invade Myrtle Beach. Black leather clad men and barely clothed women roam the city from one end to the other. There is nothing feminine about black leather, but it does the job during a Harley rally. Even in May, the night air gets really cool as you're speeding down the highway on a motorcycle. Leather is the best material for warmth. It keeps the cold out and the warmth in. This is also the reason behind leather chaps, worn by men and women over jeans. Chaps keep your legs warm while flattering your backside. Boots are a basic necessity on a Harley-Davidson because of the bike's exposed exhaust pipes. Hot pipes will burn exposed ankles before you realize you've touched them. Leather also does not melt as quickly as synthetic materials do, such as the materials many fashionable hiking boots are made of.

There is no rule that the Harley-Davidson riding apparel must be black, but it's a sensible choice. It conceals the road grime much better than any other color. During the early years of Harley-Davidsons, the only available color was black. The industry has recently undergone "a broadening of its customer base and a broadening of its product offerings" (the *Milwaukee Journal*). Harley catalogs offer brown leather apparel, as well as the traditional black. Many jackets have the rugged outdoor look of blue jean and brown leather. They realize "the people who visit Harley dealerships today are just as likely to be urban professionals in pinstripes, and a growing number of them are women" (the *Milwaukee Journal*). The "biker bitch" image Harley-Davidson women are so famous for is steadily fading into the past.

Harley-Davidson motorcycles are more popular now than they have ever been. The *Milwaukee Journal* reported "record sales and earnings" for Harley-Davidson Inc. through the third quarter of 1994. The Harley-Davidson corporation is like any other business. They want to sell their products. Reportedly, the "demand for Harley bikes still far exceeds supply" and many of those new buyers are women.

Those who do not consider themselves members of this biker society may tend to be judgmental of their character based on appearance alone. Many of our visitors during the Myrtle Beach Rally appear intimidating, but are actually doctors, lawyers, and politicians incognito. Women who ride Harley-Davidsons, either as passengers or actual motorists, appear even more alarming since society does not expect such outrageous behavior from women. Dani-Jean Stuart writes about the time she stopped at a store for some water during a ride on her Harley:

Inside, a couple and their five- or six-year old little girl were choosing sodas from the wall cooler. I excused myself as I edged by them, filling the narrow aisle with my heavy riding boots and leather gear, my jacket casually slung over my shoulder. The little girl's eyes were on me, full of awe-tinged curiosity. Her parents gave that guarded, oh-no-a-biker look. . . . The little girl pointed in my direction and started to wander over. "Hi!" I said, smiling. Her mother quickly snatched her up and hustled into the car. As I backed the bike slowly out of its space, I heard the girl say, "I'm gonna ride a motorcycle when I grow up." Her parents exchanged a look and her mother said, "No, honey, nice girls don't ride motorcycles."

Easyriders 128–29

Unfortunately, many women feel the same way. This sort of attitude is outdated. Many women riders have very successful careers—which would explain how they can afford a ten to twenty thousand dollar motorcycle as a hobby. Besides the desire to rebel against previous societal standards and live on the wild side for a while, there are practical reasons for our appearance when we ride. It's time women stopped condemning female Harley-Davidson riders simply because our hair, make-up, and clothes don't meet the standards of a conservative society. It is no longer considered taboo to be a lady biker. Once you begin to understand why we dress and look as we do, perhaps you would like to go for a ride on an "iron horse." Many of us find the sport as exhilarating as an all-day shopping spree to Charleston!

Works Cited

Fauber, John. "Hog Image Giving Way to Biker Chic." *Milwaukee Journal,* 3 July 1994.

"Harley Profits Ride to a Record." *Milwaukee Journal,* 19 October 1994.

Stuart, Dani-Jean. "A Good Day's Ride." *Easyriders,* January 1994: 128–29.

Questions

1. When do you catch on that the thesis is not expressed by the last sentence of paragraph one ("You can taste your independence . . . ") or by the last sentence of paragraph two (" . . . they may be snubbing a well-respected member of the community")? Does either of these echo the title? Turn out to forecast the rest of the essay?
2. Can you list the three main aspects of personal appearance that Weaver defends?
3. Can you mark places where she makes a strategic concession to show that she is not blind or deaf?
4. How did you interpret the tone of Weaver's last sentence? Does she partly drop her mask of patient goodwill?
5. If the "barrier of custom" (Montaigne's phrase, p. 279) were lowered for female bikers, would they appreciate such acceptance?

Consider the Themes

* In the anecdote from *Easyriders,* where do you notice communication by facial expression?
* If you have expertise with internal-combustion engines, can you suggest what noises are made by a Harley-Davidson that might sound musical to a rider?

STRETCH:
WRITE A PERSUASIVE PIECE THAT USES THE DIRECT APPROACH

Yes, this is an "opinion" paper: Try to change people's attitudes or behavior. As in your expository paper, make your purpose obvious; but instead of aiming to inform, use information to influence the reader's attitudes or behavior.

How can you make this an engaging piece to write and read? A paper-with-research instead of a research paper? Here are some guidelines:

Envision an Audience

Address your persuasion to as clear a readership as you can. You can modify your conception of the readers as you do research, discover ideas, and write a first draft.

This flexibility about audience will help you find a subject that means something to you. It does not have to be a perennial research-paper topic such as gun control, euthanasia, abortion, or capital punishment, nor does it have to concern some other national controversy. Instead it can appeal to the reader's local, professional, or personal interest. It should be narrow enough to give the reader the sense of probing rather than skimming.

Trumpet the Title, Introduction, and Thesis

Get attention and arouse interest with your title and introductory paragraph. You could begin with a quotation, a question, a brief story, a description, an example, an eye-opening fact.

Take a stand near the beginning and then support it. You might take a lesson in directness from a firecracker label: LIGHT FUSE AND RUN. If you wish to follow the conventions favored in many schools, have an introductory paragraph that leads up to a thesis at its end.

Here are a few nuts-and-bolts observations concerning the thesis statement in direct persuasion:

1. It should be phrased as a declarative sentence, not a question: *"X County should expand its airport."*
2. It can appear anywhere near the beginning, even in the title: *County Should Expand Airport.* If you state it in the title, also state it in the introduction.
3. It can appear as just part of one sentence: "Since golfing has grown into a major, year-around industry, *the county should expand the airport."*
4. It can be the sum of more than one sentence: *"The airport needs to be expanded. This project should be accomplished by next spring's Senior Tournament."*

When you read the writing of others, be aware that a thesis may add itself up from parts here and there; readers, when asked to interpret the thesis of a piece, will often come up with different phrasing.

Highlight the Parts

To provide even more up-front certainty to the reader, try following up the thesis statement with a list of points to be developed. Does it provide welcome guidance more than it dampens curiosity?

As you go, make the major sections so distinct that the reader can easily outline your paper. The safest kind of organization is to present a list of points—reasons, benefits, qualities, and so on. For instance, one student, who declared that teenagers should not work over fifteen hours a week, argued that such overwork has several negative effects:

1. It cuts into study time and social life.
2. It creates a money supply for alcohol and other drugs.
3. It accustoms the student to a lifestyle he or she can't afford after moving from home.

These points are called "proofs" or "confirmation" in the rhetorical tradition.

Don't feel, however, that the entire paper must work by points, or by points alone. For example, the hypothetical argument on Dads that began this chapter could first establish the extent of fatherless households, then develop points in favor of being a dad, and finally present someone's testimony about his experience as a dad. Such a persuasive effort might have five main *parts,* several of them *points.*

Each subdivision need not confine itself to a single paragraph. Use two or more paragraphs if you need them to develop your point adequately.

In your conclusion, consider rephrasing your thesis, perhaps reviewing your main points of support, perhaps referring to your title. You might present a quotation, suggest a wider implication of your idea, or paint a bright picture of its benefits.

Ten+ Topics

This list of possibilities and precedents may offer inspiration:

1. Support an opinion about something that evokes your passion. It can relate to your hometown, your major, your outside interests, your experiences, your projected career, your job, your college, a book or movie, a political question, or a cultural issue. One student argued that comic books are no longer for juveniles only.

2. Write on something provoked by your reading in *Stretch.* You might, for example,

   * argue that the quality of family life is jeopardized by a particular social force.

   * warn college students about the human papilloma virus, a disease as widespread and serious as it is intimate, according to the article by Gerchufsky cited in Chapter 5.

   * disagree with Chavez and Miller about immigration, or with Jing Dai about educational tracking, or with Simon J. Ortiz about the relationship between people and the earth (see the poem that closes this chapter).

   * finish the argument about fathers versus dads proposed at the beginning of this chapter.

3. Write on something you have recently learned in another course that changed your way of thinking or behaving. Persuade your readers to follow suit.

4. For a promotional brochure, introduce readers to an annual local festival or celebration in an attempt to persuade them to attend. Examples: Czech Days in Wilber, Nebraska, and Frontier Days in Cheyenne, Wyoming. Specify where illustrations would go. (For a photograph taken at the Conesus Lake Climb, a motorcycle race in western New York, see Figure 6.4.)

   You might develop your promotional text for presentation as a Web page. Tell what illustrations you would integrate, and provide a mail-to-button that allows interested viewers to e-mail for more information.

5. Offer an interpretation of an essay, short story, play, movie, or poem. Assume that your view will help the reader or viewer to get the most out of the work. State your opinion and back it up with quotations from the work, from critics, and perhaps from the author. (See Additional Readings for the example written by Margaret Fritz.)

6. Urge your readers to patronize a business, to become distributors in a network-sales company, or to do something in the line of commerce and professions. Or you could persuade them to *avoid* doing business somewhere as long as you yourself avoid charges of libel.

7. For the campus newspaper, write a persuasive piece on something of local interest. Recruit members for a martial arts class; urge attendance at a lecture, performance, or athletic contest; praise a band; urge a boycott; solicit blood donors.

8. Write a problem-solution paper. Establish the existence of a problem and, as early as is feasible, declare your solution(s). Or write a proposal to a group, religious or secular, of which you are a member. State the recommendation early, then show how it answers the needs of your group.

   You might gain extra impact toward the end by painting a detailed picture of the positive changes it will make.

9. Like Chavez and Miller, try to debunk a series of myths or a single myth. Or, like Weaver, write a defense of some practice, person, and so on.

10. Choose one of the topics suggested in an earlier chapter and turn it into direct persuasion.

REVISE TO MAKE THAT REACH

Show your paper to one or more people to take advantage of a fresh viewpoint.

Have you taken on a manageable job, or are you swimming across the Pacific? Is your thesis clear from the introduction? Is your framework easy to follow?

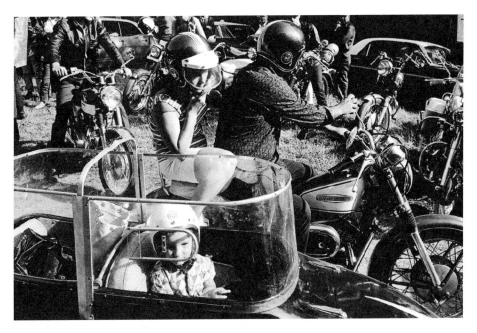

Fig. 6.4 ✳ **CONESUS LAKE CLIMB, 1969, NEW YORK**
© Steve Myers, 1996.

Do you have a sense of an audience, or are you like a speaker who gazes at the ceiling?

Can you profitably take another look at the list of discovery techniques on p. 11?

Have you developed your paragraphs adequately? Supplied transitions between them and between the main parts? Is your evidence adequate, considering your allotted number of words? Can you make one more trip to the library for one more source? Can you interview someone who would add variety, vividness, and perhaps local authenticity?

Does your tone give the reader faith in the writer's reasonableness? For instance, have you conceded any less-defensible points? Should you concede any limitations to your argument? For example, although a high school job may indeed be time-consuming, doesn't it help a teenager stay busy and out of trouble? Don't be afraid to weigh probability rather than declare certainty.

Have you appealed to the reader's feelings without relying excessively on unsubstantiated assertions or on incendiary words? Have you spent your cash of information before asking for the credit of emotion? Then, review "Explain" (Part II).

Perhaps, to the contrary, your "mask" is too bland. Just like facial expressions in speech, your writing persona can arouse interest. Make sure your style doesn't promote boredom by wordiness and slack grammar. Have you used too much redundancy in your organization? That is, have you given so many signals regarding your arrangement that they start to distract from your content?

Do you have enough variety of supporting material, or do you rely on one type? Have you tried to show that your plan is not only desirable but also feasible? In arguing cause and effect, have you acknowledged the situation's complexity? Raised other possibilities and tried to rebut them?

Have you doublechecked your facts? Take a lesson from the writer who declared that the first shots of the Civil War were fired from Fort Sumter. (They were fired *at* the fort, which was a U.S. government outpost in Charleston harbor.)

Have you given the dough of thought time to rise by leaving your paper in a warm place for a while?

EXTRA CHALLENGE

Try a bonus exercise alone or with a friend.

1. Write an exploratory essay on why you hold a certain belief. Try to plumb your cultural background, your personality, your experience, your education, and your vested interests. A valuable exercise in self-knowledge, this essay will help you appreciate the way human convictions are nourished by a rich soup of influences.

2. Recast the final draft of your direct persuasion paper as a dialogue in which one speaker seeks to convince another. Or recast your explanatory paper of Chapter 5 as direct persuasion.

3. On behalf of a restaurant, write the copy (words) for a half-page advertisement in the college newspaper. Start with this headline: "HEIMLICH'S CAN DELIVER YOU FROM THE PIZZA HUMDRUMS." Back up this claim with information about menu items, delivery policy, and so on.

4. Write your senator asking him to vote against the Indian Removal Bill (see Additional Readings). Since the year is 1830, you are a white male and so is your senator. Work directly—the best approach for political action letters—by referring to the bill, making your request, then advancing reasons for your position. For more information read the excerpt from Sen. Frelinghuysen's speech (p. 152) and do some other research.

5. Sketch a proposal for a multimedia campaign that will urge males to wait to become fathers until they can be dads. Audience: Guys at your old high school. (How about making up a bumper sticker like the one in Figure 6.2?)

Or as part of a proposal for a movie version of the biography *Andele, the Mexican Kiowa*, argue that the chapter called "Light Dawning" (see Chapter 1) could be transformed into effective film. Go into detail using technical words from movie making.

POEM: A TRADITIONAL FAMILY

The spoken language of Native American storytelling influences the poetry of Simon J. Ortiz. The following was originally published in a collection that revealed how uranium mine workers in New Mexico were forced to change their working relationship with the land.

For an interpretative framework for this poem, see Margaret Fritz, "Interdependence between the Land and the People in Simon J. Ortiz," in the Additional Readings.

WE HAVE BEEN TOLD MANY THINGS BUT WE KNOW THIS TO BE TRUE

Simon J. Ortiz

The land. The people.
They are in relation to each other.
We are in a family with each other.
The land has worked with us.
And the people have worked with it.
This is true:
Working for the land
and the people—it means life
and its continuity.
Working not just for the people,
but for the land too.
We are not alone in our life;
We cannot expect to be.
The land has given us our life,
and we must give life back to it.

The land has worked for us
to give us life—
breathe and drink and eat from it
gratefully—
and we must work for it
to give it life.
Within this relation of family,
it is possible to generate life.
This is the work involved.
Work is creative then.
It is what makes for reliance,
relying upon the relation of land and people.
The people and the land are reliant
upon each other.
This is the kind of self-reliance
that has been—
before the liars, thieves, and killers—
and this is what we must continue

to work for.
By working in this manner,
for the sake of the land and people
to be in vital relation
with each other,
we will have life,
and it will continue.

We have been told many things,
but we know this to be true:
the land and the people.

TIPS FOR PROSE

Ortiz reinforces the directness of this poem by echoing its title and thesis in the conclusion.

Indeed, the impact of this poem comes partly from its generous redundancy. It tends to use several signals where one could do, a style more reminiscent of speech than of writing. Ortiz tends to recycle words: In the title and first two verse-stanzas, in fact, only about 20 percent of the words are used just once. All this repetition may suggest the chanting of a group.

As a writer, you must judge how much repetition to supply and allow. You can use redundancy to tighten coherence by repeating key words; to reinforce comprehension by building in extra signals (i.e., second chances); and to help carry a point by making an idea familiar through repetition.

To get a sharper sense of redundancy, do one of the following exercises based on "We Have Been Told Many Things . . . ":

(1) Go through the poem to underline the words *land* and *people* to see how often they recur.

(2) Cross out every word in the title and first two verses that occurs more than once. (Consider all forms of *have* and *be* as one word, as well as *give* and *given*.)

Works Cited

Chavez, Linda, and John Miller. "The Immigration Myth." *Reader's Digest* 148.889 (May 1996): 69–73.

Landers, Ann. [Letter.] *Sun News,* [Myrtle Beach, SC], 31 May 1995: 7C.

"Number of Fatherless Kids Takes a Huge Leap." *Sun News,* [Myrtle Beach, SC], 24 April 1995: 3A. Source: *Washington Post.*

Ortiz, Simon. We Have Been Told Many Things but We Know This to Be True." *Fight Back: For the Sake of the People, for the Sake of the Land.* INAD Literary Journal 1.1 (1980): 35–36.

Tilly, Chris, and Randy Albelda. "It's Not Working: Why Many Single Mothers Can't Work Their Way out of Poverty." *Dollars & Sense,* November/December 1994: 8–10. Rpt. in *Family.* Vol. 5. Ed. Eleanor Goldstein, Art. 40. Boca Raton, FL: Social Issues Resources Ser., 1993–1994.

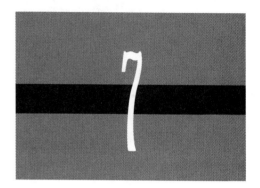

Indirect Persuasion

D ear Mom & Dad,

How are y'all doing? I hope everything is going okay. Is it hot enough for you? It sure is hot here. The college is raising tuition this coming fall. I hope they don't raise the cost of summer school along with it. Goodness, these summer sessions are costing enough!

Oh, Geep is getting married August 16 in Florida, so I'll have to get a dress while I'm home this weekend because I can't afford the dresses here. Dad, I have been looking around for a set of new tires, mine are so bumpy and roar so loud I can barely ride in the car. Maybe we can look for a sale on tires this weekend, okay? I have had to cut back on my hours at work since I have such a heavy courseload.

Well I have to go now. I just thought I'd drop a line or two to let you know how things are going. As you can tell, I am going to have to borrow money this weekend. Take care and tell everyone hello! See you this weekend—if I have enough money to buy gas! Don't worry I'll be fine.

Love,

JoAnn

P.S. Sorry about all the collect calls.

Jo Ann James hopes to reach out and put the touch on someone. She knows that her parents will decline an outright request for money—even if she supports it with reasons. So she prepares them for a request by explaining her financial problems: soaring tuition, an expensive dress, roaring tires, and shrinking hours. Like a farmer who tills the ground before sowing the seed, she presents information that appeals to her readers' logic, emotion, and regard for her credibility. She hopes that her implied thesis— "You should lend me money"—does not fall on the hard ground.

Even though this letter is simple, its leading-up approach can give you a model for more complex indirect persuasion. As a flexible writer, you will find this principle helpful with readers who will resist your message, whether it be a request, recommendation, or judgment. Their attitudes may range from the skeptical to the defiant, and their grounds from the philosophical to the practical. They will greet a directly presented thesis with crossed arms, frowns, and jaws set in opposition. So instead of announcing your point early on, you will delay revealing it—or merely imply it rather than stating it explicitly.

Think of a sailboat traveling against the wind. The sailor does not point the bow directly into the wind but instead tacks to the left and right, zig-zagging, making slow headway by indirection. Similarly, would-be persuaders often avoid confronting the reader head-on. They work inductively—that is, by furnishing details that point logically to a conclusion. First they present information or reasons in hope that the reader, by assenting to these smaller points, will accept the main proposition that follows.

The letter in Figure 7.1 offers a skillful example of the indirect approach. The writer, an accountant, judges that the Internal Revenue Service (IRS) will be more disposed to grant her request if she delays it until the end, after she has made a case.

She begins the first paragraph courteously by thanking the IRS officer, then invites sympathy with the word "struggling." By admitting guilt on behalf of her clients, she signals her peaceful intentions that invite the reader to be receptive rather than defensive. She sketches the problem in a single sentence and concludes the paragraph with a request for help—not yet specifying what kind.

The rest of the letter explains a confused tax situation in objective detail. Notice that the writer's businesslike mask maintains goodwill and credibility by avoiding recrimination. Finally she offers her courteous

PATRICIA F. MESEC, C.P.A.
5200 West Ottawa Avenue
Littleton, Colorado 80123
(303)979-5509

November 23, 19__

Ms. Linda Byrd
Internal Revenue Service
Problem Resolution Office
600 17th Street
Denver, Co. 80202-2490

Dear Ms. Byrd:

Thank you so much for taking the time to talk with me today regarding the account of Mr. and Mrs. Iam N. Bigtrouble. As I mentioned, we have been struggling for over six months to resolve several issues concerning the income taxes which they owe. They are very aware that they do, indeed, owe back taxes. Every notice they receive, however, is not only from a different office, but also shows a different amount now due. We need your help.

We sent a packet of materials to Ms. Kim Lovemywork at your Ogden office. That packet contained notarized statements from doctors and other officials, statements which substantiate legitimate reasons for the Bigtroubles' failure to file tax returns for the year 1992. We have asked that the failure to file penalties be abated for the reasons stated in the packet. We have received no response.

We have submitted a Form 1040X for the tax year 1992. This amended return reports all the income, deductions and exemptions which should have been reported originally. The IRS response to this 1040X shows no credit for the 1993 tax refund which was retained. In addition, no credit is given for the money which has been garnished from Mrs. Bigtrouble's wages every two weeks for the last six months.

Mr. and Mrs. Bigtrouble would like very much to settle their account with the IRS and to move forward with their lives. When you are considering penalties, please consider that six months have passed while we have truly been trying to settle this account. Any abatement will be greatly appreciated as will your prompt attention to this very confused tax situation.

Thank you very much.

Sincerely yours,

Patricia F. Mesec

Patricia F. Mesec

Fig. 7.1 ∗ MR. AND MRS. BIGTROUBLE VERSUS THE IRS—BUSINESS LETTER USING THE INDIRECT APPROACH

Courtesy Patricia F. Mesec.

petition for (1) a prompt resolution and (2) an abatement (a break) on the penalties.

The inductive approach can characterize a piece of writing in its entirety, in a section, or to a degree. Indirect persuasion can join narration when a story leads up to a thesis or implies it, as in Woody Guthrie's song "Talking Dust Bowl" (see Chapter 1). And whenever persuasion works obliquely—with a tone of inquiry, of uncertainty, by asking questions and seeming to reserve judgment—it can overlap with exploration.

Advertisements usually work by indirection. Often they imply a link between a product or service and something desirable: a line of clothing with cool people, a brand of mustard with a luxurious British sedan. Sometimes they lead up to a request for action:

ORDER TOLL FREE 1–800–652–0990.

Or "Visit your Such & Such dealer now!"

For a complete example of such a buildup, see Figure 7.2 on page 194. Published during World War II, this ad gets attention by integrating an illustration with eye-catching typeface. The headline declares: "Music in the National Effort!" Then the ad booms out the word **MUSIC** four times in a list of wartime capabilities. The rest of the copy (i.e., the words) vaunts the importance of music to a wartime democracy, declares a need for an organized program, explains how the council is addressing that need by recruiting local leadership, calls on the reader (as a musician) to help, and tells him or her to write for information.

Indirect persuasion, whether to sell a product or an idea, encourages the audience not to "hang up" on the caller. In fact, you will encounter this strategy in telemarketing (sales efforts by telephone). The phone rings and a friendly voice greets you by name and then, pretending not to read from a script, tries to get you involved in an interchange by asking you a question. The voice continues to bid for your good will and your interest. To deal with common objections the spiel has fallback positions and counterquestions. Finally the telemarketer asks you to do something—to give money to a school or charity, to switch phone companies, to tour a housing development, to order a credit card, and so on.

The indirect approach is one that you should be able to recognize in all communication and to employ as a rhetorically fit writer.

WARM UP FIRST

Perhaps with a partner, write a sales letter that applies the theory presented in the sidebar "The Wild Beauty of Eel Skin." Try to sell a product or service—for example, your own car or some type of lessons. You may want to specify any use of color, graphic effects, and illustrations. Perhaps rough out an attractive letterhead.

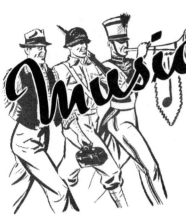

Music IN THE NATIONAL EFFORT!

MUSIC at the front inspires our fighting men.

MUSIC at home helps civilian morale.

MUSIC in the factory speeds the tempo of production.

MUSIC wherever Americans gather expresses the

SPIRIT OF AMERICA!

It is no mere theory that music is essential. It is in itself an expression of freedom characteristic of the democratic way of life for which we are now waging a battle to the finish. It cannot flourish among oppressed peoples, but even our enemies recognize that music in wartime is a stimulant which spurs soldiery and citizenry alike to greater efforts.

Participation of the people in music will not perish in America so long as America remains free and democratic. But for it to grow and flourish in wartime, for it to play a vital, living role in our war effort with maximum effectiveness, a definite program is required—a program of aims and purposes for music which are national in scope, yet dependent upon local leadership and direction in each of our country's thousands of cities, towns and villages.

To fill this need the Music Industries War Council is conducting a drive to mobilize all forms of music for the national effort, that our armed

forces, civilian workers and children may have the advantage of the recreational and educational benefits and the patriotic inspiration that music affords.

It is *your patriotic duty*, as a musical leader in your community, to enlist the musical resources, facilities and interests in your locality for participation in this national program. The part you play will automatically advance your standing in your community, but even more important to you, to us, to all Americans, it will bring music to the fore as a force for *victory*.

The Music Industries War Council will, upon request, furnish you with ideas, suggestions and practical help in organizing your local musical contribution to help win the war. Write today.

SOME OF THE WAYS YOUR LOCAL MUSIC ORGANIZATIONS CAN HELP WIN THE WAR

BANDS—DRUM CORPS—ORCHESTRAS

a. Escorting draftees to trains.
b. Playing at defense bond and stamp sale rallies.
c. Concerts at nearby cantonments.
d. Concerts at war production factories.
e. Collecting of vital materials, with small units serenading each block while materials are being collected.
f. Community concerts.
g. Patriotic rallies and parades.

CHOIRS—GLEE CLUBS

a. Singing at home defense meetings, with director leading in community singing.
b. Singing at defense plants.
c. Appearing in conjunction with instrumental groups at mass meetings and concerts.

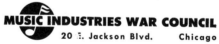

MUSIC INDUSTRIES WAR COUNCIL
20 E. Jackson Blvd.   Chicago

Fig. 7.2 ✳ ADVERTISEMENT USING THE INDIRECT APPROACH

From *Metronome: Modern Music and Its Makers* 58 (June 1942): 6.

SALES LETTER, THE WILD BEAUTY OF EEL SKIN

A sales letter tries to ease a reader's grip on his or her wallet. Traditionally in the United States it follows this sequence:

Get attention. Other things are competing for the reader's time, so an effective sales letter uses anything that will get him or her reading (including an eye-catching envelope). Typical resources are pictures, color, typeface, a testimony or other quotation, an offer, a question, a startling assertion.

Arouse interest. The letter presents information that appeals to the reader's curiosity as to what, when, who, why, and where.

Kindle desire. By connecting with the reader's needs, the letter draws on the latent power of the reader so as to achieve its purpose. It encourages the reader *to want* to do something.

Ask for action. The letter does more than to convince the reader that something is desirable: It requests concrete action. And it makes this action as easy as possible—for example, by including a card to be filled out and returned with no postage necessary.

Here is an example provided by a student.

EEL SKIN COMPANY
1099 32nd Ave.
Manhattan Beach, CA 90266
(213) 545–XXXX
FAX (213–545–ZZZZ)
e-mail ealie@aol.com

July 5, 19—

Mr. Horacio Barrera
323 Walnut, Unit 35
Huntington Beach, CA 92647

Dear Mr. Barrera:

Because of its full-grained beauty, its strength and its softness, EEL SKIN is enjoying tremendous acceptance.

EEL SKIN is 150% stronger than leather and becomes softer and more supple with use. Variations in color and other markings such as scars, scratches, bites, and stretch marks or fat wrinkles only enhance the wild beauty of EEL SKIN.

The EEL SKIN we use comes from conger eels, a popular foodstuff in the Orient. Conger eels are not an endangered species.

Feel certain your eel skin selection will bring you many admiring compliments. Please enjoy looking through the enclosed brochure and call us at (213) 545–ZZZZ to place an order.

Sincerely,

Adnan (Eddie) H. Alie

enc.

PROFESSIONAL ARGUMENT

Cristoforo Colombo in Italian, Cristóbal Colón in Spanish: In whatever version of his name, he became a cultural myth. Like a long-venerated statue in the public square, however, the image of Columbus has been much eaten away by acid in the air. Many people regard him as an invader rather than a discoverer.

About the time of the 500th anniversary of Columbus's arrival, the following essay appeared in *Time* magazine. The author takes up the ongoing controversy in the Americas over how to regard the man whose ships made the first historic connection between Europe and "these lately discovered nations" (see Montaigne in Additional Readings).

HAIL, COLUMBUS, DEAD WHITE MALE

Charles Krauthammer

The title seems equivocal: both positive ("hail") and negative ("dead white male," used to decry the emphasis on men and the past).

The political left looks pompous by this spin on Queen Victoria's "We are not amused." The quotations sound shrill. Krauthammer seems pro-Columbus. Nevertheless, will he argue that the celebration should be tempered by ambivalence?

The 500th anniversary of 1492 is approaching. Remember 1492? "In Fourteen Hundred Ninety-Two/ Columbus sailed the ocean blue." Discovery and exploration. Bolivar and Jefferson. Liberty and democracy. The last best hope for man.

The left is not amused.

In Madrid the Association of Indian Cultures announces that it will mark the occasion with acts of "sabotage." In the U.S. the Columbus in Context Coalition declares that the coming event provides "progressives" with their best political opening "since the Vietnam War." The National Council of Churches (NCC) condemns the "discovery" as "an invasion and colonization with legalized occupation, genocide, economic exploitation and a deep level of institutional racism and moral decadence." One of its leaders calls for "a year of repentance and reflection rather than a year of celebration."

For the left, the year comes just in time. The revolutions of 1989 having put a dent in the case for the degeneracy of the West, 1992 offers a welcome new point of attack. The point is the Origin. The villain is Columbus. The crime is the discovery—the rape—of America. The attack does, however, present the left with some rather exquisite problems of political correctness. After all, Columbus was an agent of Spain, and his most direct legacy is Hispanic America. The denunciation of the Spanish legacy as one of cruelty and greed has moved one Hispanic leader to call the NCC's resolution "a racist depreciation of the heritages of most of today's American peoples, especially Hispanics."

That same resolution opened an even more ancient debate between Protestants and Catholics over the colonization of the Americas. For Catholics like historian James Muldoon, the (Protestant) attack on Columbus and on the subsequent missionary work of the (Catholic) church in the Americas is little more than a resurrection, a few centuries late, of the Black Legend that was a staple of anti-Catholic propaganda during the Reformation.

The crusade continues nonetheless. Kirkpatrick Sale kicked off the anticelebration with his anti-Columbus tome, *The Conquest of Paradise*. The group Encounter plans to celebrate 1992 by sailing three ships full of Indians to "discover" Spain. Similar merriment is to be expected wherever a quorum gathers to honor 1492.

The attack on 1492 has two parts. First, establishing the villainy of Columbus and his progeny (i.e., us). Columbus is "the deadest whitest male now offered for our detestation," writes Garry Wills. "If any historical figure can appropriately be loaded up with all the heresies of our time—Eurocentrism, phallocentrism, imperialism, elitism and all-bad-things-generally-ism—Columbus is the man."

Therefore, goodbye, Columbus?

Balzac once suggested that all great fortunes are founded on a crime. So too all great civilizations. The European conquest of the Americas, like the conquest of other civilizations, was indeed accompanied by great cruelty. But that is to say nothing more than that the European conquest of America was, in this way, much like the rise of Islam, the Norman conquest of Britain and the widespread American Indian tradition of raiding, depopulating and appropriating neighboring lands.

The real question is, What eventually grew on this bloodied soil? The answer is, The great modern civilizations of the Americas—a new world of individual rights, an ever expanding circle of liberty and, twice in this century, a savior of the world from totalitarian barbarism.

Indirect Persuasion ✳ **197**

If we are to judge civilizations like individuals, they
should all be hanged, because with individuals it takes but
one murder to merit a hanging. But if one judges civilizations by what they have taken from and what they have
given the world, a non-jaundiced observer—say, one of the
millions in Central Europe and Asia whose eyes are turned
with hope toward America—would surely bless the day Columbus set sail.

Thus Part I of the anti-'92 crusade is calumny for
Columbus and his legacy. Part II is hagiography, singing of
the saintedness of the Indians in their pre-Columbian Eden,
a land of virtue, empathy and ecological harmony. With
Columbus, writes Sale, Europe "implanted its diseased and
dangerous seeds in the soils of the continents that represented the last
best hope for humankind—and destroyed them."

Last best hope? No doubt, some Indian tribes (the Hopis, for example) were tree-hugging pacifists. But the notion that pre-Columbian
America was a hemisphere of noble savages is an adolescent fantasy
(rather lushly, if ludicrously, animated in *Dances with Wolves*).

Take the Incas. Inca civilization, writes Peruvian novel-
ist Mario Vargas Llosa, was a "pyramidal and theocratic society" of "totalitarian structure" in which "the individual
had no importance and virtually no existence." Its foundation? "A state religion that took away the individual's free will and
crowned the authority's decision with the aura of a divine mandate
turned the Tawantinsuyu [Incan empire] into a beehive."

True, the beehive was wantonly destroyed by "semiliterate, im-
placable and greedy swordsmen." But they in turn represented a culture
in which "a social space of human activities had evolved that was neither legislated nor controlled by those in power." In other words, a culture of liberty that endowed the individual human being with dignity
and sovereignty.

Is it Eurocentric to believe the life of liberty is superior to the life of
the beehive? That belief does not justify the cruelty of the conquest. But
it does allow us to say that after 500 years the Columbian legacy has created a civilization that we ought not, in all humble piety and cultural rel-
ativism, declare to be no better or worse than that of the Incas. It turned
out better.

And mankind is the better for it. Infinitely better.
Reason enough to honor Columbus and bless 1492.

Questions

1. Does Krauthammer's relatively indirect approach help to carry his
   point? Suppose you were to state his thesis in the first paragraph as
   something like this: "Ditties aside, simplistic phrases overlooked,
   mankind is infinitely better for the arrival of Columbus." Would this
   shift toward directness be welcome or unwelcome to you?

2. What are Krauthammer's main proofs? Does he indulge in *ad hominem* attacks? Do they help to carry his point?

3. Do you agree that the "real question" is "What eventually grew on this bloodied soil?"

4. How much does research add to the writer's credibility, logic, and emotional appeal?

5. How would you describe his distinctive voice or mask? How does it differ from that of Chavez and Miller's in their argument about immigration?

Inductive argument can be effective in a speech: For a transcription of President Roosevelt's address to Congress on the day after the bombing of Pearl Harbor, see Additional Readings.

Consider the Themes

* Looking at the opposition between groups, what values does the cultural right seem to cherish in this issue? The left?

* How would you compare and contrast the supposed invasion of 1492 with the invasion in 1941 (i.e., by the Japanese when they attacked Pearl Harbor in Hawaii)?

STUDENT PERSUASION 1

Several hundred years *before* the landfall of Columbus in the Americas, England began its conquest of Ireland, an island lying to its northwest. (See Figure 7.3 for map.) Thus began an ugly conflict that has lasted over eight hundred years. The heavy English boot trod not only upon Irish soil but on the Irish people.

In the late 1500s Queen Elizabeth gave Irish land to English nobles, and her successor, King James, gave away even more. After the 1650s Oliver Cromwell moved large numbers of Scots Presbyterians into Ulster, the northern province of the island, creating the basis for the current problem. Northern Ireland remained a part of Great Britain when the rest of the island (overwhelmingly Catholic) became the Irish Free State in 1922.

So the island has a substantial majority of Catholics who think of themselves as Irish-Celts, and a minority of Protestants who think of themselves as British-Scots-Ulster. Most of the latter are now concentrated in Ulster, where they constitute a slight majority.

The crux of the issue is the definition of "Ireland." Is it an island country (as the Catholics would maintain), one that enjoys cultural and political homogeneity and embraces the somewhat anomalous area of Ulster? Or is it (as the Protestants and the British would maintain) a physical island that lacks a corresponding sociopolitical unity? After all, Ulster has had a long history of separateness from Ireland and of connectedness to Scotland (and in fact Belfast is closer in distance to Scotland than to Dublin).

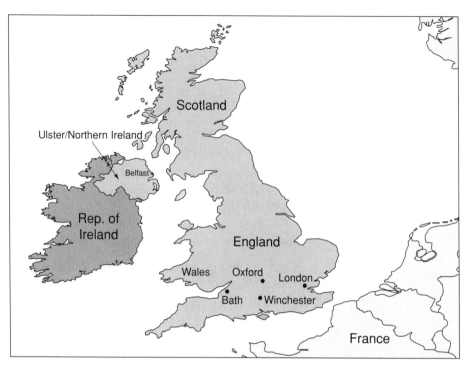

Fig. 7.3 ✳ **MAP OF GREAT BRITAIN (INCLUDING NORTHERN IRELAND) AND THE REPUBLIC OF IRELAND**

The Irish Republican Army (I.R.A.) became a notorious agent of violence in its effort to free Northern Ireland of Great Britain. How should a person regard this group? Matthew Martin's paper, written in 1990, tries to answer the question.

THE IRISH REPUBLICAN ARMY
Terrorists or Freedom Fighters?
✳

Matthew P. Martin

Audience: Anyone interested in terrorism or Ireland

Brits Kill Irish!

B It was a sunny Sunday afternoon, January 30, 1972, in Derry, Northern Ireland. Approximately 15,000 Irish people gathered for a peaceful march in protest of a law instated by the British Government. This law that was put into act on August 9 forbade all marches in Northern Ireland for a full year. There were already too many demonstrators present for the Army to stop, so they decided to confine the demonstration to the Catholic Ghettos of Derry, called the Bogside (Kelley 161–164).

At about 3:30 P.M., the demonstrators approached the edge of the Bogside, where the army had erected barriers. Some of the protestors left, but many did not. These remaining Irish Nationalists began shouting and throwing stones at the Army. At first the Army used tear gas and water hoses in retaliation, but before anybody knew what was happening the sound of gunfire rang out. The unarmed protestors ran for cover, but not all of them made it. By the day's end, 13 Catholic protestors were dead (7 of them teenagers), 29 were seriously injured. This day is known as Blood Sunday (Kelley 161–164).

Irish Kill Brits!

As the boat pulled out of port, a bomb hidden on board went off. Lord Mountbatten, a cousin of Queen Elizabeth and a war hero, was going yachting on this Monday, August 27, 1979. Mountbatten was killed instantly in the explosion. Also killed in the blast was Mountbatten's 14-year-old grandson and the Dowager Baroness of Brabourne. Paul Maxwell, who was also killed, was a 15-year-old local Irish boy serving as pilot. The I.R.A. apologized for Maxwell's death, but celebrated over the other deaths (Kelley 304–305).

The I.R.A. claims that these acts were committed in retaliation for Blood Sunday. The British do not agree; they see it as terrorism.

Who Is Wrong? Is Anyone Right?

These descriptions of events are two different views of the violence that takes place almost daily in Ireland. When describing the Irish Republican Army, it is almost impossible not to mention British acts of violence alongside Irish acts of violence. With reading these two stories, it is hard to know who the "good guys" are and who the "bad guys" are. Is the I.R.A. a group of freedom fighters struggling to free their country from an unwelcome ruler? Or are they terrorists with no reason to kill? If the latter, could they have started out with good intentions, but over the course of seventy-one years strayed from their original cause?

History of the I.R.A.

In the long history of Ireland's struggle with England there has always been an army of Irishmen who have fought to free their country from England. The Irish Republican Army (I.R.A.) is just one form of these groups. The I.R.A. was established in 1919 to fight England for Ireland's freedom. Under the Government of Ireland Act, which took effect on January 1, 1922, the Irish Free State and the British Government, the political division of the island was formally recognized. The North consisted of six counties and was to be occupied by England; the 26 counties to the south were to be free to rule themselves. This split temporarily ended the war with England, but the Irish nationalists wanted nothing less than one Irish state (Lloyd 3). In 1939 the I.R.A. declared war on England. They have continued this war and have not stopped to this day.

The I.R.A. may be fighting for the same goal as they were in 1939, but they do not have the same beliefs as they did in 1939. They have become more violent and more radical as the years have increased. Due to these changes, the I.R.A. suffered a split in 1970. The Official Irish Republican Army (OIRA) does not engage in military activity: The Provisional Irish Republican Army (PIRA or Provos) is the military group known for the present day terrorism in Ireland. [See Figure 7.4.]

The P.I.R.A. gets most of its weapons from Libya, but there are other organizations who supply them. One of these organizations is NORAID (Irish Northern Aid). This group is supposedly a fund-raising group in the United States, but some members of NORAID have been convicted by the FBI for gun-running for the I.R.A.

The I.R.A.'s support had diminished since it banded together in 1919, but it is still a very influential group.

Sinn Fein

Violence is not the only method the I.R.A. uses in the attempt to unite Ireland. The Sinn Fein Nationalist Party is the political wing of the I.R.A. This political party was quite successful and had a great deal of support up until 1970. When the I.R.A. split in 1970, so did Sinn Fein, into two separate parties: Official Sinn Fein and Provisional Sinn Fein. The Official Sinn Fein, which changed its name to the Workers Party in 1982, is a communist group with a goal to be the leading socialist party in Ireland. This Workers Party now condemns the actions of the P.I.R.A. and Sinn Fein as terrorists (Kelley 124).

The Provisional Sinn Fein is now known as Sinn Fein and, through the I.R.A., makes its mark with violence. The only similarity between these two groups now is their goal to make Ireland one nation. Nowadays these parties can only hope to gain a few seats in Parliament.

Present Day I.R.A.

The I.R.A., like any other group or person who has endured almost three-quarters of a century, is not what it started out as. One thing has endured through the times, though: They started with a nationalistic goal to free Ireland from British rule and they are still after this goal.

Most of the world's population would agree that violence is wrong. If this is so, then neither the I.R.A. nor the British government is right. Why then is there a double standard? Why is Britain's violence condoned, even by the United States, and Ireland's is terrorism? The Irish are a people who have been conquered, treated like slaves, then seen as barbaric for not wanting to be treated as such. The I.R.A.'s answer to the questions about their violence is said clearly in this quote:

Bloodshed is a cleansing and sanctifying thing, and the nation which regards it as the final horror has lost its manhood. There are many things more horrible than bloodshed; and slavery is one of them. —Pearce (O'Farrell 160)

Works Cited

Campbell, Duncan. "Carry on Spying—and Dying." *New Statesman and Society,* 20 October 1989: 12.

Kelley, Kevin J. *The Longest War.* Westport, CT: Lawrence Hill, 1988.

Lloyd, John. "The Other Island." *New Statesman,* 13 November 1987: 3.

O'Farrell, Patrick. *England and Ireland since 1800.* London: Oxford University Press, 1975.

Ogden, Christopher. "The I.R.A. Play a Deadly Game of Tit for Tat." *Time,* 19 September 1988: 32.

O'Rourke, P. J. "The Fighting Irish." *Rolling Stone,* 9 February 1989: 99.

Stanley, Alessandra. "Northern Ireland: Death after School." *Time,* 18 June 1990: 36.

Questions

1. Can you express Martin's opinion in one declarative sentence?
2. What are the main phases of his indirect approach?
3. Re-read the concluding words of Patrick Pearse, commander-in-chief of the insurgents during the Easter Rising of 1916. This quotation justifies bloodshed as a means to overthrow slavery. Krauthammer, similarly, in order to defend the European conquest, depreciates the importance of its inhumane means in comparison to its positive results. Do these judgments about means and ends convince you? Disturb you? Both?
4. What can you find about the present I.R.A. via the World Wide Web? Are there any relevant Web sites? Is the organization still making news? If using a search engine, expect confusion with an identical abbreviation for (perhaps ironically) Independent Retirement Account.
5. In the paragraph beginning "Most of the world's population," circle the seven uses of *is.* Rewrite those sentences to cut out three or four appearances of the verb.

Consider the Themes

 * How might family relationships perpetuate hostility between Catholics and Protestants in Northern Ireland?
 * During World War II, why did Ireland remain neutral, protest allied military activity in Northern Ireland, and countenance the operations of German and Japanese agents on its territory? (Yet thousands of Irishmen volunteered to serve in the British military.)

* Can you find any songs that concern the seemingly intractable conflict between Catholic Ireland and Great Britain? Venerable examples from the Catholic point of view are the ballad *The West's Awake* and *Soldiers of the Rear Guard* (O'Shea).

STUDENT PERSUASION 2

Without the help of foreign invaders or religious intolerance, a state of war seems to exist in parts of some cities of the United States. Here is the testimony of a survivor.

David Stack tells of his gang experience by presenting causes, effects, and examples. Only at the end does he state the implications to the intended reader.

DEATH BECOMES YOU!

*

David P. Stack

When the street is your only true friend, it is scary. Then you realize that there is no difference between life and death. My neighborhood was rough even when I was only a couple of years old. I remember looking out my front window and seeing a chain fight where a person was later hospitalized for severe head injuries. Later as I got older, my block became known as the block that stayed hot. There was always trouble, and my gang was always involved. We were examples of a dangerous process: "Biological, psychological, and social stresses during adolescence often lead to problems and health-endangering behaviors as adolescents try to cope with these stresses" (Ingersoll & Orr; qtd. in Gonzales et al., 701).

Everything that could happen, did. We were a gang, and everybody knew it. Other gangs always tried to take us over, but they couldn't. We were ordinary people gone totally nuts; insane, that's what everyone around us thought. My friends joined the gang for various reasons, but I joined because I was born into it. My brother also influenced me because when I was younger, he and his boys always took care of me. I remember in the very beginning of high school ten guys surrounded me and were about to do damage to me. Out of the corner of my eye I saw a group of some familiar faces come charging to save my life. Ten guys ran up the stairs so we chased up after them. They ran down the halls as everybody watched. It was a great feeling knowing that three minutes ago, I was about to get the living hell kicked out of me.

Violence came at different times. I remember fighting at 6:30 in the morning. Nevertheless, usually we fought during school, after, and late nights. At night is when everything got out of control. It is when we raged.

October 22, 1991. They arrested my friend Mike for attempted murder when he assaulted a rival gang member with brass knuckles. He had crushed part of his skull and left him brain damaged. They later sentenced Mike to one year in maximum security prison in New York.

June 1, 1992. My friends were on their way to my house when they stopped at Seven Eleven to get a snack. When they came out of the store, several other rival gang members had batted my friend down. He almost died and received 148 stitches around his head.

January 2, 1993. The windows of my house were smashed, my mother's car windows were smashed, and they spray painted on my friend's house and in front of mine. In the two weeks following that incident we raised hell. I think we could have destroyed the whole town if we wanted to. Each rival gang member was beaten up and their house destroyed.

Friday, July 17, 1993. My good friend is having a party across the street where he lived. It was his birthday, and we were having a good time drinking and dancing the night away. The whole night there were many teens in the back of the garage by kegs. They were giving people dirty looks until the cops came and broke it up. Then everything got hectic. Out in the front of the house, one of those teens acted up and everything broke out into a huge brawl. When the smoke cleared, they had stabbed two of my friends, one in the neck, the other in the chest. It was an unbearable sight. The blood oozed out and never stopped. When the heart pumped, even more blood flowed out of my friends' bodies. I thought that this would have been the end for them. The doctor said the stab wound was about one millimeter away from his jugular. If it was any closer, then he would have died. They stabbed my other friend six inches down in his chest, one inch from his heart. That night was one of the longest nights I have ever been in.

October 2, 1993. I woke up and looked at my life. What the hell was I doing? I was going to end up either dead or in jail. However, when you're in the street, death becomes you. My life changed in what seemed like minutes. I was staring into the mirror and I noticed that my eyes showed me everything. I had no conscience, no life, and no heart. Fortunately I had got into a relationship with a young woman that changed everything for me. She turned my life around. I had become legit. "Legit were those young men who had walked away from the gang. They were working hard or may have gone on to school" (Hagedorn 206).

I hope what I am saying to those hard-core gang members, new jacks, and those dope fiends sinks in. Going through life waking up thinking that today could be your last has long-term psychological effects on a person. Just remember one thing; you are a burning candle, but there is someone there that will blow you out!

Works Cited

Gonzales, Jeanette, Tiffany Field, Regina Yando, Ketty Gonzales, David Lasco, and Debra Bendell. "Adolescents' Perceptions of the Risk-Taking Behavior." *Adolescence* 29.115 (fall 1994): 701–9.

Hagedorn, John M. "Homeboys, Dope Fiends, Legits, and New Jacks." *Criminology* 32.2 (1994): 197–219.

Questions

1. Do you think Stack's indirect approach helps his warning "sink in"? Or should he have warned his intended readers at the beginning and let the rest of the paper serve as clear evidence?

2. Stack's first paragraph asserts that stress causes antisocial behavior. When do you realize his true thesis, that such antisocial behavior causes death?

3. The writer develops his paper mainly by giving examples in the form of stories. Of what is Stack himself the main example?

4. In the paragraph about Friday, July 17, the author makes a slip and uses the present tense for one verb: "My good friend *is* having a party. . . ." Would the essay benefit if all the examples employed the present tense for a sense of unfolding drama?

5. How does his conclusion clarify his ominous title? Does the candle metaphor evoke your emotions? How do the last three words derive extra power from overtones of a different context?

Consider the Themes

* For Stack's audience, is print the best medium? In a film or videotape version, what might be gained and lost?

* Do you suppose that for many young people a gang is a surrogate family?

STRETCH:
WRITE A PERSUASIVE PIECE THAT WORKS INDIRECTLY

Here are a few pointers:

* Keep your title noncommittal so as not to reveal an opinion. Use a question, a subject, even a sentence as long as it doesn't tip your hand and show the reader your cards.

* Specify your intended readers under the title. In your own mind, identify (1) those whom you will not waste your time trying to persuade, if any; (2) those whom you will try to persuade; (3) the extent to which you want to persuade them.

* In your introduction get attention and interest. Raise the subject but don't state your opinion. Avoid coming across as an advocate or a foe of something, but instead wear a mask of impartiality. Or if you do sound passionate, sardonic, or otherwise emotionally involved, delay your exact judgment, recommendation, warning, and

so on, till much later. Perhaps conclude your introduction with a question or with a promise to look into the issue.

* Firm up any assumptions that the reader might not automatically share. If you call for more money, for example, don't merely assume that dollars will do something; provide some evidence. Do you feel that the individual is pretty much responsible for his or her actions? Or do you assume that larger forces tend to control the individual? Rather than slipping over such an assumption, consider reinforcing it.

* Try to understand your readers. Find common ground with them, appeal to their needs, appeal to their emotions, and—more so than in direct persuasion—pique their curiosity. Ask questions. Supply plenty of information.

* Anticipate your reader's objections, acknowledge them, and be prepared to make strategic concessions. In the reverse order from direct persuasion, rebut opposition points before giving your thesis.

* Build credibility with your logical framework and research. Try to keep the reader's goodwill. Offer personal testimony if it will lend power.

* State your thesis at the end or somewhere after the middle; it need not confine itself to one sentence.

* Once you enjoy as much goodwill and agreement as possible, consider stating a claim. End with a "conclusion" in a double sense:

    1. An indication of finality. With it you round off the subject artistically, just as you would want to do in the direct approach.
    2. A logical climax. It brings out the implication of the evidence—like the "therefore" in a geometric proof that caps a series of steps.

* Or imply your thesis by the information you select, the tone you adopt, the wording you use, and the points that you make.

As with the direct approach, you can write a problem-solution paper, but delay expressing your judgment as to either the problem or the solution, or both. To limit your scope, expend most of your argument on either the problem or the solution, whichever is more controversial. Be sure that you have established the existence of the problem; what are the latest developments?

You can also write a proposal that calls for a specific action. Delay your recommendation until the end.

With both of these formats, you might use the process of elimination: Raise alternative solutions or directions, dismiss each for well-substantiated reasons, and end up with the one you favor.

Ten+ Topics

You might look at the list of subjects in Chapter 6 (p. 183) and then develop one of them by the indirect approach. Here are some others:

1. Recast your direct persuasion argument by using the inductive approach. Make any necessary changes from start to finish.
2. Argue that Columbus should not be hailed. Or take up one of Krauthammer's points and refute it inductively.
3. Condemn the I.R.A. without making an explicit judgment until late in your paper—if ever.
4. Look back over the writing models in this book, find an issue that provokes you, and take a stand, delaying the revelation of your thesis.
5. Write an inductive opinion piece for the college newspaper. Examples of "therefores" that could follow a discreetly built-up case:

   * Students should consider taking a break from education after high school rather than going to school for seventeen years straight. (Besides doing library research, you would interview students and perhaps career counselors.)
   * Students should consider going into the Peace Corps when they graduate.
   * Students should live in another country for a semester or more.
   * Today's couples should sign a prenuptial agreement.
   * Students should consider pursuing X career.

   For a newspaper editorial that ends by expressing serious reservations about a national trend, see "Nomads at Work" in the Additional Readings.

6. Argue that a particular kind of technology poses a threat to family cohesion.
7. Write a problem-solution argument. Keep the reader curious as to the exact problem, or the solution, or perhaps both. You might investigate the day's news for a local, state, or national situation that arouses your concern.
8. Make a proposal. Keep your recommendation under wraps at least until the halfway point of your paper.
9. Write a dialogue between two people. Have them argue two sides of an issue, and let one interlocutor have the edge over the other.
10. Compare X to Y and finally conclude (or imply) that one is superior.

REVISE TO MAKE THAT REACH

For a timely review of theory, scan "Persuade" (introduction to Part III). Have you led up to your proposition by easy increments? Dared to use a little art? Consider these possibilities:

   * An experimental mask. Try an unfamiliar persona that offers new possibilities: a sardonic, mocking one; an inspirational one; or one that is meditative, conciliatory or even genial.

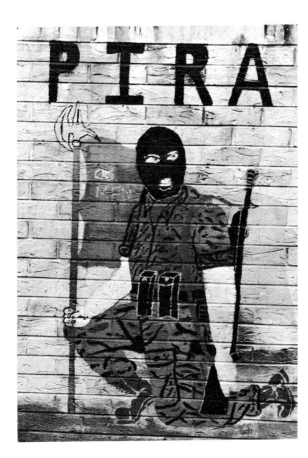

Fig. 7.4 ✳ **PHOTOGRAPH OF P.I.R.A. MURAL IN BELFAST, NORTHERN IRELAND**

Courtesy Richard O. Collin.

✳ Questions. Instead of making statements, provoke thought; involve the reader by asking questions. You may ask one and answer it, or ask one and let it imply the answer.

✳ Anaphora. Repeat the same initial word in a series: "Music . . . Music" in Figure 7.2 and "Last night . . . Last night" in Roosevelt's speech to Congress (see Additional Readings). This technique gives an impression of expansive emphasis.

✳ A one-sentence paragraph such as Krauthammer's "The left is not amused." Surprise the reader and accentuate an idea.

✳ A sentence fragment. Depart from the expected grammar when terseness will add elasticity.

✳ Figurative language. Depart from the literal now and then if a metaphor or simile will enlist the reader's imagination to help carry your point.

✳ An inductively developed paragraph. Compose a miniature version of your paper by moving from specifics to the point they suggest. (See Tips for Prose at the end of this chapter.)

Have you used a variety of persuasive sources—a story, a testimony, a pungent quotation, a law, an example, statistics, other explanatory techniques, an illustration? Can you find "numbers"—that is, quantified information? How about making one more trip to the library, electronic encyclopedia, or Web?

NO JAUNT TO HOUSTON: BAD-NEWS MEMO

Indirection can tactfully convey bad news. In a sense, this aim is persuasive because it encourages the reader to be less unreceptive to unwelcome information.

Here is a memorandum that uses a doubly indirect approach. (1) It delays the news by phrasing the subject uncontroversially, then giving reasons for the decision. (2) It merely implies the bad news—You can't take a business trip to Texas—rather than explicitly denying the reader's request.

In real estate jargon, an "outparcel" is property situated between a shopping center and a road and valued as a location for (typically) a fast-food restaurant.

> **DATE:** Feb. 19, 19—
> **TO:** C. Kissos, Associate
> **FROM:** T. Detweiler, Manager
> **SUBJECT:** Travel request

Chris, I appreciate the special interest you have in the area of out-parcels. Since the National Realtors Convention will be held in S.F. next year (a lot closer than the one in Houston), why don't you put in a request to attend that meeting? In the meantime you can use the slack time we have this winter to study up on the subject. I've called Karen over at RDF and she said she would be glad to steer you toward some articles and other information. Just give her a call at 7092.

Notice how Detweiler praises the reader and shifts quickly to positive alternatives. His tactful indirection helps to ensure Kissos' goodwill and good work.

EXTRA CHALLENGE

Enjoy working your creative muscles, perhaps with another student, by trying an unexpected use of indirect persuasion:

1. Using Roosevelt's speech to the Congress as a model (Additional Readings), lead up to a request for a declaration of war, or maybe peace. Follow each phase of his speech closely. Perhaps you must rally earthlings to fend off invaders from space; or to resist a more insidious enemy like illegal drugs.

2. Write a proclamation that advances a series of "whereas" clauses leading up to a "therefore." As a model, here is the record of the Cherokee council held on August 1, 1838; the tribe, already impounded, was about to be expelled from its homeland by federal soldiers:

WHEREAS the title of the Cherokee people to their lands is the most ancient, pure, and absolute known to man its date is beyond the reach of human record; its validity confirmed and illustrated by possession and enjoyment antecedent to all pretense of claims by any other portion of the human race . . .

And WHEREAS the natural, political and moral relations existing among the citizens of the Cherokee nation toward each other and toward the body politic; cannot in reason and justice be dissolved by the expulsion of the nation from its own territory by the power of the United States Government.

Resolved therefore by the National Committee and Council and people of the Cherokee nation, in General Council assembled, that the inherent sovereignty of the Cherokee nation, together with the Constitution, laws and usages of the same, are, and by the authority aforesaid, hereby declared to be in full force . . . and shall continue so to be in perpetuity subject to such modification as the general welfare may render expedient.

Woodward 214

3. Write a letter that refuses Joann's implied request for money (p. 190). Give your reasons *before* your refusal to prepare her to accept it. Do *not* use the thesis-and-support method. Other hints: offer alternatives, avoid negative words, and end positively. You might even *imply* the bad news rather than stating it explicitly. For a model of indirectness, see the sidebar "No Jaunt to Houston."

4. Create a print advertisement that works by indirection to sell a product. Integrate the copy with the illustration (which you need only rough out). Specify other visual appeals such as typography, layout, and color. Get attention, arouse interest, associate the product with something positive in the mind of the reader.

5. Compose a form letter that will be sent to members of your organization (whether collegiate, professional, religious, political, etc.). Working indirectly, persuade the reader to attend a function, or join an excursion, or contribute money, or help with a project, or recruit new members, and so on. Using a little artfulness, write the kind of letter that would get your own attention, interest, desire, and action. Keep in mind sources of probable resistance and try to overcome them. Appeal to the reader's needs.

You may omit the inside address and even the traditional "Dear" salutation in favor of a quick attention-getter. Make up a letterhead with the name of the organization, the street address (including zip code), the post office box (if necessary), and the telephone number. Why not draw in a logo or an illustration?

A few pointers for numbers 4 and 5:

In practical writing, favor short paragraphs and sentences; they encourage brevity and emphasize the fairly simple content. In sales letters, use an occasional sentence fragment if it adds surprise, conciseness, and the flavor of speech. Be sure to use visual emphasis techniques and graphics when they serve your aim.

SONG LYRICS

These lyrics come from the album *Free to Move,* performed by the group Israel Vibration. Although the title might seem to express the thesis, the statement "life is real" probably suggests a harsher judgment of African American life in the inner city.

The song, working indirectly, does more than to cite the burdens of harassment, societal indifference, physical and cultural oppression, cruelty, and unfairness: it offers hope.

"Life Is Real" shows some of the Rastafarian influences on reggae explained by Gregory Salter in Chapter 5. "Babylon" is the oppressive system; "I" means we or us; "his majesty" refers to Haile Selassie I of Ethiopia–Lion of Judah, descendant of King Solomon. The song tries to persuade listeners that Rastas will overcome Babylon.

Other definitions: Rudolph W. Giuliani was elected mayor of New York City in 1994; "comely" means attractive.

LIFE IS REAL

Albert Craig

A me man checking out the block
A me man staying with the flock
You see man gathering the facts
Mister big tree I am the small axe

Apple is my name, the burning flame
Harassing this lion won't make I tame

You see, man, they just don't care
More Babylon force
Giuliani swear
War in the street system on the attack
And they targeting me did Solomon say him black.

They give us Columbus and Marco Polo
And fight 'gainst we great Africano.
Life is real. Black people treated differently
Iya feel rejected by society.
A search man find my identity

Reverse man protected by his majesty
I'm saying

Hey, life is real and it's the way I feel.

Hey, you treat I with cruelty
You treat I with impunity
You treat I with partiality
Said I'ma Black but I'ma comely

Hey, 'cause I'm the apple of father eye

TIPS FOR PROSE

Add some art to your writing with an occasional understatement. For practice, use the song lyrics by Albert Craig as a partial model: Write a handful of sentences that list related hardships, and end with the understatement "—is real." Fill in the blank with a topic of your choice such as Life, College, Dating, Work, or Single parenthood.

Works Cited

Craig, Albert. "Life is Real." *Free to Move*. Ras Records, 1996.

Krauthammer, Charles. "Hail, Columbus: Dead White Male." *Time* 27 May 1991: 74.

Woodward, Grace Steele. *The Cherokees*. Norman: University of Oklahoma Press, 1963. The quotation is from the papers of John Ross. (Woodward's ellipses.)

Additional Readings

These selections range from the ancient to the day before yesterday. They illustrate a wide variety of types and forms:

double-voice format

essay

five-paragraph theme

meditation

dialogue

question and answer

stream of consciousness

instructions (for print and videotape)

editorial

chain letter

profile (in prose and verse)

news article

informal report

literary analysis

argument (scientific and general)

public law

speech transcription

poem

story (single and serial; true, fictional, and dreamed; original and rewritten)

Readings are followed by questions that invite you to analyze them, evaluate them, relate them to other pieces, and see how they illustrate the writing theory and thematic material in *Stretch*.

Alcott, Louisa May (1832–88)

Here is the beginning of Chapter 14 of *Little Women,* published in 1869. After Jo finishes some writing in her attic, she ventures out to submit it to an editor, whereupon she meets her love-interest, a boy named Laurie.

CHAPTER XIV.
SECRETS

—✳—

Jo was very busy in the garret, for the October days began to grow chilly, and the afternoons were short. For two or three hours the sun lay warmly in the high window, showing Jo seated on the old sofa, writing busily, with her papers spread out upon a trunk before her, while Scrabble, the pet rat, promenaded the beams overhead, accompanied by his oldest son, a fine young fellow, who was evidently very proud of his whiskers. Quite absorbed in her work, Jo scribbled away till the last page was filled, when she signed her name with a flourish, and threw down her pen, exclaiming,—

"There, I've done my best! If this won't suit I shall have to wait till I can do better."

Lying back on the sofa, she read the manuscript carefully through, making dashes here and there, and putting in many exclamation points, which looked like little balloons; then she tied it up with a smart red ribbon, and sat a minute looking at it with a sober, wistful expression, which plainly showed how earnest her work had been. Jo's desk up here was an old tin kitchen, which hung against the wall. In it she kept her papers and a few books, safely shut away from Scrabble, who, being likewise of a literary turn, was fond of making a circulating library of such books as were left in his way, by eating the leaves. From this tin receptacle Jo produced another manuscript; and, putting both in her pocket, crept quietly down stairs, leaving her friends to nibble her pens and taste her ink.

She put on her hat and jacket as noiselessly as possible, and, going to the back entry window, got out upon the roof of a low porch, swung herself down to the grassy bank, and took a roundabout way to the road. Once there, she composed herself, hailed a passing omnibus, and rolled away to town, looking very merry and mysterious.

If any one had been watching her, he would have thought her movements decidedly peculiar; for, on alighting, she went off at a great pace till she reached a certain number in a certain busy street; having found the place with some difficulty, she went into the door-way, looked up the dirty stairs, and, after standing stock still a minute, suddenly dived into the street, and walked away as rapidly as she came. This manoeuver she repeated several times, to the great amusement of a black-eyed young gentleman lounging in the window of a building opposite. On returning for the third time, Jo gave herself a shake, pulled her hat over her eyes, and walked up the stairs, looking as if she were going to have all her teeth out.

There was a dentist's sign, among others, which adorned the entrance, and, after staring a moment at the pair of artificial jaws which slowly opened and shut to draw attention to a fine set of teeth, the young gentleman put on his coat, took his hat, and went down to post himself in the opposite doorway, saying, with a smile and a shiver,—

"It's like her to come alone, but if she has a bad time she'll need some one to help her home."

In ten minutes Jo came running down stairs with a very red face, and the general appearance of a person who had just passed through a trying ordeal of some sort. When she saw the young gentleman she looked anything but pleased, and passed him with a nod; but he followed, asking, with an air of sympathy,—

"Did you have a bad time?"

"Not very."

"You got through quickly."

"Yes, thank goodness!"

"Why did you go alone?"

"Didn't want any one to know."

"You're the oddest fellow [i.e., character] I ever saw. How many did you have out?"

Jo looked at her friend as if she did not understand him; then began to laugh, as if mightily amused at something.

"There are two which I want to have come out, but I must wait a week." (165–67)

Questions

1. Laurie comically misunderstands Jo's errand. Why does he misread her nonverbal signals?

2. How would you describe the author's mask or voice in this excerpt?

Anonymous

This chain letter tries to persuade the reader to take an action. Apparently much-photocopied, the sheet is illegible in spots.

WITH LOVE ALL THINGS ARE POSSIBLE

❊

This paper has been sent to you for good luck. The original is in New England. It has been around the world nine times. The luck has been sent to you. You will receive good luck within four days of receiving the letter. Provided, in turn, you send it on. This is no joke. You will receive good luck in the mail. Send no money. Send copies to people you think need good luck. Do not send money as faith has no price. Do not keep this letter. It must leave your hands within 96 hours. An R.A.F. officer received $470,000. Joe Elliot received $40,000 and lost it because he broke the chain. While in the Philippines, George Welsh lost his wife 51 days after receiving the letter. He failed to circulate the letter. However, before her death, he received $7,755,000. Please send twenty copies and see what happens in four days. The chain comes from Venezuela [and] was written by Saul Anthony De Groul, a missionary from South America. Since this copy must tour the world, you must make twenty copies and send them to friends and associates. After a few days, you will get a surprise. This is true even if you are not superstitious. Do note the following: Constantine Dias received the chain in 1953. He asked his secretary to make twenty copies and send them. A few days later he won a Lottery of $2,000,000. Carlo Daddit, an office employee, received the letter and forgot it had to leave his hands within 96 hours. He lost his job. After finding the letter again he mailed twenty copies. A few days later he got a better job. Dallan Fairchild received the letter and not believing, he threw the letter away. Nine days later, he died. In 1987, the letter was received by a young woman in California. It was very faded and barely readable. She promised herself she would re-type the letter and send it on, but she put it aside to do later. She was plagued with various problems, including expensive car repairs; the letter did not leave her hands in 96 hours. She finally typed the letter as promised and got a new car.

Remember, send no money. Do not ignore this, it works.
ST. JUDE

Questions

1. What exact action does this letter solicit? Where does the letter tell the reader what *not* to do?

2. What kind of logical support does the letter offer to encourage the recipient to keep it circulating?

3. The letter relies heavily on capitalized proper nouns to establish authenticity. Underline the names of people and places: How many do you find?

4. Can you mark where paragraph indentations would clarify the organization?

5. To what human needs might a chain letter appeal?

Anseaume, Pat, Jenny D. Gasque, and Kevan White (students)

Much writing is done collaboratively. One or more people may bring wider expertise, different viewpoints, and more time to a project. The following was written by three students in Advanced Composition and published in *Alternatives* (Myrtle Beach, S.C.) in 1992.

ALTERNATIVE MUSIC: ANTIDOTE FOR STRESS

Are you stressed out? If so, you might alleviate your stress-related problems by listening to Alternative music.

Music of the Soul

Consisting of soft, melodious sounds and vibrations, Alternative music, an effective soothing and healing alternative to stress-related problems, especially ones linked to noise exposure, offers beneficial results. As simply more than relaxing music, Alternative music offers an art form that reduces anxiety and tension. The instrumentation includes natural sounds, like that of rain, or artificial sounds, like those of synthesizers or other musical instruments. Alternative music can be purchased for the same price that you would ordinarily pay for any other type music. For example, Solaris Universalis by Patrick Bernhardt and Spectrum Suite by Steven Halpern are particularly interesting because these composers have also authored books regarding the healing effects of listening to Alternative music. For instance, Patrick Bernhardt has written The Secret Music of the Soul (Harper and Row) endorsing the music's therapeutic functions and spiritual effects. Steven Halpern has written Tuning the Human Instrument and Sound Health, both touting the balance and harmony of body, mind and spirit. Halpern is also the composer, performer and producer of the internationally-acclaimed "Anti-Frantic Alternative" series of recordings for Sound RX Productions.

You may purchase Alternatives music locally at Rainforest Music Store, or you might just listen to a demonstration and decide to compose your own.

Metaphysical Journey

Noise exposure, the cause of nearly one-quarter of all mental illnesses, creates an imbalance within the human mind as well as physiological illnesses, thus producing an imbalance within the human body, according to Bernhardt. Stressful both psychological and physiologically, noise attacks the nervous system, causing fatigue, dizziness, ulcers, cardiovascular problems, unhealthy behavioral patterns, hormonal imbalances, depression and headaches, Bernhardt contends. Taking a metaphysical trip or journey offers an artful, therapeutic and alternative approach toward stress-reduction. By exerting a calming effect on the renal glands where imbalances result as an overproduction of adrenalin, by regulating the heart rate, and by lowering arterial pressure a metaphysical journey as a therapeutic approach to stress-reduction also provides a less expensive one. Abstract pictures of sounds, like Stephen Crane's synesthesia or word-painting in his literary art forms, aid by balancing the harmony of the human body, according to Halpern.

Elevator Sans Elavil

As an alternative to prescriptive and over-the-counter medications, Alternative music provides a holistic approach rather than a strictly medical one. For instance, many medical professionals endorse Alternative music's therapeutic purposes because of its subliminal, meditative, hypnotic and tranquilizing effect on their patients. Many dentists, psychiatrists, surgeons, nurses, physical therapists, anesthesiologists, counselors and psychotherapists rely on this unique methodology, addressing the issue of stress-reduction as the end result.

On a local level, many hospital and health care facilities use this holistic approach, involving terminally ill patients, their families and clergy as well as for the medical staff, i.e., physicians, nurses, counselors, and volunteers.

On an international scale, Cecile Beaudet and Richard Belfer's research and resulting article, published in *L'Impatient,* June 1989, No. 139, led to the successful use of Alternative music with pregnant women (as a preparation for delivery), with people suffering from hypertension (to help them relax), and with individuals who suffer from backaches (to correct both their breathing and their posture) under the direction of Dr. Desikachar in India. Dr. Desikachar points out: Our ancestors had classified the letters of the alphabet in different categories. Certain sounds, HA with an aspirated H, for example, have a stimulating effect. Others, like MA, sung softly on a low-pitched note, have a calming effect.

Local Aesthetics

Not only do medical professionals use Alternative music as a remedy for stress, but other experts in the fields of art, music and literature also support this belief. The healing benefits are discussed by two local experts. One is Lacy Richardson, an award-winning artist, musician, writer, member of the Waccamaw Arts and Crafts Guild, a graduate of Ringling Institute of Art and Design and a continuing student at USC–Coastal Carolina College. Tom Zuke, an artist, musician, and a former student at Paier Art Institute, is the owner of the Rainforest in Surfside Beach.

Richardson first became interested in this unique antidote for stress after his divorce. Citing Alternative music as a type of "after divorce therapy," Richardson explains that it offers "a mind-expanding, tranquil, hypnotic and meditative art form, like taking a trip without actually leaving." In a literary sense, Richardson compares Alternative music to the lyrical poetry of William Butler Yeats because of its unexpected syncopation of beat or rhythm. He describes Alternative music as "an aesthetic art form containing its individual Gestalt: that is, the artist and the listener both become the sole creator or composers."

Tom Zuke believes that the antidote for stress relies entirely on sounds to express ideas and to reflect different psychological modes and moods. He explains that "it allows you to see sounds and to hear colors. As instrumental music, it allows you to become a part of the art, without words being sung. It allows a personal response rather than just memorization of words." Zuke also says "it draws out bad things, such as anger and frustration. It is music that makes you feel good!" Because the musicians are classically-trained, Zuke maintains "they are highly specialized." Requiring different responses and interpretations on behalf of the listener, Alternative music embodies "a universal language," Zuke says. He concludes: "Music touches our souls."

Influential Exposure

Researchers suggest that repeated exposure to messages in visual media can result in desensitization to violence or disinhibition of aggressive effects. Toward this end, it seems probable that exposure to auditory media might do the same. For example, criminal charges have been filed against certain heavy-metal rock groups. Some of these charges claim that repeated exposure to messages in particular songs have led teen-agers to commit suicide. Another study on sound and hearing by S. S. Stevens and Fred Warnshofsky shows that sounds above 130 decibels become physically painful. Consider that the sound systems at a rock concert are boosted to the limit. This is beyond the pain threshold and could result in hearing loss or other disorders. Research conducted in the United States indicates that the noise levels should not go beyond 10 decibels over a period of ten minutes after the exposure. Otherwise, permanent deafness will ensue. Teen-agers 16–18 years old exhibit a hearing loss when exposed to 30 decibels, according to this research.

Because stress causes many serious psychological and physiological illnesses, anyone who experiences stress should reap the rewards of Alternative music, an acoustical, softer and more ethereal antidote. "It is a sound that traverses ether. The vibratory energy justifies the results obtained by using the therapeutic power of Alternative music," according to the Bhagavad-Gita.

Try Alternative music as a healthy alternative instead of a medical approach to your health and well-being.

Questions

1. Does the introduction start the paper with the clutch out? In other words, does it start off too abruptly? Should the first paragraph be omitted?

2. Does this paper convince you that alternative music is an effective antidote to stress? Does a reader have to be convinced about all the alleged benefits to assent to some of them?

3. Are you inclined to agree with Bernhardt that noise exposure causes nearly one-fourth of mental illnesses? Do you see noise as a problem?

4. Where do the authors use five of the cubing techniques of description, contrast, analysis, application, and evaluation? (See sidebar on cubing, p. 14.)

5. Where does the paper try to connect with a local audience?

Bancroft, Ann

This news article, distributed by the Associated Press, appeared in the Myrtle Beach, S.C., *Sun News*, 4 May 1996: 5A.

CALIFORNIA UNWED MOM COUNT HAS A PROBLEM WITH ACCURACY

———————————— ✳ ————————————

SACRAMENTO, Calif.—California's "epidemic" of unwed mothers includes some women who would be startled to find themselves counted—married mothers who elect to keep their maiden names.

As a result, hundreds, perhaps thousands, of babies born to married women are counted in the anonymous tally of births to unwed mothers.

California is one of five states in which birth certificates do not include the marital status of parents. So state and federal number counters trying to determine how many California babies are born out of wedlock use what they call an "inferential method."

"If [new mothers] sign the certificates with their maiden name, and the baby has the father's name, they're presumed not married," explained Debbie Rhea, supervisor in the state Office of Vital Records. "There's not a box where we can add that 'the names are different but they're married.' "

Rhea's office sends photocopied birth certificates to the National Center for Health Statistics, the data-gathering arm of the Health and Human Services Department, which reports demographic trends in all states. The center's analysis suggested that 35 percent of all babies born in California in 1993, the last year with full statistics, had unmarried parents.

The count of unwed mothers is important in setting spending on social programs such as welfare and health care for children. Many unwed mothers are poor and unable to work without child care; they are less prone to seek prenatal advice; and their infants are frequently born under-weight and sickly.

California's figure, interestingly, does not take into account the number of unwed mothers who are financially stable and have adequate means to care for their out-of-wedlock children.

Gov. Pete Wilson, in his January State of the State address, declared that children of unwed mothers are "overwhelmingly more likely to drop out of school, to abuse drugs, to land in jail, to have their own children out of wedlock and to become trapped in welfare dependency."

There's no way to know how many married California women keep their own last names. Demographers at the state Finance Department and the Los Angeles office of the U.S. Census Bureau declined to guess.

But John Rolph, a statistician at the University of Southern California, said that the formula for determining the number of unwed mothers seems deeply flawed. "I would expect it to be quite unreliable," Rolph said.

Assemblywoman Jackie Speier has written a bill to require marital status in the confidential section of California birth certificates. The Burlingame Democrat, who never took her husband's last name, has two children.

When the national center put California's out-of-wedlock births at 35 percent of all births in 1993, it was the ninth-highest rate in the country, behind the District of Columbia, Mississippi, Louisiana, New Mexico, Arizona, New York, South Carolina and Georgia.

There are signs that the National Center for Health Statistics is re-thinking its methodology. In a March letter supporting Speier's bill, an official expressed concern about accuracy.

"We feel that a direct question on the mother's marital status on the California birth certificate would be of great value . . . because California accounts for 15 percent of U.S. births," wrote Mary Anne Freedman, director of the center's Division of Vital Statistics.

Questions

1. What are the two confused meanings for the symbol "unwed"?
2. Would you say that unwed status itself is the major reason why unmarried mothers seek less prenatal advice and have more underpar babies?

Barry, Dave

Dave Barry is syndicated humor columnist working out of the *Miami Herald*. He is fond of hyperbole (exaggeration), allusions to popular culture, surprising juxtapositions, unpredictable organization, tonal shifts, buildups and letdowns, made-up information, and all things weird and vulgar.

Here he applies his virtuoso wit to a common subject. (His reference to Einstein's hair refers to its rather bouffant appearance in photographs.) From the Myrtle Beach, S.C., *Sun News,* 8 December 1996.

BALD TRUTH ABOUT HAIR

✳

Today's Topic is: Your hairstyle.

Is your hairstyle important? To answer that question, let's consider the starkly different career paths of two individuals: Albert Einstein and Tori Spelling.

Tori Spelling is a top celebrity and highly successful television star, despite having the natural acting prowess of a Salad Shooter. Why? Because she always has a neat, modern hairstyle. Also her father produces every show on television except the test pattern. But her hair is surely a factor.

In contrast, Albert Einstein—despite being a brilliant genius who not only discovered the Theory of Relativity ("E equals H_2O") but also prepared his own tax returns—never so much as appeared on "Hollywood Squares." He auditioned repeatedly, but the talent coordinators always turned him down.

"What was that on his head?" they'd ask each other, after he left the studio. "A yak?"

So we see that hairstyle is very important. This is true even in the animal kingdom. Baboons, for example, spend countless hours grooming each other, applying conditioners, combing fur over the bald spots on their butts, and using all the other little styling tricks that make them the confident, successful and cosmopolitan creatures they are, equally at home on a rotting zebra carcass as on a rotting giraffe carcass.

It is no different with humans. If you have a lunch meeting with an important client, you are definitely going to make a strong impression if you reach over and pick a live insect out of his or her hair. But it also helps if you have a nice hairstyle. Unfortunately, a lot of people—and here I am thinking of women—hate their own hair. In my experience, when a woman looks at herself in a mirror, even if her hairstyle is really nice, she sees Chewbacca.

Men, on the other hand, tend to feel positive about their hair. Even if a man has a grand total of only four hairs left, he will grow them to the length of extension cords and carefully arrange them so they are running exactly parallel, two inches apart, across his otherwise stark naked skull, and he will look at himself and think, "Whoa, these four hairs are looking GOOD."

But whether you're a woman or a man, you should know the basics of hairstyle management presented here in the popular Q and A format:

Q. How can I have really nice hair?

A. If you look at the models in commercials for hair-care products, you'll notice that their hair is thick, glossy, lustrous and manageable. What's their secret? It's simple: They were born with nice hair. That's why they are professional hair models, whereas you and the late Albert Einstein are not.

Q. Should balding white men shave their heads, the way many African-American men, such as Michael Jordan, do?

A. No. It's not fair, but the simple truth is that balding African-American men look cool when they shave their heads, whereas balding white men look like giant thumbs.

Q. Why is it that some older women, when their hair starts to turn gray, instead of dyeing it back to whatever natural-looking shade it originally was, decide to dye it roofing-tar black or traffic-cone orange, which are colors normally associated with Halloween?

A. Apparently it is some kind of sorority initiation.

Q. What is the best way to style my hair?

A. You are asking the wrong person. I've been trying for more than 40 years, with absolutely no success, to get my hair to form a simple part. All I want is a basic straight line, such as can be found on Al Gore, the vice president, and Ken, the doll. So every morning, right after my shower, I attempt to style my hair with a brush and a hair dryer. I cannot begin to tell you how hilarious my hair thinks this is. You've heard of "free-range" chicken, right? Well, I have "free-range" hair. It laughs gaily and dances in the blow-dryer breeze, humming "Born Free." When I'm done, it looks exactly the same as when I started. It is no closer to forming a part than Dom DeLuise is to winning the Olympic pole vault.

Q. When you were in New York on a book tour several years ago, did you briefly find yourself in the same television-studio makeup room as Barbara Walters?

A. Yes.

Q. What is her styling secret?

A. Enough hair spray to immobilize a buffalo.

Q. Speaking of famous celebrities, did Madonna discuss any hair-related issues in her diary as published in the November issue of Vanity Fair?

A. Yes. On Page 224, Madonna had this to say about acting in the movies: "People sit around all day scrutinizing you, turning you from left to right, whispering behind the camera, cutting your nose hairs. . . ."

Q. Madonna has *nose hairs?*

A. You wouldn't believe. Sometimes she requires a machete.

Q. In conclusion, what is the one word that describes the key to a successful hair style?

A. "Hat."

1. How does Barry play off the usual expectations set up by his first sentence? By the question-and-answer format? Where might a straightforward version of this discussion be published?

2. What does the first half of the essay pretend to establish?

3. In part 1, where does Barry use comparison-contrast four times for comic effect?

4. "So we see that hairstyle is very important" (paragraph 6): Does the conclusion follow the evidence? From what kind of logical fallacy is Barry tickling laughter?

5. Where does Barry reintroduce earlier material of the essay in a surprising context?

6. What kinds of writing allow at least touches of wit? What kinds do not?

Bjorklund, Melissa (student)

Two views of Catholic boarding school, positive and negative, interact like counterpoint in polyphonic music.

This double-voice format can also be achieved by setting up two columns on the computer.

CATHOLIC SCHOOL

—✳—

Nearly all adults tell of their glory days in high school, the joys,
Most high school students take for granted being a
the thrills and the carefree ambience. How quickly they forget
typical all-American teenager. They live at home, have
about the pain of growing up—the problems with grades and academics,
the freedom to date and socialize, and participate in normal
the disappointments of broken friendships and hopeful infatuations, the
activities of a public high school. These freedoms are not
difficulties of peer-pressure, and the troubles regarding decision-making
those of a Catholic boarding school. At a Catholic boarding
and setting goals. Because of all these stresses on young people, I think a
school there is a lack of privacy, a limited amount of
Catholic boarding school is an excellent alternative to a public high
independence, and the setting is in an unnatural social
school education.
environment.

Catholic boarding schools in all cases offer a strict disciplinary envi-
Privacy is always limited at any boarding school, owing
ronment. This sometimes scares a teenager off, not knowing that this sort
to the fact that there are no private rooms since students
of atmosphere can be most helpful. Catholic boarding schools are often
must share dormitories with two to three other persons.
misunderstood. There were never harsh beating sessions. The sisters, who
The doors of the rooms are not to be locked because roll
are the disciplinarians, never treat the students as less than mature adults.
is taken every two hours by nuns who walk into dorm rooms
When a student is punished, it is usually by a cleanup duty assignment or
unannounced. Meals at Catholic boarding schools are mandatory
a restriction from going on outings. Mandatory study periods are held
and attendance is required because roll is again taken.
every weeknight, but if a student's G.P.A. falls below a 2.0 extra time will
Sometimes it would make one think that there was really a
be added to his or her study hall. The sisters are not only teachers but are
maximum security prison.
more than willing to help you with your school assignments.

The development of high personal morals and values is an impor-
Independence is curbed at a Catholic boarding
tant part of any religious school. Religion classes are required and are con-
school. Students are physically restricted from
sidered as important as math and English. Being exposed to religion, in
coming and going off school campus as they please.
any case, cannot be harmful; the student has the option to accept or re-
Decisions on clothing, activities, classes, travel,
ject it. These classes concern themselves not only with God, yourself and
and time management are decided by others so
others. These classes concern themselves not only with God but also is-
students exercise little if any independence.
sues of morality and self-esteem; e.g., how to love God, yourself and oth-

ers. These classes teach religion from an objective point of view, but they

teach students about their inner selves on a personal basis.

The friendships students make at any boarding school are very
Students of a Catholic boarding school are usually pawns of an
close ones. Boarders learn to live with diverse types of people. Students
unnatural social environment. Students do not come into social
are exposed to not only other students from all around the United States
contact daily with members of the opposite sex; consequently, the
but all over the world! Their friends become their family and the school
surroundings are not conducive to the development of a well-rounded

becomes their home. Students learn to accept others for what they are,

individual. Another problem with an all-male or all-female school is

they learn how to love and how to be loved. At boarding school it is not

the absence of normal high school activities such as homecoming

their mothers' shoulders they cry on but those of their close friends.

festivities and sports that interact with both males and females.

At the age of fourteen I accepted the opportunity to attend Notre

I attended a catholic boarding school for my

Dame Academy, a Catholic boarding school in Middleburg, Virginia.

freshman and sophomore years in high school. When I

Before going, I had only two priorities: myself and fun. My G.P.A. was a

was faced with the decision to finish my junior and

1.7, I had no knowledge of the world, and I really didn't care. I attended

senior years at Notre Dame Academy or return home and

Notre Dame Academy for two years, but that short period of time was the

finish school, I decided to return home because I felt

more important to my self-improvement than any period of my life. I

I was missing a big part of an average teenager's life.

came out of Notre Dame with a 3.7 G.P.A., I gained many life-long

I wanted to sleep in my own room and eat when I

friends, my mind was enriched with the cultures to which I was exposed,

wanted. I wanted to lead a normal social life, be

I had organized priorities, and most of all, I now loved God. I recommend

a cheerleader, and have a boyfriend. These privileges

a Catholic boarding school to any high school student to insure that their

you can only attain by living at home, and attending

high school years really *are* glory years.

a public highschool.

Missy McDuffie Bjorklund

Questions

1. How does the double-viewpoint format resemble a dialogue?
2. What is yet another viewpoint that could be given in place of the one in handwriting? A fourth?

Chaucer, Geoffrey (ca. 1342–1400)

The Knight" and "The Miller" are two character sketches in which Chaucer makes use of some literary traditions, as the notes to *The Riverside Chaucer* point out, but he made great poetry of them. Let him coach you as a prose writer. Notice the lavish, varied, and vivid details presented. And notice the directness of the first portrait—which works by thesis and support—as compared to the indirectness of the second, which nowhere makes an overall judgment about the Miller.

The six-hundred-year-old English will seem less daunting if you read the poems twice. To decipher a word, think of its modern spelling or define it tentatively by its context. You don't have to understand each word to get the general meaning of the poem.

From *The General Prologue to The Canterbury Tales. The Riverside Chaucer,* 3rd ed. Ed. Larry D. Benson. Boston: Houghton Mifflin, 1987.

THE KNIGHT

A KNYGHT ther was, and that a worthy man,
That fro the tyme that he first bigan
To riden out, he loved chivalrie,
Trouthe and honour, fredom and curtisie.
Ful worthy was he in his lordes werre,
And therto hadde he riden, no man ferre,
As wel in cristendom as in hethenesse,
And evere honoured for his worthynesse;
At Alisaundre he was whan it was wonne.
Ful ofte tyme he hadde the bord bigonne
Aboven alle nacions in Pruce;
In Lettow hadde he reysed and in Ruce,
No Cristen man so ofte of his degree.
In Gernade at the seege eek hadde he be
Of Algezir, and riden in Belmarye.
At Lyeys was he and at Satalye,
Whan they were wonne, and in the Grete See
At many a noble armee hadde he be.
At mortail batailles hadde he been fiftene,
And foughten for oure feith at Tramyssene
In lystes thries, and ay slayn his foo.
This ilke worthy knyght hadde been also
Somtyme with the lord of Palatye
Agayn another hethen in Turkye;
And everemoore he hadde a sovereyn prys.
And though that he were worthy, he was wys,
And of his port as meeke as is a mayde.
He nevere yet no vileynye ne sayde
In al his lyf unto no maner wight.
He was a verray, parfit gentil knyght.
But for to tellen yow of his array,
His hors were goode, but he was nat gay.
Of fustian he wered a gypon
Al bismotered with his habergeon,
For he was late ycome from his viage,
And wente for to doon his pilgrymage.

THE MILLER

The MILLERE was a stout carl for the nones;
Ful byg he was of brawn, and eek of bones.

That proved wel, for over al ther he cam,
At wrastlynge he wolde have alwey the ram.
He was short-sholdred, brood, a thikke knarre;
Ther was no dore that he nolde heve of harre,
Or breke it at a rennyng with his heed.
His berd as any sowe or fox was reed,
And therto brood, as though it were a spade.
Upon the cop right of his nose he hade
A werte, and theron stood a toft of herys,
Reed as the brustles of a sowes erys;
His nosethirles blake were and wyde.
A swerd and a bokeler bar he by his syde.
His mouth as greet was as a greet forneys.
He was a janglere and a goliardeys,
And that was moost of synne and harlotries.
Wel koude he stelen corn and tollen thries;
And yet he hadde a thombe of gold, pardee.
A whit cote and a blew hood wered he.
A baggepipe wel koude he blowe and sowne,
And therwithal he broghte us out of towne.

Questions

1. Can you supply a first-line summary of the Miller as Chaucer does for the Knight? What is appealing about him? Appalling? Both?

2. In what ways do the Knight and Miller contrast?

3. Which character seems of more social value, the chivalric crusader or the cheating Miller? In Chaucer's eyes? In yours?

4. What kinds of nonverbal details help to make up the portraits?

5. Suppose you were to try a film adaptation of these portraits. What information about these figures would be challenging or impossible to get across? What judgments? What details would "translate" well?

Donne, John (d. 1631)

Devotions upon Emergent Occasions (1624) was written during the course of John Donne's near-fatal illness. Each of the twenty-three devotions begins with a meditation on the human condition, makes an expostulation (an attempt to persuade), and concludes with a prayer. The following excerpt is the first part of such a devotion.

From J. William Hebel et al., *Prose of the English Renaissance* (New York: Appleton-Century-Crofts, 1952): 641–42.

X VII. *Nunc lento sonitu dicunt, Morieris: Now, this bell tolling softly for another, says to me, thou must die.*

17. MEDITATION

———— ✳ ————

Perchance he for whom this bell tolls may be so ill as that he knows not it tolls for him. And perchance I may think my self so much better than I am, as that they who are about me, and see my state, may have caused it to toll for me, and I know not that. The church is catholic, universal; so are all her actions. All that she does, belongs to all. When she baptizes a child, that action concerns me; for that child is thereby connected to that head which is my head too, and engraffed into that body, whereof I am a member. And when she buries a man, that action concerns me. All mankind is of one author, and is one volume; when one man dies, one chapter is not torn out of the book, but translated into a better language; and every chapter must be so translated. God employs several translators; some pieces are translated by age, some by sickness, some by war, some by justice; but God's hand is in every translation; and his hand shall bind up all our scattered leaves again for that library where every book shall lie open to one another.

As therefore the bell that rings to a sermon calls not upon the preacher only, but upon the congregation to come; so this bell calls us all. But how much more me, who am brought so near the door by this sickness. There was a contention as far as a suit (in which both piety and dignity, religion and estimation, were mingled), which of the religious orders should ring to prayers first in the morning; and it was determined that they should ring first that rose earliest. If we understand aright the dignity of this bell that tolls for our evening prayer, we would be glad to make it ours by rising early, in that application that it might be ours, as well as His, whose indeed it is. The bell doth toll for him that thinks it doth; and though it intermit [stops ringing temporarily] again, yet from that minute that that occasion wrought upon him, he is united to God. Who casts not up his eye to the sun when it rises? but who takes off his eye from a comet when that breaks out; Who bends not his ear to any bell, which upon any occasion rings; but who can remove it from that bell which is passing a piece of himself out of this world? No man is an island, entire of itself; every man is a piece of the continent, a part of the main; if a clod be washed away by the sea, Europe is the less, as well as if a promontory were, as well as if a manor of thy friend's or of thine own were. Any man's death diminishes me, because I am involved in mankind. And therefore never send to know for whom the bell tolls. It tolls for thee.

Questions

1. Is this a meditation as defined in Chapter 2? (Could the tolling bell make a brief composition of place—one already fused with the internal colloquy?)

2. Does the first paragraph represent an internal colloquy? (The first two sentences do have a questioning tone—"Perchance"—and they lead by association to the subject of human unity.)

3. Can you explain the "book" analogy in the first paragraph?

4. Where does Donne refer to himself? Address the reader?

5. How does Donne's conclusion compare to Hurston's?

Fritz, Margaret (student)

This paper was written in a course on Native American literature at the University of South Dakota. Margaret Fritz gently presses her view that readers of Simon J. Ortiz, an Acoma Pueblo Indian poet born in 1941, should be aware of an important theme. (For the full text of the poem "We Have Been Told Many Things . . .," see Chapter 6.)

INTERDEPENDENCE BETWEEN THE LAND AND THE PEOPLE

✳

The native people of North America speak of their relationship to the earth in terms of family. This family relationship is rarely understood by those preaching progress, those who view land as just another commodity to be bought and sold. But to the Native Americans the land was more than just another commodity; it was their life! The land was their final resting place and the source of their spiritual power. All of its features—the rivers, the mountains, the rocks, and the valleys—are dynamic; every part is living and vital. Everything, from the smallest firefly to the largest mountain, belonged to one earth. Life was seen as a great circle . . . each person had a place on that circle and was related to everyone and everything. They saw their role on this earth, not as rulers, but as caretakers.

Of course, being human, not every native person acknowledges this all of the time. That is why the spoken and written word is so crucial. The poetry of Simon J. Ortiz powerfully portrays the American Indian's relationship to the earth, and all things of the earth. Ortiz's words not only paint a picture of wonder and beauty, but they often, directly and indirectly, teach us a valuable lesson. I've decided to focus on one aspect of this family relationship—the interdependence between the land and the people.

This love of the land is vividly illustrated in Simon Ortiz's book, *Woven Stone* (1992), a collection of poetry and prose from three earlier books. In his introduction, Ortiz explains the relationship between Native Americans and the earth:

Native Americans had a religious belief that depended upon a spiritual and material relationship with creation and the earth. People got what they needed to live from the land-earth, and they gave back, with their work, responsibility, and careful use of natural resources, what the land needed. Their creators gave them life, and they, with prayer, meditation, and ritual, gave back life; they received and gave. (29)

This philosophy explains the sacred relationship that the Native Americans had with the "land-earth"—a reciprocal relationship of love, respect and responsibility.

In an earlier exchange when asked what the main theme of his poetry is, Ortiz replied, " . . . to recognize the relationship I share with everything" (Jaffe 406). This theme of shared relationships underlies much of his past and present work.

In "Old Hills," from *Woven Stone,* Ortiz's words convey a sense of timelessness:

> West of Ocotillo Wells,
> the hills are pretty old.
> In fact, they're older than any signs
> telling tourists where they're at,
> older than all of millennium's signpainters. (69)

This poem is a story within a story. Quite simply, it's about life. On the surface it describes the everyday events that shape and form our brief existence. However, below the surface it describes the everlastingness and permanence of the land, the ancient hills and sculpted valleys carved by ancient seas of long ago.

The "land-earth," I feel, is also depicted as maternal. In "Mid-America Prayer," from *Woven Stone,* Ortiz speaks of this motherly bond:

> Standing again
> with and among all items of life,
> the land, rivers, the mountains, plants, animals . . .
> and the earth mother which sustains us. (289)

The "land-earth," like a mother, brings forth life—from the tiniest ant to the mightiest oak. From her, we and all other living things come. We shall soon pass . . . but the mother-child relationship will endure with respect, devotion, and responsibility. It coddles and unconditionally accepts us: "The rocks and cacti tolerate us/very quietly" (69). The land, like a mother, is patient and understanding. It forgives us for our ignorance, and waits patiently for the day when we give thanks for all that the land, our mother, has done for us.

In poems such as "We Have Been Told Many Things but We Know This to Be True" and "Returning It Back, You Will Go On," both from *Woven Stone,* Ortiz sends a clear message to the people. A message imploring the people to care for the land. The land is not something to be bought and sold . . . something to be used and mistreated. The land is, quite simply, the center of existence—the ultimate source of our very lives.

We see the importance of this bond in "We Have Been Told Many Things but We Know This to Be True," from *Woven Stone.* This poem poignantly expresses the sacred relationship between the land and the people:

> This is true:
>> Working for the land
> and the people—it means life
> and its continuity.
> Working not just for the people,
> but for the land too.
> We are not alone in our life;
> we cannot expect to be.
> The land has given us our life,
> and we must give life back to it. (325)

These words vividly illustrate the family relationship. We are all together in this land. We are all together in this world. Humans are not alone, nor are they destined to "rule" over the earth. The land is more than lifeless dirt and clay. It is pulsating and shifting—eternally giving us life, and it is our responsibility to nurture the earth, as it so unfailingly nurtures us.

Likewise in his poem, "Returning It Back, You Will Go On," from *Woven Stone,* this sacred relationship between the land and the people is expressed again:

> When you plant something,
> watch it grow, nourish it,
> so carefully, so gently, sing, talk,
> watch it grow, harvest it,
> prepare it, pray, speak about it
> to others, remind them, watch your children grow,
> use and eat it and return it back . . .
> Returning it back, returning
> it back, you will go on, life will go on. (331)

These words eloquently express the deep connection Native Americans have with the land—the home in which they live, die and are buried. They beautifully remind us that the land is not inactive, but alive and dynamic. Its lifeblood pulses through the fruitful soil, carrying nourishment to all that flourishes upon it.

In Ortiz's latest book, *After and Before the Lightning* (1994), the theme concerning relationships appears again. In his introduction, Ortiz explains that one purpose of this book was to help him prepare for, and face, the reality of a South Dakota winter:

The winter prairie surrounded me totally . . . I could not put on enough warm clothing nor be prepared enough nor was there a way to avoid it. The reality of a South Dakota winter demanded to be dealt with. So I was compelled to write the poetry in *After and Before the Lightning.* (Preface xiii)

But his poems also subtly portray a hidden relationship between the land and the people, a relationship strengthened by beauty and wonder.

What I like about *After and Before the Lightning* is how the words paint a clear picture of life on the prairie during the winter season. A clear picture, I feel, regardless of whether the reader is a native of South Dakota or not. His poetry reinforces this reality and acknowledges both the ferociousness and the miraculousness of nature. The words make me remember that even though winter is bleak and never-ending, it's also beautiful. And sometimes before we can see the beauty, we must live through the reality. I think his poems flow this way—from experiencing and accepting the reality of the winter season, to finally seeing the beauty beneath the bitter cold.

In his poem, "Earth Mother, She Cares," we can imagine the "snow which doesn't melt," and the fact that "We can do nothing else/but pray, pray hard" (3). Yes, this is true, for we cannot capture and tame the awesome forces of nature, we can only hope and pray that nature will be kind. Likewise in his poem, "Driving, the Snowy Wind," we see reality once again: "The snowy wind is fierce,/insistent, unrelenting" (5). The winds are legendary on the plains. They blow over the prairie, slowly gaining strength with neither woods nor mountains to slow their fury. And finally, in "Destined," we begin to accept the inevitable: "Bitter cold and endless/it is this South Dakota wind and snow,/a destiny we cannot deny" (14). These poems create an image of the dark side of nature. A side that is cruel and unselective in her destruction.

Yet, this dark side is necessary, for it forces us to admit that we are helpless against the powers of nature. We have no say. We can only weather the storm as best we can. Once we accept this reality we are more able to appreciate the beauty beneath the harshness.

This beauty is evident in his poem, "Beauty Unmatched": "Beauty without question, unable/to be described, simply accepted" (48). We also see this reference in "Beauty All Around: Borrowed From Dineh," in the words, "Now the sun is so low on the horizon./Now there is beauty all around" (52). This beauty does exist. It's there in the early morning when I awaken to a strikingly brilliant light, a picture post-card scene. The trees, usually so lifeless and bare, sparkle with life. Even my old, rusty automobile has been transformed into a glittering chariot. The clear blue sky. The fathomless starry nights. The strengthless sun glides across the heavens and we are often unaware of its presence until evening when it magically awakens and takes on a splendor which is undescribable. Out of all the beauty that winter brings I like the sunsets best. The brilliant hues of violet set against the pale, blue sky . . . the miracle of ordinary things.

Ortiz's poetry powerfully portrays the American Indian's relationship to the earth and all things of the earth. His poems eloquently paint a picture of wonder, beauty, and interdependence. In a 1985 interview Ortiz commented that his poems are "prayers as well," and indeed they are. They are prayers of hope and beauty. But most importantly, they are prayers imploring us to care for the land, the mother of us all.

Works Cited

Jaffe, Harold. "Speaking Memory." *The Nation,* 3 April 1982: 406–8.

Ortiz, Simon J. *After and before the Lightning.* Tucson: University of Arizona Press, 1994.

———. Interview. *The Circle: Hocoka.* By Shirley Sneve. South Dakota Public Television. KUSD, Vermillion, 1985.

———. *Woven Stone.* Tucson: University of Arizona Press, 1992.

Questions

1. What is Fritz's thesis? Does she persuade you to accept it?

2. Look again at paragraph 6, which begins "The 'land-earth,' I feel. . . . " The first quotation from Ortiz was added to a previous draft after Fritz did some more reading. Does the change improve the paper?

3. In your impression, does the writer's testimony about the winter add or detract from her undertaking?

4. Fritz, who is part German, part Norwegian, and part Yankton Sioux, writes: "I don't know that much about my 'Indian-ness' "? How might her response to Ortiz compare to yours?

5. Can you define your attitude toward the land? How might it differ from that of Ortiz?

Frost, Robert (1874–1963)

The speaker in this poem expresses skepticism about an unexamined practice and the hand-me-down adage used to support it.

From *Complete Poems of Robert Frost* (New York: Holt, Rinehart and Winston, 1964): 47–48.

MENDING WALL

Something there is that doesn't love a wall,
That sends the frozen-ground-swell under it,
And spills the upper boulders in the sun;
And makes gaps even two can pass abreast.
The work of hunters is another thing:
I have come after them and made repair
Where they have left not one stone on a stone,
But they would have the rabbit out of hiding,
To please the yelping dogs. The gaps I mean,
No one has seen them made or heard them made,
But at spring mending-time we find them there.
I let my neighbor know beyond the hill;
And on a day we meet to walk the line
And set the wall between us once again.

We keep the wall between us as we go.
To each the boulders that have fallen to each.
And some are loaves and some so nearly balls
We have to use a spell to make them balance:
'Stay where you are until our backs are turned!'
We wear our fingers rough with handling them.
Oh, just another kind of outdoor game,
One on a side. It comes to little more:
There where it is we do not need the wall:
He is all pine and I am apple orchard.
My apple trees will never get across
And eat the cones under his pines, I tell him
He only says, 'Good fences make good neighbors.'
Spring is the mischief in me, and I wonder
If I could put a notion in his head:
'*Why* do they make good neighbors? Isn't it
Where there are cows? But here there are no cows.
Before I built a wall I'd ask to know
What I was walling in or walling out,
And to whom I was like to give offense.
Something there is that doesn't love a wall,
That wants it down.' I could say 'Elves' to him,
But it's not elves exactly, and I'd rather
He said it for himself. I see him there
Bringing a stone grasped firmly by the top
In each hand, like an old-stone savage armed.
He moves in darkness as it seems to me,
Not of woods only and the shade of trees
He will not go behind his father's saying,
And he likes having thought of it so well
He says again, 'Good fences make good neighbors.'

Questions

1. From whom did the neighbor learn the saying?
2. When is a wall a "barrier of custom" (Montaigne) and when is it a means of safety?
3. How do the speaker's descriptions of nonverbal communication affect your judgment of his neighbor?
4. How would you describe the "mask" that the speaker wears?
5. How close does the first line come to expressing a thesis? What might be the "something"?

Fullwood, Becky (student)

Whereas Frost's "Mending Wall" includes a hint of dialogue, this piece presents an entire one-on-one exchange in the question-and-answer format.

For Socrates' use of the dialogue in the service of philosophical inquiry, see the excerpt from "Phaedrus."

Tips on How to Be a Cashier

Q: What does a cashier in a grocery store do? What are the job's duties?

A: A cashier rings up the purchases, either by hand or scanner. The cashier collects the purchase price and makes change. Cashiers see that the orders are bagged properly and that the customers are satisfied.

Q: That doesn't sound too difficult.

A: It isn't.

Q: What are some of the skills that are needed to do this work?

A: Good hand and eye coordination is necessary so that the items are rung up properly and not too slowly. Customers don't want to stand in line a long time. They don't want their groceries thrown around or damaged. Experienced cashiers should be able to tell when a price is incorrect. They should call for assistance to correct the problem. It is important for the store to collect the right amount of money, and no customer wants to be overcharged. Good cashiers can't guess at the price or take the customer's word.

Q: Why can't you take the customer's word? Wouldn't it be rude not to?

A: It is not the customer's job to remember the prices: they are not always paying attention; they could just be dishonest.

Q: What else do cashiers have to be able to do?

A: Cashiers have to know how to count money correctly and to make change. This is most important. Thousands of dollars pass through a cashier's hands during a shift. The counting has to be right! The groceries have to be bagged well, too: no one wants mashed bread. People want a quality product for their money. Since they have made their choices, they regard these items as their property. The bags should not be too heavy. Some people are not able to carry heavy packages, or overfilled bags may break. A cashier should treat every customer's groceries as if they were their own.Most important of all, the cashier has to be courteous and helpful. He or she should always be polite, no matter what the customer does or says. If a customer has a problem that the clerk can't handle, a member of management should be called. A good cashier always expresses willingness to help. Answer all questions, do not make the customer feel stupid or silly for asking. This is not what you are here for. The customer really is always right.

Q: Why is it important to know how to make change? Don't the registers tell how much money to give back?

A: Yes, they do. But they have to be told how much money is being given. Sometimes clerks count wrong, or the customers change their minds and give a different amount of money than was keyed in. For example—a bill is $12.07. One customer may give the cashier $13.00. Someone else may decide after the cashier has keyed in $13.00 to give $13.07, or even $20.07. This customer either wants a specific amount of change back, or just wants to give this amount of change. The customers don't care if it is easy or hard to figure their change. They just want it to be correct. The store cannot afford to have a clerk who makes mistakes. Mistakes like this cost money. A cashier who gives out improper change will not be kept for long. No customer will stand for being shorted.

Q: Why does a cashier have to bag groceries? Aren't there baggers for this?

A: Yes, but sometimes they have other duties. When it is not very busy a cashier does all his or her own bagging. When finished ringing up an order, one can always turn around and help the bagger.

Q: If a cashier can operate the register, bag groceries, and make change—what else needs to be done?

A: The work area has to be kept clean. Cashiers need to be able to get along with other store employees. Cashiering is a cooperative job. You will need to be helpful to everyone, not just to the customers.

Q: Tell us about this cleaning. Why should cashiers need to clean? Aren't they busy enough just ringing up groceries?

A: Each store has varied duties for all its employees. There may be some stores in which a cashier will help stock shelves or bag produce to fill in the time. There may be stores in which a cashier only runs a register, but I have never worked in one.

Q: You must think cashiers are pretty important.

A: I think cashiers are the most important employees in a grocery store. Many times they will be the only people that the customers come in contact with directly. They are the ones that give the store's patrons an overall impression of the store. Make this impression a positive one. Make people want to come back.

Questions

1. What advantage can the dialogue form have over the usual monologue approach to exposition? What disadvantage? Would it help you as a writer to imagine carrying on a dialogue with your reader?

2. The questioner in this dialogue is only vaguely defined. Suppose Becky Fullwood were to identify the person as a cashier-trainee in order to define her intended reader more clearly? Would the teacher then address the learner as *you?*

3. Can you employ the pronoun "you" to rewrite the tangled grammar of this sentence? "A cashier should treat every customer's groceries as if they were their own."

4. Could Fullwood's dialogue (or a revision) work as the script for a video-taped job-description? Or is it too wordy and not dramatic enough?

Gilbert, Jeffery (student)

Jeffery Gilbert, who grew up in Oregon, wrote this group of related stories as a twenty-four-year-old freshman. He tells about watching and taking part in the dances of Pacific Indians. What feelings come through to you about his experiences with people of a different race and culture?

CONVERSATIONS WITH LEHLOOSKAH
❋

Coyote's the one who taught people how to dance. He's the pinhead who started this, it's all his fault.

—Chief Lehlooskah

The First Circle

I met Lehlooskah for the first time when I was in the fourth grade. My class attended a performance that he and his tribe offered to elementary school students. Lehlooskah was a story teller. Maybe he was one of the last. He had learned the craft from his father, who in turn had learned the tradition from his father and so on all the way down the line. Lehlooskah, wanting to preserve his culture, took his stories to children.

My class filed into the traditional Longhouse by pairs. The air smelled of cedar and smoke. The corners of the long building were supported by brightly painted totem poles. The floor was covered with soft dirt. Three or four other classes had already taken seats on the expansive benches lining the walls in rows. We hurried to find space for ourselves. When we were finally settled, Lehlooskah entered and began to speak.

His voice was rich and deep. He welcomed us into his house and began to tell stories. Wonderful stories: He spoke of brave warriors and foolish clowns. He told us tales of brave and wise Bear and silly, lucky Coyote who is loved best by man because he is closest to him. The old chief related myths of ancient monsters and mysterious beings, Sasquatch and Wendigo, who hunt man with the howl of the winter winds.

Lehlooskah, through the easy power of his voice alone, created love, magic, and friendship. But it was the dancers who brought it all to life.

They spun around the room like dervishes. Each kicking up clouds of dust and sparks from the fire. A mask on one's head turned him into another person, or an animal, or even an element. It was as if the wind itself was being born on the back of a man in a mask.

My classmates and I sat transfixed by the whirling dancers. We were reluctant to breathe. I was afraid that any wrong move I made would destroy the atmosphere of the dance. Everything about the ceremony seemed so delicate. We could sense its age.

All of the world's cultures have incorporated some form of communicative dance into their society. Assuming that dance is a universal language is, however, misleading. Dance is a cultural experience. Any information that is conveyed by dance must be understood culturally within religious or social contexts before any communication will take place.

I had the cultural exposure of a white middle class brat who goes to a private suburban school and whose father managed a trailer park. The dance itself made very little sense to me culturally. Without Lehlooskah's verbal interpretations I would have been completely lost.

Later, after the dancers had wound down, towards the end of the program, Lehlooskah spoke of eagles. He told us that their power was the gift of young warriors. He told us how their down, if carried, would protect one against any and all challenges one would encounter and keep you safe within his tribe. At the end of his story the totem poles surrounding us coughed thousands of downy feathers into the air. As Lehlooskah and his tribe said goodbye to us we were surrounded by a flurry of soft white feathers.

Years later I had an opportunity to speak with Lehlooskah again. I told him that I still had the eagle down he gave us so long ago in a little box at the foot of my bed. "Eagle down?" asked Lehlooskah. "Yes," I said, "It came out of the totem poles at the end of your show, I've kept it."

Lehlooskah put his arm around my shoulders and patted my back, "Goose," he said. "We get them from old pillows." He had the most infectious laugh of any man I have ever met.

Second Circle

A few months later, when I was about 19, Lehlooskah invited me to a ceremony he and "the boys" were having. He knew that I was interested in his culture and I think took pride that he had played such a large part in creating that interest in me. He wanted to show me part of his culture without the distraction of having a herd of school kids around to water it down. I gladly accepted.

We were seated around the fire. The dancers stomped around the perimeter of the circle just as I remembered them doing so long ago. I clapped along with the drummers. It was so easy to find yourself trapped in the engaging energy of the dance. Lehlooskah, at my side, laughed his deep wonderful laugh, "So, how's it feel to be a redskin, whiteboy?" "Pretty dang good, Squanto," I replied. I guess Lehlooskah was pleased with my answer because he shoved me up into the circle. A few of the dancers surrounded me and, against my protests, showed me the simple steps that were necessary to execute the dance. Great stomping fun steps they were. I never did quite get the hang of them, but spinning around the fire one could easily forget that he was screwing up the rhythm and that those weird marks on the ground were being caused by his tennis shoes. It just didn't matter. It was fun and inclusive. The other dancers had a way of putting the "Newbies" through the wringer in such a way that it made you feel right at home. They'd start to trip you up then reach out and catch you before you really start to fall. One dancer was exceptionally good at aping the other's dance steps. He loved to imitate me. He'd stomp really hard and look straight at the ground with a look of such intense concentration that it was impossible not to laugh. I don't think there was any insult meant. There was none taken anyway. Instead it was as though by making light of my unfamiliarity with the dance they were accepting me into their circle.

Specifically, all I really remember about the dance is a scattering of visual images. I can see laughing faces, sparks from the fire, and one pretty Chinook girl who wasn't really part of the dance, but believe me, I remember her anyway.

The simple dance step that was used by the Indians was based on a simple two-time drum rhythm. Once I was able to relax into it the movement came easy. The dancers and I orbited the campfire together, each following the same basic step but exploding into a more personal series of movements and gestures as the mood would strike him. This was a very free dance style. It was also a very exhausting one.

After I had finished dancing I sat back down next to Lehlooskah. My face was flushed red from my close proximity to the fire and there were smudges of dirt on my chin. He gave me one of his bear-like hug-pats and handed me a beer, "Don't tell your mother about this part, kid."

Third Circle

I remember one dance very specifically. A man entered the firepit dressed in a very elaborate mask. The mask was carved from the bark of a tree and was very brightly painted. The outside of the mask resembled a large demonic looking bird. It was ingeniously constructed so that the beak of the bird could open and close creating a loud clapping sound. The dancer used this effect to punctuate the rhythms of the drummers as he danced. Another aspect of this mask was that it opened up to reveal another mask beneath it: A character of a man in great pain. Lehlooskah whispered to me, "That's Disease."

Disease danced around the circle in an unusual way. He moved with a peculiar gaiting step, opposite that of the other dancers. Along the way he kept threatening the audience by darting close to them and revealing the hidden face underneath the outer most mask. As he passed the other dancers he reached out and touched some of them. The dancers he had touched soon began to fall motionless to the ground. Then another dancer in a mask entered. This mask was of a human face surrounded by the image of a bear. This new dancer carried a short decorated stick and had an elaborately decorated pouch slung over one shoulder.

"The medicine man," Lehlooskah explained.

One by one the other dancers left the circle leaving the medicine man and disease alone in the center of the pit. The two danced each other around the circle, jumping through the flames of the fire and circling one another. The music was quiet but intense. The staccato clapping of Disease's bill was the loudest noise in the circle.

Finally, the medicine man began to dance in concentric rings around his opponent. He twirled his stick above his head and made great leaps into the air. On one of these leaps he swung the stick through the fire and then brandished it as a torch. Disease tried to fight back but he was no match for the shaman. The Medicine Man whirled his flaming baton over and around his head and shoulders. Sparks flew about him like angry hornets. He threatened Disease with the flame. After about three minutes the conflict was over. Disease ran off into the night. The dancers returned and followed the medicine man about in a dance of thanks. Eventually, the medicine man thanked the dancers and left the circle.

I later learned that this was a performance dance. A dance of this type is typically very coordinated, not at all like the free stepping individualized dance that I had participated in earlier. A performance dance must be based upon a specific story or event and the dancers will take upon themselves characters or forces separate from themselves. Masks are often used as a means of expressing character. This dance style is used for entertainment, thanksgiving, boasting of one's personal prowess, or infrequently as a means of appealing to spirits for help or guidance.

Fourth Circle

"The sun dance," said Lehlooskah, "is a hell of a lot of fun." I had over the past three or four years visited my friend Lehlooskah a number of times and participated in a few of the dances they had annually. More often than not, however, I remained a spectator. On this day Lehlooskah had invited me to join in a ritual called the Sun Dance.

"It's really not part of our culture," explained the chief. "It was used more often by the Plains Indians, but we like it anyway."

"What's it for?" I asked.

"Oh, probably just the hell of it."

"You aren't going to stick me with anything are you?"

"Yep, antler right through your chest, need another beer?"

"Um, an antler, you say?"

"Nah, just kidding with you, whitey. We use bungee cords these days, hurts less."

The sun dance was held around a pole stuck into the ground. The cords were tied to the top and the ends were fastened to five or six different members of the tribe. A fire was lit at the base of the pole and we were simply to jump and dance around the pole using the cord for leverage and to jump and fly.

I remember the feel of the taut cord as I leaped into the sky, how it connected me to everything, I imagined that it really was attached to my flesh, I saw other dancers connected to the same pole and I realized that, for the moment, we were all connected, all part of the same organism.

Fifth Circle

The friendship dance was my favorite. Everyone in the circle was involved. You would dance across the floor and give a small gift to another member of the circle. Then you would take his or her seat and they, in turn, would dance over to somebody else and give them a gift.

Lehlooskah liked to hand out beer during this dance. He gave the children candy, of course but I think he liked handing out beer a bit more. It's funny, I can't ever remember seeing that guy drunk.

The friendship dance was a wonderful experience. I remember dancing my way across the circle of faces to deliver my gift of a small pebble to a young girl whom I had befriended. She smiled and stood up, then twirled her way across the fire ring to give a feather to someone else. Everybody was smiling and most were pounding on some sort of percussion instrument. People were singing and yelling at each other. The yellow light of the fire played across every face.

Eventually, people stopped waiting to receive a gift before they entered the dance and they just started moving out onto the floor. The entire pit was awash with people. Everyone dancing away long into the night.

The friendship dance really had no ending that I could ever decipher. It just went on until everybody had left for home. Like friendship, it really had no temporal constraints.

Indian dance is a structured and elaborate art form. In order to fully understand the communicative aspects of it we must be exposed to it directly. Communication, without a recipient able to understand what is being conveyed, is useless. If the audience available to the Pacific Indians continues to decline, then the dance of these people will be relegated to a Hollywood stereotype.

Works Consulted

Folklore, Cultural Performances, and Popular Entertainments: A Communications-Centered Handbook. Ed. Richard Bauman. New York: Oxford University Press, 1992: 41–49.

Mason, Bernard S. *Dances and Stories of the American Indian.* New York: Ronald Press Company, 1944.

Questions

1. Do you agree with Gilbert's classmates that the title should be more accurate and inviting? If so, can you suggest an alternative?
2. Can you write in a subtitle for each of the five "circle" headings to indicate their subjects?
3. What do the reported conversations with Chief Lehlooskah add to the piece?
4. Where do the stories gain vivacity from nonverbal details about voice, touch, appearance, motion, and setting?
5. What does the writer's library research add? Should it be compressed, eliminated, or tied in more subtly anywhere?

Goodman, Ellen

In this column, published in 1985, Ellen Goodman uses the full meditation sequence including composition of place, internal colloquy, and resolution. The series of questions sets it apart from her informal essay on letter-writing (Chapter 3) which, though meditative in a broader sense, is not a formal meditation.

PLANNING ON THE LUXURY OF REST

※

CASCO BAY, Maine—The light has already changed. The soft air-brushed quality of August has lifted and everything—the prematurely red branch of the sumac, the wilting jewel weed, the over-ripe rosehips—is outlined in September clarity.

Lying on the porch with my prop (the book that accompanies my nap), I try to postpone the new year, to fend off the lists that lurk right outside my vacation consciousness. I want to sink for just a few more hours into that state of timelessness and ease that is as comfortable and unrestrained as the rope of the hammock beneath my body.

Like most of those whose biorhythms were imprinted by the school calendar, I know that summer doesn't last until the 22nd. Already this "Dear Parent" is being urged back into seasonal harness.

Leisure—not that American oxymoron "leisure-time activity" but real leisure—is being replaced by alarm clocks and time frames and schedules. There is a foreign hand at the metronome and as the temperature goes down, its tempo goes up. By some unnatural order, we are given more to do just as the days get shorter.

What do I want to take home from my summer vacation? I close my eyes and think. Time. That is what I would like. The wonderful luxury of being at rest. The days when you shut down the mental machinery that keeps life on track and let life simply wander. The days when you stop planning, analyzing, thinking and just are.

I don't know why it is so hard to find the same piece of time during the rest of the year. Life is more frenzied, I am told by friends. They say this philosophically, as if "it" were in charge and we had lost control.

The people I know live within the confines of their weeks-at-a-glance. When more is demanded of us, we get larger datebooks with more elaborate planners. We fit things in. We schedule—family, work, friendships. We organize with a fury of split-second timing. But we almost never pencil in time to do nothing.

It gets harder every year to figure out what separates our own lives from those of the creature frantically working the goldenrod beside me against a deadline of frost. What is the difference? A soul, the theologians say, a sense of mortality, a sabbath. Maybe it is the last, a day of rest, that we have lost first.

One of the advantages of this summer retreat is that I truly vacate both the workplace and the marketplace. But soon, at home, I will be again subject to Shopping Sundays, and to Washing Sundays, Cleaning Refrigerator Sundays, Driving the Car Sundays. There is no empty day in my weeks-at-a-glance.

My father, my grandfathers, I don't know how many generations back, worked six days and had one off. I don't at all envy their work life. But most of us work five days at one job, then thank God it is Friday and proceed to work two days at another.

Our mothers and grandmothers, for their part, labored for their families full-time. Now we hold two jobs, moonlighting every week, and then consider Sunday shopping to be a wonderful modern convenience, a sure sign of progress.

What, I wonder from my post in a hammock, would happen if we reclaimed a private Sabbath? What if we obeyed that most humane of the old religious injunctions: a day of rest?

I wonder if there might not be some freedom in the restriction. The freedom to not chauffeur, shop, clean. The freedom to spend time in the most profligate way, whole hours of it in leisure and pleasure, instead of frittering away the coinage in errands and obligations.

I don't know if I can reclaim the secular Sabbath, even for sanity. At the door to a summer cottage the chores of fall already knock, demanding attention. It is remarkably hard to transfer chunks of time from doing to being, to give ourselves as much time as our laundry. But this new year, I resolve to try.

What will I take home from my summer vacation? A bit of nothing. One day a week, maybe. With luck, it may even take root in the cool September weekends.

Questions

1. How do Goodman's sequence and tone seem to express the "being" that she wants to rescue from "doing"?

2. Would you agree that her resolution comes in the last paragraph?

Gore, Shayla S. (student)

Written for a freshman English course, this profile was published in the Coastal Carolina University newspaper, *The Chanticleer,* on November 12, 1996. Notice how the author tries to get the attention and interest of a well-defined readership.

TRIP AROUND THE WORLD
PROVES TO BE ENLIGHTENING

✳

Have you ever thought about traveling? How about Anchorage, Alaska? Or maybe Tokyo, Japan? Can you imagine renting a convertible and exploring Hawaii Kai, Hawaii? Everyone would like to do traveling like that at some point in their life, but can you imagine doing it all in one year?

Coastal Carolina's own Tricia Smietana, teacher of English 101, basically traveled around the world in 354 days. Her journey began shortly after she completed graduate school at Clemson University. Smietana felt really burned out after receiving her master's degree in one year. After seeing an ad in the newspaper, she decided to apply for a job with World Airways.

When asked about her experiences, Smietana replied, "My favorite place was Anchorage, Alaska. When we first arrived, we saw a moose at the airport. We also got to ride with a team that participated in the Ididerod, which is the great dog-sled race that takes place every year." She also spoke of the beautiful salt water pools in Tel Aviv, Israel.

Although there were several places that she enjoyed throughout her flying days, there were also a few that were not so pleasant. "I hated Brazil; it was smelly, nasty, and the people were very rude. I remember, once, I was on a flight trying to serve food, and a guy grabbed me and asked me, "Do you want to learn to samba?"

She explained that she really appreciates the U.S. in relation to the way that women are treated. "Other countries treat women like sex objects. You are a second-class citizen if you are a woman. In Paris, if you are a woman walking down the street with your legs shaved, and you have on panty-hose, then you are assumed to be a prostitute." Smietana went on to explain that Frankfurt, Germany, and Paris were amongst Brazil in the "hated" category.

"I wasn't really impressed with Japan. I expected more high-tech and everything seemed not up-to-date." She also laughed when she thought of how low everything was because of the height of the Japanese. When they walked down the street in their uniforms, they felt like famous celebrities because people pointed, whispered, and stared with fascination because of how tall they were and the way they were dressed.

Smietana also mentioned that she met a lot of people all over the world, and they still keep in touch. She is currently on leave from World Airlines and can go back at any time.

When asked if she will ever go back, she replied, "I don't think I will. I enjoy teaching and it's really what I want to do."

Questions

1. In the margin, can you label each paragraph with the topic it discusses?

2. Which paragraph(s) might be expanded to satisfy the reader's curiosity?

3. In the paragraph on Japan, can you replace the confusing pronoun in "When they walked" with a noun phrase?

4. Would you expect a photograph to go along with the words of this interview?

5. What might someone from another culture dislike about the United States?

Goshow, Brian (student)

This story announces its point in the title and unfolds by strict chronology. For a radically different version, see the piece that follows it.

THE MISTAKE
—✳—

It was a warm, sunny, early-spring day. There was a winter chill in the air yet, which required a jacket to be worn. I had just turned 16 so I was in the process of looking for a car. On this day, my father and I decided we would look at a car that a neighbor was selling—a 93-year-old neighbor. The car was a 1951 Chevrolet two-door sedan—unique.

I always wanted a car that was different than everybody else's. I had spent weeks searching used car lots everywhere. I looked at everything from hearse ambulances to Volkswagen buses. It was this 1951 Chevy that intrigued me, though, and I inspected it from a distance every day as I passed. On this day, though, I was going to be able to touch it, sit in the driver's seat, and maybe even start it up.

We drove up the road and stopped at the house and after about five minutes of looking at it, the door to the house swung open and out came Mr. Nyce. It took him a considerable amount of time to get to where he parked the car on the lawn, but for 93 years old he was still in pretty good shape. He greeted us with his Pennsylvania Dutch accent and proceeded to tell us about the car. From the tone of his voice I could tell that he had a soft spot in his heart for this car. I inspected the car checking everything out. I checked the frame which seemed to be in pretty good shape. The body had some rust in the fenders but I figured I could patch that up.

As I looked at it thoughts kept going through my head. I had visions of what a great hot rod it would make, and how big it was and how much my friends would like it and everything. All these thoughts probably made the rust look a little bit better than it was.

My father warned me but since it was my money, it was my decision. Mr. Nyce continued to tell how good of a car it was and the great gas mileage that it got. I now realize how good of a salesman he was, but it made me feel like there was something special about it. Then he told me that he would drop the price to $1100 from the original $1500 because I was "such a nice neighbor boy." Now I had to buy it.

After a few months of driving I realized the mistake I made. First of all, the gas gauge didn't work, which was responsible for a number of good workouts in pushing a car. In the next two years it needed a new transmission as well, which wasn't easy to find for such an old car. When I crossed railroad tracks the road would get showered with rust pouring from the fenders and undercarriage. A short circuit somewhere caused the battery to drain causing me to have to take the battery cable off every day when I got to school. Finally, as I drove home from school one day, my brakes suddenly failed and I had to use the emergency brake to stop. After this incident I decided to put it in my yard and forget about it.

I had a lot of fun times in that car but for many reasons I have to admit it was a big mistake.

Questions

1. The title bathes most of the story in dramatic irony, for the reader, unlike sixteen-year-old Brian, already knows that the car will be a bad purchase. If the writer had wanted to preserve suspense, what title could he have used?

2. About half the story recalls one scene: What is it?

3. The next-to-the-last paragraph begins with a topic sentence, "After a few months of driving I realized the mistake I had made." To support it, how many details does Brian present about the car's disintegration?

4. In a revision, where could Brian share more details about the whole experience? Of appearances? Thoughts? Spoken words?

5. How does the writer deflect potential criticism from his father?

Here is a psychological, rather than chronological, version of events in Brian Goshow's story. It was inspired by techniques used in the novel *La Jalousie* by Alain Robbe-Grillet (Paris: Les Éditions de Minuit, 1954).

"THE MISTAKE" SCRAMBLED

✳

by Randall A. Wells

No brakes!
93 years old, Chevy
Always wanted a car that was different, good workouts pushing it, no gas gauge, still in pretty good shape for 93, still a winter chill in the air, needed a jacket, Dad & I

It's your money, your decision. 1951, two-door sedan what a great hot rod when I crossed the railroad tracks the road got showered with rust, Mr. Nyce neighbor body had some rust in the fenders but I could patch that up it took him considerable time to get to where he parked the car on the lawn, the hearse-ambulance, weeks searching used car lots, the Volkswagen bus, but this Chevy intrigued me, I inspected it every day as I passed

Mr. Nyce

"What a good car it has been, what great mileage," Pennsylvania Dutch accent, had to put in a new transmission within two years, rust pouring from the fenders and undercarriage onto the railroad tracks, a soft spot in his heart for the car from the tone of his voice, '51 Chevy, unique, the door swung open at the house after five minutes of looking at it, how much my friends would like it and everything, took him a considerable amount of time, frame seemed to be in pretty good shape, some rust, Pennsylvania Dutch accent

Every day when I got to school having to take the battery cable off a short circuit somewhere in the car caused the battery to drain rust, 93

Sorry to see it go, and maybe he was, -sylvania Dutch, he would drop the price from the original $1500 to $1100, 93 to 16 years old, neighbor boy, now I had to buy it's your money, 51, I was going to be able to touch it, Dutch, good workouts, transmission hard to find for it took a considerable amount of time, a lot of fun times in that car, after this incident I decided to put it in my yard and forget about it, sit in the driver's seat and maybe even start it up

emergency brake!

Questions

1. What habits of mind does this version try to approximate?
2. In the apparent chaos, what indications of order do you spot?
3. How do the grammar and punctuation serve the intended effect?
4. If you were to scramble the story you wrote for Chapter 1, what would you try to highlight?
5. Could Brian Goshow borrow anything from this version to enrich his fourth paragraph (" . . . thoughts kept going through my head")?

Graham, Tracy Kolb (student)

This paper was written in Business/Professional English. The assignment: Observe nonverbal communication somewhere and then report on it to other students.

FLIRTING NONVERBALLY
———————————*———————————

This report examines the types of nonverbal behavior that play a part in flirting. The setting for my examination was the Spanish Galleon, a nightclub that caters to men and women who want to meet people of the opposite sex. Obviously, this is an appropriate setting for observation of flirting.

The most immediately observed type of nonverbal flirting is style of dress. Many people who come to the Spanish Galleon dress with flirting in mind. Many women wear tight, revealing clothing. This type of dress is not typical of only the young adults. Even those that people would classify as older, mature women often dress in this manner. Most women who dress this way are single. Women who come in with husbands or boyfriends tend to dress more conservatively, probably because they have less reason to advertise their bodies. Men's styles also can be flirtatious. For example, a man might wear tight jeans and a tight T-shirt with the sleeves rolled up to emphasize his muscles. Other men might wear expensive looking clothes or jackets and ties to make women think they are wealthy and/or successful.

People at the Galleon also flirt by their movements. Women especially, though not exclusively, sometimes try to accentuate their features when walking by putting an extra swing into their hips. Some men almost "strut" across the floor so as to put on an air of confidence and masculinity. Some women intentionally lean over so that their cleavage is in view. Likewise, some men flex their muscles at every opportunity. All of these movements are most likely to attract the opposite sex.

Dancing is something nonverbal that caters to the art of flirtation. How close together people stand when they dance can usually give an observer a better idea of the relationship between the two dancers. The closer two people stand, the more affection is being shown. However, as much and even more can be revealed by dance partners that stand without touching their partners. This distance gives a person an opportunity to put on a show for the other person, taking pains to accentuate their body and their ability to move sexily and invitingly.

Dress and full body movement are not the only forms of flirtatious nonverbal behavior. Things as basic as how a person holds a drink or cigarette can be forms of flirtation. For instance, a man may let his cigarette dangle out of his mouth; a woman may run her finger around the mouth of a beer bottle. Eye contact is also used in flirting. It can establish interest in another person possibly even all the way across a crowded room. However, eye contact as well as all of the other types of nonverbal behavior previously discussed can also be used to show disinterest. This is simply another part of flirtation. For example, a stern glare might scare someone away. After all, an important part of flirting is demonstrating to the ones you like that you are not interested in the others. Of course, a person could always be playing hard to get!

Questions

1. Does this report seem clear and complete? Incisive?

2. To connect with readers of, say, *Cosmopolitan* magazine, how would you rewrite the title? The introduction? What kind of illustration would you use?

3. Should Tracy Graham forecast her main points in the introduction? Use headings? At what point would you find such redundancy intrusive rather than helpful?

4. What purposes are achieved by the first sentence of the last paragraph ("Dress and full body movement are not the only forms . . . ")? Should the last paragraph be divided into two parts at "However, eye contact . . ."?

5. Why might the name "Spanish Galleon" appeal to customers? Is it one of the "new Spanish sails" decried by Paul Rice in Chapter 3?

Greene, Christina D. (student)

In the report by Tracy Graham, appearance suggests reality. But the relationship between the two is often problematical. This tension is a frequent one in life and literature.

For example, in the book *Andele,* the fierce Kiowa who goes on plundering expeditions and wants to be a chief conceals a gentle Hispanic boy inside himself (see Chapter 1, "Light Dawning"). What about that big, rough-looking girl on the school playground?

LACRETIA

<hr/>

Her name was Lacretia. We called her "the creature." She was two years older and stood six inches taller than anyone else in my class. She walked around with a mean look on her face that would convince anyone that she was a creature. All of my classmates seemed to be afraid of her. If she asked for anything they gave it to her, although they sometimes wanted it for themselves.

To me she did not act like a mean person. I often saw her standing on the fence alone while waiting for the bus after school. Although she looked lonely, I would not talk to her because I was afraid of what everyone else would think.

One day I went home and told my family about Lacretia. My brother said that she was lonely because all of her friends were at Jr. High with him. It was true, but I got upset with my brother for even talking about her. Maybe I was upset because I felt sorry for Lacretia. My mother said that we probably made her feel lonely and left out. She said that we should try to become friends. This sounded sensible to me but I still did not want to be her friend because I thought that my other friends wouldn't like me.

That night I dreamed that Lacretia was chasing me around the school with a stick. I looked back and saw that she was catching up. Then I tripped, slowly falling to the ground. I thought Lacretia was going to beat me with that stick. I closed my eyes and prepared myself. Then I heard her say "Here, you dropped your pencil." What I had imagined to be a stick was merely a pencil. Lacretia smiled as she helped me get up.

The next morning when I got to school I was determined to at least speak to her. After school when I saw Lacretia I went up to her and began to talk. I stood on the fence and talked to her until her bus came. She knew me very well because she had been in my brother's class before. She explained that her mother had been sick and she often stayed out of school to make sure she was all right. When she did this she missed days in school and was denied credit. The next year she went to school the kids picked at her, she got into trouble, and was suspended from school many times. She never caught up with her work and was held back again. She said that she was now determined to get out of the seventh grade even if it meant leaving everyone else alone and keeping to herself.

I found that Lacretia was a nice girl. We became friends and later graduated from high school together. Yet the name "the creature" followed her through high school. I often felt sorry for her when I heard people call her that because I knew she was not a creature at all, but instead a kind person.

Questions

1. Can you trace distinct phases in this narration? Background? Complication? Rising action? Crisis? Climax? Resolution? Is there suspense? Surprise? Irony? Does the story offer a deeper understanding of human beings?

2. Where do you notice a story-within-a-story? Another? (For a more extended example, see "Designer Genes." And for a fully elaborated dream, with people dancing to no beat and rooms defined by no walls, see the untitled piece by Andrew Karns.)

3. Where does nonverbal communication as pictured in this story seem unreliable as a source of information? Reliable? Where does Christina Greene, as a character in her story, use verbal communication to explore a situation?

4. What role does the writer's family play in defining her conflict?

5. In a revision, where could the author develop the story further?

Gregory, Dick

According to the *Almanac of Famous People* (4th ed.), Dick Gregory was born in 1932. He was a comedian who became a writer and political activist.

FROM *NIGGER: AN AUTOBIOGRAPHY*

—✳—

I never learned hate at home, or shame. I had to go to school for that. I was about seven years old when I got my first big lesson. I was in love with a little girl named Helene Tucker, a light-complected little girl with pigtails and nice manners. She was always clean and she was smart in school. I think I went to school mostly to look at her. I brushed my hair and even got me a little old handkerchief. It was a lady's handkerchief, but I didn't want Helene to see me wipe my nose on my hand. The pipes were frozen again, there was no water in the house, but I washed my socks and shirt every night. I'd get a pot, and go over to Mr. Ben's grocery store, and stick my pot down into his soda machine. Scoop out some chopped ice. By evening the ice melted to water for washing. I got sick a lot that winter because the fire would go out at night before the clothes were dry. In the morning I'd put them on, wet or dry, because they were the only clothes I had.

Everybody's got a Helene Tucker, a symbol of everything you want. I loved her for her goodness, her cleanliness, her popularity. She'd walk down my street and my brothers and sisters would yell, "Here comes Helene," and I'd rub my tennis sneakers on the back of my pants and wish my hair wasn't so nappy and the white folks' shirt fit me better. I'd run out on the street. If I knew my place and didn't come too close, she'd wink at me and say hello. That was a good feeling. Sometimes I'd follow her all the way home, and shovel the snow off her walk and try to make friends with her Momma and her aunts. I'd drop money on her stoop late at night on my way back from shining shoes in the taverns. And she had a Daddy, and he had a good job. He was a paper hanger.

I guess I would have gotten over Helene by summertime, but something happened in that classroom that made her face hang in front of me for the next twenty-two years. When I played the drums in high school it was for Helene and when I broke track records in college it was for Helene and when I started standing behind microphones and heard applause I wished Helene could hear it, too. It wasn't until I was twenty-nine years old and married and making money that I really got her out of my system. Helene was sitting in that classroom when I learned to be ashamed of myself.

It was on a Thursday. I was sitting in the back of the room, in a seat with a chalk circle drawn around it. The idiot's seat, the troublemaker's seat.

The teacher thought I was stupid. Couldn't spell, couldn't read, couldn't do arithmetic. Just stupid. Teachers were never interested in finding out that you couldn't concentrate because you were so hungry, because you hadn't had any breakfast. All you could think about was noon-time, would it ever come? Maybe you could sneak into the cloakroom and steal a bit of some kid's lunch out of a coat pocket. A bite of something. Paste. You can't really make a meal out of paste, or put it on bread for a sandwich, but sometimes I'd scoop a few spoonfuls out of the paste jar in the back of the room. Pregnant people get strange tastes. I was pregnant with poverty. Pregnant with dirt and pregnant with smells that made people turn away, pregnant with cold and pregnant with shoes that were never bought for me, pregnant with five other people in my bed and no Daddy in the next room, and pregnant with hunger. Paste doesn't taste too bad when you're hungry.

The teacher thought I was a troublemaker. All she saw from the front of the room was a little black boy who squirmed in his idiot's seat and made noises and poked the kids around him. I guess she couldn't see a kid who made noises because he wanted someone to know he was there.

It was on a Thursday, the day before the Negro payday. The eagle always flew on Friday. The teacher was asking each student how much his father would give to the Community Chest. On Friday night, each kid would get the money from his father, and on Monday he would bring it to the school. I decided I was going to buy me a Daddy right then. I had money in my pocket from shining shoes and selling papers, and whatever Helene Tucker pledged for her Daddy I was going to top it. And I'd hand the money right in. I wasn't going to wait until Monday to buy me a Daddy.

I was shaking, scared to death. The teacher opened her book and started calling out names alphabetically.

"Helene Tucker?"

"My daddy said he'd give two dollars and fifty cents."

"That's very nice, Helene. Very, very nice indeed."

That made me feel pretty good. It wouldn't take too much to top that. I had almost three dollars in dimes and quarters in my pocket and held onto the money, waiting for her to call my name. But the teacher closed her book after she called everybody else in the class.

I stood up and raised my hand.

"What is it now?"

"You forgot me."

She turned toward the blackboard. "I don't have time to be playing with you, Richard."

"My Daddy said he'd . . . "

"Sit down, Richard, you're disturbing the class."

"My Daddy said he'd give . . . fifteen dollars."

She turned and looked mad. "We are collecting this money for you and your kind, Richard Gregory. If your Daddy can give fifteen dollars you have no business being on relief."

"I got it right now, I got it right now, my Daddy gave it to me to turn in today, my Daddy said . . . "

"And furthermore," she said, looking right at me, her nostrils getting big and her lips getting thin and her eyes opening wide, "we know you don't have a Daddy."

Helene Tucker turned around, her eyes full of tears. She felt sorry for me. Then I couldn't see her too well because I was crying, too.

"Sit down, Richard."

And I always thought the teacher kind of liked me. She always picked me to wash the blackboard on Friday, after school. That was a big thrill, it made me feel important. If I didn't wash it, come Monday the school might not function right.

"Where are you going, Richard?"

I walked out of school that day, and for a long time I didn't go back very often. There was shame there.

Now there was shame everywhere. It seemed like the whole world had been inside that classroom, everyone had heard what the teacher had said, everyone had turned around and felt sorry for me. There was shame in going to the Worthy Boys Annual Christmas Dinner for you and your kind, because everybody knew what a worthy boy was. Why couldn't they just call it the Boys Annual Dinner, why'd they have to give it a name? There was shame in wearing the brown and orange and white plaid mackinaw the welfare gave to 3,000 boys. Why'd it have to be the same for everybody so when you walked down the street the people could see you were on relief? It was a nice warm mackinaw and it had a hood, and my Momma beat me and called me a little rat when she found out I stuffed it in the bottom of a pail full of garbage way over on Cottage Street. There was shame in running over to Mister Ben's at the end of the day and asking for his rotten peaches, there was shame in asking Mrs. Simmons for a spoonful of sugar, there was shame in running out to meet the relief truck. I hated that truck, full of food for you and your kind. I ran into the house and hid when it came. And then I started to sneak through alleys, to take the long way home so the people going into White's Eat Shop wouldn't see me. Yeah, the whole world heard the teacher that day, we all know you don't have a Daddy.

Questions

1. Does this story have a sort of thesis at the beginning?

2. Where does Gregory use generalized narration? Dramatized? Why? Does he follow strict chronology?

3. The use of dialogue is not the only sound of the spoken word. What do you notice about Gregory's "voice"?

4. Since Gregory was born in 1932, his teacher was probably of what race? What does he gain by conceding that she had at least some reason for her actions?

5. At the story's climax, how do the teacher's verbal and nonverbal communication interact?

Horn, John

This newspaper article offers a perspective on an upcoming event, the Academy Awards. With a slightly argumentative edge, Horn explains that what most filmgoers regard as background music can be a vital part of the movie, even a new language with which to communicate.

"Scores" appeared on the Associated Press wire in February 1996.

SCORES MORE THAN BACKGROUND
Composers translate movie plot into music

LOS ANGELES—Want to see a movie without any wallop? Just turn off the film's score.

Turn off the screeching strings in "Psycho." Shut out the orchestral triumph in "Star Wars." Skip the bittersweet piano from "Love Story." Miss the majestic theme of "Born Free."

Most people—including many executives in the film business—don't give movie scores much thought. Yet a good score can make an average film nearly great, and a bad score can make a polished work seem inept.

Under slightly new rules for the 68th Academy Awards, 10 film scores have been nominated for Oscars. The scores, judged by the composers' peers as 1995's best, are distinctly different, united only by a common accomplishment. All of the scores have translated plot, character, and setting into a new language—music.

Good scores, like nice wallpaper, not only cover the crack, but make the room look beautiful. At the same time, too much music can yield too many distractions—movies can drown in a sea of violins, oboes and flutes.

"All of us have the inclination to want to stand out—to want to be special," says composer Thomas Newman, whose "Unstrung Heroes" score was nominated in the newly named original music or comedy score category. "But if you call too much attention to yourself, it's not special."

"When you're selling an emotion, you have to push all the buttons an audience is expecting to have pushed," says James Horner, nominated for "Apollo 13" and "Braveheart" in the newly named original dramatic score category. "But it all has to be very gentle."

Almost every movie's story line suggests appropriate music—that's why the Oscar-nominated "Pocahontas" score (by Alan Menken and Stephen Schwartz) has recurrent themes plucked from Native-American melodies. Sometimes, though, the most obvious music is the least workable.

The plot of "Unstrung Heroes" follows an eccentric Jewish family. Newman started his research listening to klezmer, clarinet-heavy Jewish folk music, looking for hints of where the score might go. It didn't go anywhere.

"It just seemed pandering—it seemed to parody the movie," Newman said.

Newman then looked at the film's title, and started playing on the word "unstrung." He toyed with zithers, mandolins and banjos—all of them detuned, or unstrung.

"The instruments gave me some clues," Newman says. "The characters were so neurotic, it was like strings snapping."

For "Braveheart," Mel Gibson's epic set in 13th-century Scotland, Horner first listened to Middle Age music, plainsong and the chants of Benedictine monks. It was interesting, evocative—and, in a movie setting, totally unbearable.

"Mel wanted to take a lot of chances, but he left me to do it. It was my conservatism that kept the score from being too different, too unapproachable," Horner says.

The composer built the score around primitive instruments such as small Irish bagpipes and medieval flutes, using less of the familiar tones of a 20th-century orchestra. Horner had to carefully manage the film's explicit violence: Too serious a score would be overkill, and anything too light would make the bloodshed laughable.

"How do you score a disembowelment? That's very tricky," Horner says. "I told Mel, 'Let's score it like a lullaby.' By using a boy's choir and softening it acoustically, it makes the scene more dreamlike—it softens the whole thing."

For "Apollo 13," the plot suggested standard Hollywood action movie music. Horner and director Ron Howard went in a different direction.

"I wanted to get at the idealism of all these young men," Horner says. "I just didn't want it to be a traditional movie score." The movie's score is dominated by a hymn sung by children; it is loudest when the astronauts step onto the deck of the aircraft carrier.

"The hymn is like Shaker music—an early American harmony that you might hear in a small turn-of-the-century church," Horner says.

Compared to "Braveheart" and "Apollo 13," not a lot happens in "Sense and Sensibility." Director Ang Lee's movie version of Jane Austen's 19th-century romance is about feelings, not actions—when emotions change, they do so subtly.

"Ang was very keen to have a gentle feel—he wanted a very intimate score, one that reflected the suppressed emotions of that society," says Patrick Doyle, the nominated composer of the "Sense and Sensibility" score. That intimacy carries into the movie's incidental music—several piano pieces in the film were composed by Doyle, too.

Attentive listeners will notice definite but minor shifts in the film's score as the story unfolds. The music surrounding the character of Marianne Dashwood (played by Kate Winslet) is at first innocent, young. When she nearly dies from a fever, the music changes.

"There's a maturity and an emotional catharsis," Doyle says. "The music becomes a little more grown up."

The "Toy Story" score is hardly grown-up. That made for a good fit for Randy Newman, a composer with a child's fascination for whimsy.

Randy Newman is probably best known for "I Love L.A." and "Short People," but he has scored many films, including "The Natural," "Avalon," "Maverick" and "The Paper."

Questions

1. How does the writer's introduction try to "sell" his article?
2. Although primarily informative, the article does have a thesis that promises substantiation. What is it?
3. What quality seems most likely to define a good score?
4. Can you make out several main sections following the claim about "new language"? Which is the longest section? How is it developed?
5. Do you agree that music can be a language? If so, how?

Hurston, Zora Neale (1891–1960)

Zora Neale Hurston died penniless and obscure but left a rich legacy.

Raised in Florida, Hurston then attended Howard University in Washington, D.C., later becoming the first black student to attend Barnard College in Manhattan. She helped to create the "Harlem Renaissance," a group of young African-American artists that flourished in the 1920s and 1930s.

This personal essay was published in the magazine *World Tomorrow,* which specialized in writing by and about African-Americans. You might compare this buoyant piece to the graver "Explaining Race to a Child," by Leonard Pitts, Jr.

HOW IT FEELS TO BE COLORED ME (1928)

❋

I

I am colored but I offer nothing in the way of extenuating circumstances except the fact that I am the only Negro in the United States whose grandfather on the mother's side was not an Indian chief.

I remember the very day that I became colored. Up to my thirteenth year I lived in the little Negro town of Eatonville, Florida. It is exclusively a colored town. The only white people I knew passed through the town going to or coming from Orlando. The native whites rode dusty horses, the Northern tourists chugged down the sandy village road in automobiles. The town knew the Southerners and never stopped cane chewing when they passed. But the Northerners were something else again. They were peered at cautiously from behind curtains by the timid. The more venturesome would come out on the porch to watch them go past and got just as much pleasure out of the tourists as the tourists got out of the village.

The front porch might seem a daring place for the rest of the town, but it was a gallery seat for me. My favorite place was atop the gate-post. Proscenium box for a born first-nighter. Not only did I enjoy the show, but I didn't mind the actors knowing that I liked it. I usually spoke to them in passing. I'd wave at them and when they returned my salute, I would say something like this: "Howdy-do-well-I-thank-you-where-you-goin'?" Usually the automobile or the horse paused at this, and after a queer exchange of compliments, I would probably "go a piece of the way" with them, as we say in farthest Florida. If one of my family happened to come to the front in time to see me, of course negotiations would be rudely broken off. But even so, it is clear that I was the first "welcome-to-our-state" Floridian, and I hope the Miami Chamber of Commerce will please take notice.

During this period, white people differed from colored to me only in that they rode through town and never lived there. They liked to hear me "speak pieces" and sing and wanted to see me dance the parse-me-la, and gave me generously of their small silver for doing these things, which seemed strange to me for I wanted to do them so much that I needed bribing to stop. Only they didn't know it. The colored people gave no dimes. They deplored any joyful tendencies in me, but I was their Zora nevertheless. I belonged to them, to the nearby hotels, to the county—everybody's Zora.

But changes came in the family when I was thirteen, and I was sent to school in Jacksonville. I left Eatonville, the town of the oleanders, as Zora. When I disembarked from the riverboat at Jacksonville, she was no more. It seemed that I had suffered a sea change. I was not Zora of Orange County any more. I was now a little colored girl. I found it out in certain ways. In my heart as well as in the mirror. I became a fast brown—warranted not to rub nor run.

II

But I am not tragically colored. There is no great sorrow dammed up in my soul, nor lurking behind my eyes. I do not mind at all. I do not belong to the sobbing school of Negrohood who hold that nature somehow has given them a lowdown dirty deal and whose feelings are all hurt about it. Even in the helter-skelter skirmish that is my life, I have seen that the world is to the strong regardless of a little pigmentation more or less. No, I do not weep at the world—I am too busy sharpening my oyster knife.

Someone is always at my elbow reminding me that I am the grand-daughter of slaves. It fails to register depression with me. Slavery is sixty years in the past. The operation was successful and the patient is doing well, thank you. The terrible struggle that made me an American out of a potential slave said "On the line!" The Reconstruction said "Get set!" and the generation before said "Go!" I am off to a flying start and I must not halt in the stretch to look behind and weep. Slavery is the price I paid for civilization, and the choice was not with me. It is a bully adventure and worth all that I have paid through any ancestors for it. No one on earth ever had a greater chance for glory. The world to be won and nothing to be lost. It is thrilling to think—to know that for any act of mine, I shall get twice as much praise or twice as much blame. It is quite exciting to hold the center of the national stage, with the spectators not knowing whether to laugh or to weep.

The position of my white neighbors is much more difficult. No brown specter pulls up a chair beside me when I am down to eat. No dark ghost thrusts its leg against mine in bed. The game of keeping what one has is never so exciting as the game of getting.

III

Sometimes it is the other way around. A white person is set down in our midst, but the contrast is just as sharp for me. For instance, when I sit in the drafty basement that is The New World Cabaret with a white person, my color comes. We enter chatting about any little nothing that we have in common and are seated by the jazz waiters. In the abrupt way that jazz orchestras have, this one plunges into a number. It loses no time in circumlocutions, but gets right down to business. It constricts the thorax and splits the heart with its tempo and narcotic harmonies. This orchestra grows rambunctious, rears on its hind legs and attacks the tonal veil with primitive fury, rending it, clawing it until it breaks through to the jungle beyond. I follow those heathen—follow them exultingly. I dance wildly in-side myself; I yell within, I whoop; I shake my assegai above my head. I hurl it true to the mark yeeeooww! I am in the jungle and living in the jungle way. My face is painted red and yellow and my body is painted blue. My pulse is throbbing like a war drum. I want to slaughter some-thing—give pain, give death to what, I do not know. But the piece ends. The men of the orchestra wipe their lips and rest their fingers. I creep back slowly to the veneer we call civilization with the last tone and find the white friend sitting motionless in his seat, smoking calmly.

"Good music they have here," he remarks, drumming the table with his fingertips.

Music. The great blobs of purple and red emotions have not touched him. He has only heard what I felt. He is far away and I see him but dimly across the ocean and the continent that have fallen between us. He is so pale with his whiteness then and I am *so* colored.

I do not always feel colored. Even now I often achieve the uncon-scious Zora of Eatonville before the Hegira. I feel most colored when I am thrown against a sharp white background.

For instance at Barnard. "Beside the waters of the Hudson" I feel my race. Among the thousand white persons, I am a dark rock surged upon, and overswept, but through it all, I remain myself. When covered by the waters, I am; and the ebb but reveals me again.

IV

At certain times I have no race, I am *me*. When I set my hat at a certain angle and saunter down Seventh Avenue, Harlem City, feeling as sooty as the lions in front the Forty-Second Street Library, for instance. So far as my feelings are concerned, Peggy Hopkins Joyce on the Boule Mich with her gorgeous raiment, stately carriage, knees knocking together in a most aristocratic manner, has nothing on me. The cosmic Zora emerges. I belong to no race nor time. I am the eternal feminine with its string of beads.

I have no separate feeling about being an American citizen and colored. I am merely a fragment of the Great Soul that surges within the boundaries. My country, right or wrong.

Sometimes, I feel discriminated against, but it does not make me angry. It merely astonishes me. How *can* any deny themselves the pleasure of my company? It's beyond me.

But in the main, I feel like a brown bag of miscellany propped against a wall. Against a wall in company with other bags, white, red and yellow. Pour out the contents, and there is discovered a jumble of small things priceless and worthless. A first-water diamond, an empty spool, bits of broken glass, lengths of string, a key to a door long since crumbled away, a rusty knife-blade, old shoes saved for a road that never was and never will be, a nail bent under the weight of things too heavy for any nail, a dried flower or two still a little fragrant. In your hand is the brown bag. On the ground before you is the jumble it held—so much like the jumble in the bags, could they be emptied, that all might be dumped in a single heap and the bags refilled without altering the content of any greatly. A bit of colored glass more or less would not matter. Perhaps that is how the Great Stuffer of Bags filled them in the first place—who knows?

Questions

1. Hurston rather severely divides her essay into four sections marked by Roman numerals. But played off against this formality is unpredictability. How well can you forecast the content of any section from the introduction? From the preceding section or sections? From the way each begins?

2. How would you describe the personality of the writer as it seems to manifest itself? The first part of her essay alludes to a "sea change" that took place when she moved to Jacksonville. Do you suspect that, like Gregory, she experienced something traumatic? If so, why might she downplay it?

3. Hurston uses an abundance of writing techniques to define "how it feels." Where does she draw on figurative language? Dialogue? Narration? Contrast? Argumentation? Description? Allusion? A list?

4. "No dark ghost thrusts its leg against mine in bed": This figurative image of nonverbal behavior suggests what literal fear?

5. If this piece were expressed as music, where would the moods change?

INDIAN REMOVAL ACT

———————*———————

The following document, abridged, is Public Law 148 (28 May 1830), 4 *United States Statutes at Large*, pp. 411–12. It illustrates the incongruity that can exist between law and justice. (For thoughts on the law that helped enthrone Jim Crow, see Leonard Pitts, Jr., "Explaining Race to a Child".)

This bill passed in the administration of Andrew Jackson. Figuring in its motivation were racism, cultural prejudice (including Puritanism), states' rights, land, and gold. It forced about sixty thousand Native Americans to migrate to lands west of the Mississippi River; in 1838 four thousand Cherokees—about one-third—died along the way. (For an excerpt from a senator's speech against the Indian Removal Bill, see p. 152, and for the declaration of the Cherokee council, see p. 211.)

Chap. CXLVIII.—*An Act to provide for an exchange of lands with the Indians residing in any of the states or territories, and for their removal west of the river Mississippi.*

Be it enacted by the Senate and House of Representatives of the United States of America, in Congress assembled, That it shall and may be lawful for the President of the United States to cause so much of any territory belonging to the United States, west of the river Mississippi, not included in any state or organized territory, and to which the Indian title has been extinguished, as he may judge necessary, to be divided into a suitable number of districts, for the reception of such tribes or nations of Indians as may choose to exchange the lands where they now reside, and remove there; and to cause each of said districts to be so described by natural or artificial marks, as to be easily distinguished from every other.

Sec. 2. *And be it further enacted,* That it shall and may be lawful for the President to exchange any or all of such districts, so to be laid off and described, with any tribe or nation of Indians now residing within the limits of any of the states or territories, and with which the United States have existing treaties, for the whole or any part or portion of the territory claimed and occupied by such tribe or nation, within the bounds of any one or more of the states or territories, where the land claimed and occupied by such tribe or nation, within the bounds of any one or more of the states or territories, where the land claimed and occupied by the Indians, is owned by the United States, or the United States are bound to the state within which it lies to extinguish the Indian claim thereto.

Sec. 3. *And be it further enacted,* That in the making of any such exchange or exchanges, it shall and may be lawful for the President solemnly to assure the tribe or nation with which the exchange is made, that the United States will forever secure and guaranty to them, and their heirs or successors, the country so exchanged with them; and if they prefer it, that the United States will cause a patent or grant to be made and executed to them for the same: Provided always, That such lands shall revert to the United States, if the Indians become extinct, or abandon the same.

Sect. 4. *And be it further enacted.* . . . [The President may reimburse the Indians for improvements they made to their present land.]

Sec. 5. *And be if further enacted,* That upon the making of any such exchange as is contemplated by this act, it shall and may be lawful for the President to cause such aid and assistance to be furnished to the emigrants as may be necessary and proper to enable them to remove to, and settle in, the country for which they may have exchanged; and also, to give them such aid and assistance as may be necessary for their support and subsistence for the first year after their removal.

Sec. 6. *And be it further enacted,* That it shall and may be lawful for the President to cause such tribe or nation to be protected, at their new residence, against all interruption or disturbance from any other tribe or nation of Indians, or from any other person or persons whatever.

Sec. 7. *And be it further enacted.* . . . [The President may still govern the Indians.]

Sec. 8. *And be it further enacted,* That for the purpose of giving effect to the provisions of this act, the sum of five hundred thousand dollars is hereby appropriated, to be paid out of any money in the treasury, not otherwise appropriated.

Approved, May 28, 1830.

Questions

1. How would you describe the mask or voice of this law? How does it clash with the law's content?
2. Can you boil down each section into one short sentence? Begin it with "The President may," as in the summary of Sections 4 and 7.
3. Was this forced removal an example of "ethnic cleansing"?

Kape, Salomea

Born in Lodz, Poland, in 1926, Salomea Kape came to the United States in 1966 and lives in Brooklyn, New York. She is an anesthesiologist.

DESIGNER GENES

———————— ✳ ————————

"**W**ho's the girl in the red dress?" I asked Hannah as we walked the poorly lit corridor of the Pathology Building.

The year was 1947, my first year in medical school, in Lodz, Poland. I was not in the best physical shape since I was covered with small abscesses, which disappeared and reappeared with a mind of their own. My doctor stated that the multiple purulent craters were a minor cosmetic disease, which he treated with a tar-like pungent ointment. The ancient remedy didn't help, but it always provided a free space around me in the most crowded places. I saw a weak interest in the doctor's eye while he had examined my bleeding gums.

"Oho! Scurvy! Eat fruits, child," he announced in an almost cheerful tone.

Fruits! In the winter? In 1947?

I shook my head. "I have a peptic ulcer and fruits cause a stomach ache," I said in a thin voice.

The good doctor was irritated with the litany of minor illnesses and moved impatiently in the chair.

"Drink milk, child. Next patient, please."

But I was still better off than Hannah who had lost a good deal of her hair in the concentration camp and whose scalp shone through the thin remaining strands. I was lucky to have survived the war and I shouldn't have bothered the doctor with furunculosis, shaky teeth, and a dull pain in the belly.

I was too thin and Hannah was too bloated. We carried the memories of the ghettos and death camps and we smiled uneasy smiles or rather half-smiles or else we were boringly, deadly serious. We wore expressions as if to say, "Don't-be-too-happy-expect-a-disaster-every-minute-of-your-life." We were odd looking specimens dressed in a hodgepodge of clothing, handed down by the United Nations Relief and Rehabilitation Agency.

But the student in the red dress was different. The golden tan of her unblemished face matched the smiling, sky-blue eyes and the blond, straight, thick hair that formed a golden cask around her head. It was a glorious head untouched by powder, lipstick, or make-up. She smiled and listened attentively to an assistant in pathology and he in turn couldn't take his eyes off her. Other students had paused in their conversations to look at her.

"Who's she? What's her name? Is she an actress playing a medical student?" I again asked the well informed Hannah.

"That's Ola Kohn. She's the youngest student in the school and so far she has the best grades. The hospital of internal diseases was named after her grandfather, Dr. Jacob Kohn. Her father was a well known criminal lawyer and Ola inherited her mother's beauty." All these facts Hannah delivered in one breath.

"It figures." I said, a high dose of jealousy in my voice. "She has the perfect genes."

My interest in Ola remained high and I accosted her in the cinema house, 'Polonia.'

"Servus Ola. I'm Sally," I said holding out my hand, "I missed inorganic chemistry classes and I'd like to borrow your notes."

"Sure." She smiled a smile that disappeared slowly and lingered in her eyes. "But my notes are short. I'm sick and tired of these lectures given in movie houses. Yesterday we had physiology classes in the Symphony Hall and our professor, with his long hair, looked like a Toscanini talking about thyroid disease. At least the hall is warm and bright, but the movie houses are damp, dark, dirty, and cold. Will they ever build a university with real lecture halls?"

"First the government must rebuild Warsaw, then Gdansk, later Wroclaw, and Stetin. Our grandchildren will attend chemistry classes in the 'Polonia'."

"You're a real optimist." She tilted her head and smiled.

"Let's study together," I said using all my social grace. "I am a speedwriter and I make excellent notes. I have some textbooks, too, and we might form a terrific team."

"Fine, fine. Fantastic." Ola clasped her hands and in that moment of her childish delight, I was struck by the sweetness and innocence of her seventeen years. I was only three years older but inside me was a worried oldness and I could never smile the way Ola did.

Soon we were an inseparable duo. I made tons of notes while Ola wrote a few sentences, for she remembered most of the lecture.

"Ola," I said with unmasked envy, "did the gift of 'oral' memory pass along to you with your paternal chromosomes?"

"It's not hereditary. It's an acquired quality. A long time ago I learned to listen and to remember," she said and smiled.

Between the second and third year of medical school, the furuncles and scurvy made a quick exit precipitated by Ola's decisive action. She ordered, "Stop taking the antediluvian ointment, I'll buy penicillin on the black market."

The injection of the thick, yellowish, glue-like antibiotic into my glutei was like a red-hot nail penetrating my muscles and many times I preferred to be left alone with the painless furuncles. But when they vanished leaving silvery, star-like scars, I said to Ola, "I can't pay you back, but all the stars belong to you."

"It is a good omen for my future practice, stars instead of money." She touched the big scar on the back of my neck and declared, "My necklace will conceal it nicely."

Ola graduated from medical school summa cum laude, I without any "laude." We both chose internal medicine as our specialty.

In the vernacular of the time, we expressed our ultimate disgust or contempt in a single word, "cholera." And "cholera" we said to the political system in Poland in 1957 when we had decided to leave. Our ways parted; hers led to Israel and mine to the USA.

"You'll write letters to me?" I asked a moronic question for I knew well that she'd never write. "I'm going to miss you very much." I understated my feelings with this banal phrase.

"I'll miss you too," she said smiling.

I wrote letters. "Ola; 'the' is an unpronounceable nightmare. My lips, tongue, and vocal cords refuse to make this 'the' sound. Kind Americans say that I have a charming accent while at the same time they are tilting one ear toward me in order to understand the cacophony of English coming from my Polish-oriented mouth. Don't condemn me, for I abandoned internal medicine for anesthesia."

The phone rang as soon as Ola could afford to pay for long distance calls.

"Sally?" An echo was dancing on the old wire, ". . ally . . ally . . Don't cry over an accent. I started from scratch with a new alphabet. The kingdom of internal medicine is divided into many provinces and I am now specializing in the wonder of the 'pump.' I love you from the bottom of my 'pump'."

Over the years, the wire lost the echo and Ola's voice became gravelly and raspy. During the wars and many military actions in Israel, my telephone bills raised husband's eyebrows, but in time of peace I was driven by guilt of the unwritten letters I composed in my head but never sent out.

In the mid-seventies the phone rang and the familiar voice, without the troubling echo said, "We're coming to New York for a year. Ignaz took a sabbatical at New York University."

"Great, great." I said. I had waited a long time for her visit.

I mapped out in my head a tour of New York for them. No, I decided, not the triviality of the Empire State Building or the faded symbolism of the Statue of Liberty. We'd start at the triangle of Lincoln Center with the Metropolitan Opera at its apex. Then we'd walk to the Museum of Modern Art and I'd show them Central Park, the Plaza Hotel, the Metropolitan Museum. I'd take Ola to the weekly meeting of the cardiology section in my hospital and I saw us sitting in the hospital cafeteria during the lunch hours. I already smelled the familiar aroma of the hospital meals.

In a state of elation, I greeted her at the Kennedy airport. I scanned her face which wasn't very much affected by age. Its fine structure and good features remained unchanged, but her dark glasses somehow divided us like a heavy curtain.

"I have an allergy to dust and the glasses protect my eyes. I slept poorly in the plane. Do you have a sleeping pill?" she asked. I replied: "No, I don't. Since when did you start smoking?" I looked at the cigarette in her hand.

"Everyone smokes in Israel. We're all living in a war zone. Do you have any Valium?" she asked. "No, I don't."

"I'll call you soon." She hurried out of the airport and promised to call. But she didn't. I kept calling but in the morning she was asleep, in the afternoon she was taking a nap, and at night she was too tired to meet me. After a week of futile efforts to see her, I finally reached her by phone.

"Cholera! You owe me an explanation. Did I do something wrong?"

We arranged to meet in an obscure luncheonette on the Upper East Side. I disliked the place as soon as I pushed open the dirty door, but I ordered a cup of coffee from the waitress who kept a toothpick in her mouth.

"Ola," I said without pausing for small talk, "what's wrong?"

"Nothing is wrong," she started hesitantly, stopped and started again, "but I'm not feeling well lately and I'm an insomniac. I think more and more about the past. Why didn't we ever talk of the war?"

"I couldn't. You made a smooth transition after war . ."

She interrupted sharply. "None of us survived the war 'smoothly.' I was on the Aryan side, in a little village, near Warsaw. Our lives on the Aryan side hinged on the color of our hair, shape of our nose, intonation of our voices, and a thousand little factors of which the most important was luck. I was the lucky eleven year old blond girl with blue eyes and a snub nose. I blended well among the Poles. My aunt and uncle weren't so lucky, since they had the kind of a pale skin which turns brown with the first rays of sun and their hair was and eyes were black. They were hidden by the Poles in the attic, a windowless cubbyhole with a camouflaged entrance. Their one year old daughter was separated from the high risk parents and adopted by a childless Polish family. My blond, beautiful, and fearless mother was the master-mind of this elaborate plan of survival and every Sunday she brought money to the Poles for our upkeep. I was supposed to be a war orphan and I called her Mrs. Rolsky. Every night I visited my aunt and uncle in the attic and they gave me lessons in math, history, Latin, and physics. We didn't have pencils or paper and I did my homework in my head while I worked in the fields, milked the cows or cleaned the house. For three years they continued the oral teaching and slowly they replaced my parents. Mrs. Rolsky faded away as my mother. A few months before the liberation, the Gestapo came straight to the attic and shot my uncle and my aunt in the courtyard. I saw the execution from the window and crawled under the bed. The Polish woman told my mother when she came for her usual Sunday visit, 'Take the girl with you. NOW! She's crying and she looks like a Jewish child. I can't help you anymore. The Gestapo arrested my husband.' My mother wiped the tears from my eyes and said imploringly 'Ola, you have some chance to survive. The end of the war is near. Smile, smile. You must look livelier and merrier. Your eyes should give nothing away about yourself. I promise that we'll cry together after the war and we'll take the baby home.' After the war, my mother left the baby with the adopted parents for she believed that the little girl would be better off not knowing of her Jewish origins and the parents' fate. I kept smiling till I couldn't smile anymore."

Two rivulets of tears came down her cheeks and I instinctively removed her dark glasses. The whites of her eyes were crisscrossed by a fine net of tortuous red vessels, the iris had a glazed blue color and the pupils: I recognized the familiar pin-pointed pupils of the overdosed patients in the emergency rooms into whose collapsed lungs I pumped liters of oxygen. A glassy eyed junkie named Ola was looking at me. I turned my gaze from her face and said, "I have to go home."

I drove home hunched over the steering wheel and I noticed from the corner of my eyes the dirty papers flying high in the wind. I saw people in rags poking in the trash cans with sticks and drinking from brown paper bags. I looked at the hostile faces of the rush-hour drivers and I felt acid regurgitating in my mouth. A concentrated hate exploded inside me.

"Cholera at you, New York."

"Cholera with you, Ola."

Two days later the phone rang.

"Sally," she said "I wanted to tell you . . . "

"I'm on call." I stopped her in the mid-sentence, ice in my voice. I listened to her and all I could think was, "junkie, junkie."

"I'll call you some other time," Ola said.

Several days later somebody called and without giving a name left a message.

"Ola committed suicide. No funeral services. She donated her body to medical research." I was then on call again and I was very busy all night in the operating room, but the next day I didn't recall the cases. I went to see Ola's husband.

"Ignaz," I said and I had to squeeze the words through a constricted throat. "I failed her. She called and I didn't let her talk to me. I could have saved her if I hadn't been such a damn righteous person. I didn't let her talk." I repeated it again and again, for the click of the phone and the silence hanging on the wire still sounded in my ears.

"No, Sally, nobody could have saved Ola," he said and I noticed a deadly tiredness in his face. "She was depressed and was hospitalized and treated. She warded off the depression by intoxicating herself with Demerol, Valium, and Nembutal. Death was for her a better solution, more desired than her present existence. She left a letter for you."

"Sally," she wrote. "It took years to find my cousin's address, but I was too much of a wreck to write a letter. Give her my ring and ask her to forgive me." The ring was lost during the police investigation and the letters Sally sent to Poland came back stamped "Addressee unknown."

Questions

1. Where does her appearance conceal, and where reveal, Ola's true self?

2. Would you agree that Nazi Germany has claimed another victim?

3. What is the significance of the returned letters?

4. What do Dr. Kape's "brown paper bags" in New York City bring out in the story? In what ways do they differ from Hurston's "brown bag" of miscellany?

5. Since its two central characters are adults, why was this story printed in the *Newsletter of the International Study of Organized Persecution of Children* (2.1, Spring-Summer 1994, published by Child Development Research)?

Karns, Andrew S. (student)

Here is a tale spun out by the unconscious. Karns has been able to share its sensory details, incongruities, contradictions, and non sequiturs through the power of verbal symbols.

UNTITLED STORY

As I enter the house that has no egress I notice the surroundings: An old white picket fence missing a few boards, a tall pine tree that seems to be humming a deep and thoughtless tone as the wind passes through, and the sun as it gets swallowed by the extremely large and unhappy, dark clouds. I become scared because there are no lights on in the house and I know that by the time I enter it the sun will be gone. There are no windows in the house; there aren't even any walls in the interior (which seems odd to me because somehow there are many different rooms).

I don't ever remember there being a door or any entrance of some kind, but I still end up inside the house. The first room I enter is a cold and dark one, but the floor seems almost hot underneath my toes. I can't see the floor and I can't even see my hands in front of my face. I catch a scent of a certain smell that cannot be explained, but I recognize that smell and realize where I am. I grow more afraid and yet, at the same time, I remain calm. I keep walking without a clue of where I am going, but I do know what lies ahead.

Suddenly the floor turns cold and slippery: I guess it is ice, but now the room itself has become extremely hot. I do not sweat, for I cannot, because I am not sure whether I am too hot or too cold. Without warning a green light shines from nowhere. It fills the room so now I can actually see. I still can't see myself which sort of confuses me, but I do not stop to ponder. There are other people in this room, but they don't have any faces. They are really short or maybe I am just really tall. They are dancing slowly to no beat at all. This doesn't seem strange to me even though this is not normal and it is strange.

I then enter the room of the gamblers, which is filled with the stench of cheap cigars and pipe tobacco. I can only really see one person because the black light illuminates his shirt, but I can still see the others moving around. I want to stop and play but I cannot because I feel that I have work to do, so I keep walking past them as they don't even acknowledge that I am there.

At this point I am really scared. I want to find a way out and find it fast, but I can't run nor can I see anything anymore. I hear a noise in the distance and it sounds like music being played on a record player at a super low speed. The music fills the room with melancholy and I try to whistle a tune to block out the music but I can't hear myself. I then try to talk or even hum but I find out that I can't make any noise at all. My feet become heavy which in turn makes me tired of walking. I cannot stop, though, because I am afraid that I might never get out of the room filled with the infinite sadness.

Suddenly the music stops or maybe it is just blocked out by the sound of a train going along a smooth track. This sound is sort of soothing to me but I am still frightened, for I cannot see any trains. All I see is a moving picture above me that looks like the inside of a lava lamp that fills the ceiling that is as large as the sky. Darkness surrounds me except from above where the lava remains. It is red with a maroon background.

The lava sky sort of puts me in a trance and makes me forget about my intent of finding a way out of the house and instead tires me even more than before. I now search for a mattress of a bed to comfort my tiredness as I keep walking through the everlasting lava room.

After a long time of walking I notice that the lava is gone. It is now completely dark except for a bright white light shining off in the distance. I walk towards the incandescence which slowly rises to the sky and shines a ray on something white on the ground. I slowly walk towards the object which appears to be a bed. I feel relieved when I see this, but as I approach I notice that it is occupied. I look at the person lying there asleep and I know that I have seen him somewhere before. He awakens with a jerk and sits up in an instant. He looks at me as I look at him: with a face full of confusion. He mumbles something to me which I don't understand at first, but then I realize what he said. "It is all just a dream."

Questions

1. Where do you notice unrealistic features that are characteristic of dreams?

2. Where is the dreamlike atmosphere made vivid by appeals to the senses of sight (including color), sound, smell, texture, temperature, and weight? What do the details about music add?

3. Where do the only spoken words occur?

4. Where in your reading do you remember works, passages, or images that seem to draw on the irrational nature of dreams for their power?

5. Can you create a dream for Jo March? Read the beginning of Chapter XIV of *Little Women* (see Alcott, above), where Jo encounters a pet rat, an undescribed editor, the young man Laurie, and a dentist's sign with a "pair of artificial jaws which slowly opened and shut to draw attention to a fine set of teeth." Perhaps weave these details into the dream along with her ambition as a writer. You might read Gary Walker and Diana Jo Wilson's version (Readings).

McCall, Stephanie Owens (student)

An informal essay can lean heavily on personal experiences, or it can express personality by thought and style rather than by references to the writer. Or it can do both, like the following, in which a country girl reflects on her community.

PLEASANT HILL

—— ✳ ——

I think anyone who lives in one place for any number of years must be observant of the changes that occur in just one small, tiny block of the world.

Stick barns that house snakes in their rafters turn into gas-powered, easy-curing tobacco barns. A tractor pulling a wooden cart with men cropping by hand turns into a one-man powered machine that winds through the rows in minutes.

The old dirt roads that have been paved, and the new ones that have been cut through what used to be lush forest or even corn fields.

I recall the new church being built and the older members refusing to attend because it just wasn't the same.

Old people dying, new babies being born. The community just replenishes itself. New people with the same last name. Everyone knows everyone else.

Cox's grocery stands in its original place, passed on from father to son. Men and women returning home to carry on the tradition of keeping farms in the same family for generations.

I wonder if anyone else thinks about all the changes in our community and how everything appears to move in a cycle?

A stranger would have to see this as a quiet place, but is it really? Gathering at church on Sunday. Going to R.L.'s any night of the week for the best coffee and the best conversation. One can sit around to discuss the War Between the States and Donald Trump all in a night.

People get up at sunrise to garden and farm. I believe Dalmar and Vernice have the cleanest garden I have ever seen. Never a weed in sight.

Mrs. Cribb moved out of her little white house, and I moved into it. Always people moving, but they never seem to leave, and if they do, they always come back home.

I've seen the changes of the last twenty years, and it makes me so curious as to what will be in the next twenty years.

I've found someplace that I never want to leave, and I believe this is fortunate, since some people never know where they want to be.

No shopping malls, no movie theaters, not even a big grocery store.

Land, trees, farms, family, longevity, heritage.

Questions

1. In your response to "Pleasant Hill," do the sentence fragments and short paragraphs help create an impression of thoughts caught on-the-fly? An "inner rhythm" (Goodman)? What would be lost if all or most of the fragments were revised as complete sentences?

2. Although the piece starts off with the theme of "changes," it comes upon the different idea of a "cycle" in paragraph seven. If revised for more unity, what would be lost?

Stephanie Owens McCall did rework her essay to settle on "changes" and to add details. As an experiment, two of her classmates then recast her second version in a way that will help you appreciate the charm of the informal essay:

"PLEASANT HILL" AS A FIVE-PARAGRAPH THEME

※

by Freda Green and Renee Michau

Have you ever stopped to think about changes that silently and subtly take place in your individual space, the space of your home and your community? No matter where a person lives, he or she can witness change. In most cases, change is not instantly obvious. Reflection and a time line are needed for the observation. The change in individual space from last week, last month or even six months can barely be noticed. But those of a longer period can be drastic, particularly if a twenty year time frame is used. I have seen changes occur in three major areas. There is the change in population, in the lifestyle of the people, and in the structure of the land.

Over the past twenty years, my small community has practically doubled in size. Because of the dramatic population increase, it was necessary four years ago to build a new school. The lonely stretch of road that just a few years ago had only a single farm house is now scattered with several homes. In addition it now has many dogs and children. People live closer together than they once did, and the neighbors are more plentiful.

Along with the population changes, time has also modified lifestyles. The population is now very mobile. Residents who used to make the fifteen mile trip once a week into the nearest town now make this trip an everyday event. In addition, technology has made electronic goods such as television sets, radios, and V.C.R.'s more readily available and affordable. Stories have been told as to how the whole community would gather at the home of the family who owned the only radio. They would listen to the "Grand Ole Opry." Now, people enjoy their own radio and television along with many other appliances. Convenience has become important for the new lifestyle of the majority.

The largest change has occurred in the structure of the land. Farms have been split up to make room for new homes, and land has been cleared for the sale of timber. New churches have been built, and old schools have been torn down. New highways are being built. They are connecting new houses, and new bridges. Road number 261 used to run fifty feet away from my front door, but today it runs five hundred feet away from it.

No matter where a person goes, he or she can witness change. People can especially see this if they live in one place for a number of years. Whether we are for or against change, evolution of a small community is inevitable.

Questions

1. What is lost or gained in this tightly and conspicuously ordered version?

2. Does a three-point development serve this material best? McCall's instructor and one of her fellow students rewrote this rewrite to focus on two causes of change: the development of technology and the growth of population. For another variation, two students rewrote her expanded essay as an interview made up of questions and answers. Stephanie also rewrote it in the double-voice format: The typed lines told how the community changes and the handwritten lines, below them, how things stay the same. Stephanie's instructor then rewrote her essay as the following:

"PLEASANT HILL" AS A STREAM OF CONSCIOUSNESS

by Randall A. Wells

Used to run by my front door, 261, trucks woke me up at night, could wave, knew who was going where when, tobacco leaves wafted onto yard from truck now runs five hundred feet from my front door, change, change, lonely stretch of road one house now scattered with them, dogs, kids, closer together now, twice as many people, new school, daily, decade, change, I have seen it, children once went away for college, travel, returned to retire or raise their families, more neighbors, nearest town fifteen miles away, women used to make the trip once a week, now everyday happening, new houses where farms were, now split up, land cleared for sale of timber, new technology, new churches, VCR's, television sets, radios, stories of whole community gathering at home of family who had the only radio listening to *Grand Ole Opry,* old schools have been torn down, used to run fifty feet from my door, brand new highways being cut through everywhere, connecting new houses, new bridges, new appliances, convenience is the key word, metamorphosis, I have been fortunate to see the differences in one rural community, has practically doubled in size, a sort of "newness," someone transplanted from twenty years ago to today might have a little trouble finding their way around, Grand Ole Evolution

Questions

1. Does this version have any redeeming social value?

2. With this long series of grammatical patches, do you get a sense of a mind working by association? Of any surprising juxtapositions?

Méndez, Concha

These lines are expressed by someone who did not quite become a mother. They were published in *Niño y sombras* (Madrid: Ediciones Héroe, 1936): 7–8.

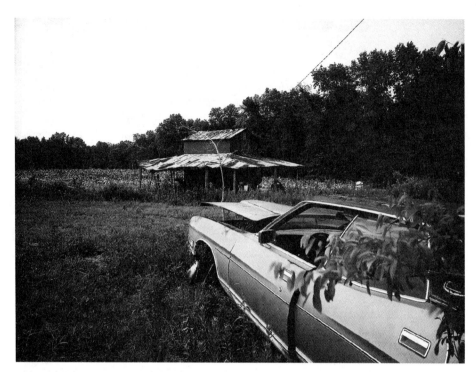

PLEASANT HILL, S.C.
Tim Dillinger

Untitled Poem

Translation by Gregory K. Cole

¿Hacia qué cielo, niño,
pasaste por mi sombra
dejando en mis entrañas
en dolor, el recuerdo?
No vieron luz tus ojos.
Yo sí te vi en mi sueño
a luz de cien auroras.
Yo sí te vi sin verte.
Tú, sangre de mi sangre,
centro de mi universo,
llenando con tu ausencia
mis horas desiguales.
Y después, tu partida
sin caricia posible
de tu mano chiquita,
sin conocer siquiera
la sonrisa del ángel.

Toward what heaven, child,
you passed through my shadow
leaving the memory
in my entrails in sorrow?
Your eyes did not see light.
Yes, I saw you in my dream
in the light of a hundred dawns.
Yes, I saw you without seeing you.
You, blood of my blood,
center of my universe,
filling with your absence
my unequal hours.
And afterwards, your departure
without a possible caress
of your little hand,
without even knowing
your angel's smile.

¡Qué vacío dejaste,	On leaving
al partir, en mis manos!	what emptiness you left in my hands!
¡Qué silencio en mi sangre!	What silence in my blood!
Ahora esa voz, que vence,	Now, that voice that overcomes,
del más allá me llama	calls me imperiously
más imperiosamente	from the great beyond
porque estás tú, mi niño.	because, my child, you are there.

Questions

1. To whom is this poem addressed?
2. Can you interpret these paradoxes: "I saw without seeing you"; "Filling with your absence/ my unequal hours"?
3. In line 1, the word *cielo* can have what two meanings in Spanish?

Miller, Brian (student)

Here is a traditional set of instructions for print. A two-column video-script version appears immediately after it. For an introduction to such a script and the abbreviations it may use, see Chapter 4.

CHOOSING THE RIGHT KNEEBOARD:
Print Version

———————————— ✳ ————————————

It isn't hard to get hooked on kneeboarding, because the number of tricks you can do are endless. The ultimate decision in kneeboarding is choosing the right board. Different boards are designed to aid different styles of riding. When choosing a board you should take note of the different characteristics of each make and model.

Most kneeboarding tricks stem from three different categories: cutting, spinning, and getting air. A good board is capable of handling combinations of each of these three categories while some more specialized boards give optimum performance in one category or the other. Different board characteristics determine how the board will handle different types of tricks.

Ted Bevelacqua, known as "Ted the Shred" in kneeboarding circles, has been innovating kneeboard tricks and techniques for the last eighteen years. According to him, "parallel channels, a contoured kneepad, and a convex bottom" [Figure 1 omitted] are all desirable attributes to have if you would like your board to perform flawless cutting maneuvers. Ted explains that the channels are necessary to hold the board in the water during razor sharp turns. According to Ted a contoured kneepad offers more control than a standard flat kneepad and this additional control is necessary when making a rapid change of direction. Ted also feels that a convex bottom is necessary for optimal cutting, "With a spoon-like bottom you can easily roll from edge to edge on your board" (88–89).

David Jennings, the defending world kneeboarding champion, lists "a wide body, a smooth bottom, and a beveled edge" [Figure 2 omitted] as the attributes necessary if you would like your board to perform well during spinning maneuvers. Jennings describes how a wide board offers "stability and balance at all times. This is especially true during spins when you are not sure exactly how you will be landing."A smooth bottom, according to Jennings, is necessary so that "the board runs across the water in whatever direction you want it to go." A beveled edge allows the board to spin. Jennings remarks, "A round edge on the board tends to stick to the wake. It's more forgiving, but if you're glued to the wake you aren't going to be spinning" (91).

Getting air, or leaving the water, on a kneeboard is the heart of many tricks and is also a trick in itself. Kneeboarding legend Mario Fossa believes that "a wide tail, sharp rails, and a convex bottom" [Figure 3 omitted] are the key attributes to look for in a kneeboard if you are looking to get big air. A convex bottom shape is necessary for the same reasons it is helpful when cutting. Fossa adds that a convex shape "will dampen landings too." Fossa also likes a wide tail. "For a kneeboard you ideally want more of a square tail. The wider the better. This puts more of the board's surface on the water, creating more leverage." Fossa also feels that sharp rails are a good attribute to have on a kneeboard: "A board with sharp rails simply rides higher in the water. This makes it much easier for the board to leave the water" (93).

A good all around kneeboard will balance each of these attributes and allow the rider to do tricks in each of these categories. More specialized equipment may vastly improve cutting, spinning, or jumping but will rarely give the maximum performance in all three categories. When purchasing a kneeboard, keep in mind the tricks you would like to achieve and the attributes that make them possible.

Work Cited

Bevelacqua, Ted, David Jennings, and Mario Fossa. "Bent out of Shape." *WaterSki,* June 1995: 88–93.

CHOOSING THE RIGHT KNEEBOARD:
Video-Script Version

✳

by Brian Miller

VIDEO	AUDIO
CU host	Kneeboarding has become one of the most popular water sports in America. Before you hit the water here are a few suggestions about how to choose the right board.

LS Kneeboarding doing tricks	**Host (VO):** Kneeboards come in all shapes and sizes and each different shape and size is suited to different types of performance. Each different type of board is suited to excel in one type of maneuver or another. Most kneeboarding maneuvers can be categorized as cutting maneuvers, spinning maneuvers, or maneuvers to get air.
CU Ted Bevelacqua:	Hi, I'm Ted Bevelacqua, I've been innovating and perfecting kneeboard tricks for the last eighteen years and I'm here to help you choose a kneeboard that will be right for you.
LS Ted cutting hard, sending up spray a mile high	**Ted (VO):** If you are looking for a kneeboard that will cut on a dime then there are a few features you should look for when choosing a kneeboard.
CU kneepad	Check to make sure that the board has a thick, contoured kneepad. This will give you the extra control that is necessary to pull off quick changes in direction.
CU board: bottom	Also if the board has a convex bottom it will give you more stability and control, something which is a necessity for most kneeboarders.
CU board: strap and channels	Other features that you should look for in a board that will cut are a thick, comfortable strap and parallel channels. The strap helps hold you on the board and the channels keep the board on water.
LS David Jennings completing a big 720-degree air	**David Jennings (VO):** I'm David Jennings, the defending kneeboard world champion. If you're looking for a board that will perform flawless spinning maneuvers, you should try to find one with a wide body, a smooth bottom, and a beveled edge.
CU board: top	A wide body will give you stability and balance, both of which are necessary during big spins when you are unsure of exactly how you are going to land.
CU board: bottom	Also a board with a smooth bottom will run across the water in whatever direction you want it to go.
CU board: edge	Look for a board with a beveled edge. A rounded edge may be more forgiving, but rounded edges tend to stick to the wake and if you're glued to the wake you're not going to be spinning.

LS Mario Fossa getting big air	**Mario Fossa (VO):** I'm Mario Fossa, head instructor at Mario Fossa's Kneeboarding School in Tampa, FL. If you are looking for a board that will get big air, choose one with a convex bottom, a wide square tail, and sharp rails.
CU board: convex bottom	A convex bottom will give you stability and control and also help cushion your landings.
CU board: back	A large amount of leverage is necessary if you want to catch big air, so look for a kneeboard that has a wide square tail. This puts more of the board's surface on the water.
CU board: rails	Also look for a board with sharp rails. These help the board ride higher in the water, and if the board is riding higher in the water then it is easier for it to leave the water.
CU host:	Our three experts have given use some good advice on choosing specialized kneeboards by looking at their features and how they perform. It is also important, however, to look at other less specialized equipment.
LS kneeboarders doing tricks	**Host (VO):** The majority of the moderately priced kneeboards on the market are not designed to do only one type of maneuver. Many boards have attributes that allow them to perform any of the three categories of tricks. You should keep this in mind when you choose your kneeboard.

Questions

1. What advantages does each version have? Limitations?
2. Where could Miller use the abbreviation **SOT** (sound on tape)?

Montaigne, Michel de (1533–92)

This essay was probably written between 1572 and 1574. Michel de Montaigne wonders about a cultural assumption, declares a hypothesis, and defends his somewhat outrageous idea.

Like his temperament, his style is more open, inclusive, and exploratory. The translator describes it as "free, oral, informal, personal, concrete, luxuriant in images, organic and spontaneous in order, ranging from the epigrammatic to the rambling and associative . . . " (vi).

From *The Complete Essays of Montaigne*, trans. Donald M. Frame (Stanford University Press, 1958): 81–84.

OF THE CUSTOM OF WEARING CLOTHES

W herever I want to turn, I have to force some barrier of custom, so carefully has it blocked all our approaches. I was wondering in this shivery season whether the fashion of going stark naked in these lately discovered nations is forced on them by the warm temperature of the air, as we say of the Indians and Moors, or whether it is the original way of mankind. Inasmuch as all things under heaven, as Holy Writ says, are subject to the same laws, men of understanding, in considerations like these (where we much distinguish natural from artificial laws), are wont to have recourse to the general order of the world, in which there can be nothing counterfeit.

Now, since everything else is furnished with the exact amount of thread and needle required to maintain its being, it is in truth incredible that we alone should be brought into the world in a defective and indigent state, in a state such that we cannot maintain ourselves without external aid. Thus I hold that, just as plants, trees, animals, all things that live, are naturally equipped with sufficient covering to defend themselves against the injury of the weather,

And therefore everything is covered o'er
With either hide, silk, shells, thick skin, or bark,

LUCRETIUS

so were we; but like those who by artificial light extinguish the light of day, we have extinguished our own means by borrowed means. And it is easy to see that it is custom that makes impossible for us what is not impossible in itself; for of those nations that have no knowledge of clothes, there are some situated under much the same sky as ours; and besides, our most delicate parts are those that are always kept uncovered: eyes, mouth, nose, ears; with our peasants, as with our ancestors, the chest and belly. If we had been born with natural petticoats and breeches, there can be no doubt but that Nature would have armed with a thicker skin the parts she intended to expose to the beating of the seasons, as she has done for the fingertips and the soles of the feet.

Why does this seem hard to believe? Between my way of dressing and that of a peasant of my region I find far more distance than there is between his way and that of a man dressed only in his skin.

How many men, especially in Turkey, go naked as a matter of religion!

Someone or other was asking one of our beggars whom he saw in the depth of winter as cheering in his shirt as someone muffled to the ears in sables, how he could endure it. "And you, sir," he answered, "you have your face uncovered; now, I am all face." The Italians tell this story of the duke of Florence's fool, I think it was: that on his master's inquiring how, so poorly clad, he could bear the cold which he himself had trouble bearing, the fool replied, "Follow my rule, and pile on you all the garments you have, as I do, and you won't suffer from the cold any more than I do." King Massinissa, even in his extreme old age, could not be induced to go with his head covered, however cold, stormy, or rainy it might be. This is also said of the Emperor Severus.

In the battles fought between the Egyptians and the Persians, Herodotus says it was remarked both by others and by himself that of those who remained dead on the field, the skulls of the Egyptians were incomparably harder than those of the Persians, because the latter kept their heads always covered, first with caps and then with turbans, whereas the former kept theirs shaven and bare from infancy.

And King Agesilaus observed until his decrepitude the habit of wearing the same clothing in winter as in summer. Caesar, says Suetonius, always marched at the head of his army, most of the time on foot, head bare, whether it was sunny or raining; and they say as much of Hannibal:

Then with bare head
He met the frenzy of the storm, the falling sky.

SILIUS ITALICUS

A Venetian who stayed in the kingdom of Pegu a long time and has only just come back writes that the men and women there always go barefoot, even on horseback, and with the other parts of the body clothed.

And Plato gives this wonderful advice, for the health of the whole body: to give the head and feet no other covering than that which nature has provided.

The man whom the Poles chose for their kind after ours, and who is in truth one of the greatest princes of our century, never wears gloves, or changes for winter or any weather whatever, the bonnet that he wears indoors.

Whereas I cannot bear to go unbuttoned and untied, the laborers in my neighborhood would feel fettered if they were otherwise. Varro maintains that when it was ordained that we should keep our head uncovered in the presence of the gods or the magistrate, it was done more for our health, and to harden us against the attacks of the weather, than on account of reverence.

And since we are on the subject of cold, and Frenchmen, accustomed to array ourselves in varied colors (not I, for I scarcely wear anything but black or white, in imitation of my father), let us add in another connection that Martin du Bellay says he saw, on the march to Luxemburg, frosts so severe that the supply of wine was cut with hatchets and axes, distributed to the soldiers by weight, and carried away in baskets. And Ovid, very close:

Uncasked, the wines retain the shape of casks,
And lumps are passed around instead of flasks.

OVID

The frosts are so bitter at the mouth of Lake Maeotis that in the same place where Mithridates' lieutenant had fought the enemy dry-footed and defeated them in the winter, he won a naval battle against them the next summer.

The Romans suffered a great disadvantage in their combat with the Carthaginians near Placentia, because they went to the charge with their blood congealed and limbs benumbed with cold, whereas Hannibal had passed out fire throughout his host to warm his soldiers, and distributed oil among each company, so that by anointing themselves they might render their sinews more supple and limber, and encrust their pores against the assault of the air and the freezing wind that was blowing.

The retreat of the Greeks from Babylon into their country is famous for the difficulties and hardships that they had to overcome. This was one: they were met by a terrible blizzard in the mountains of Armenia, and lost all knowledge of the country and the roads. Being quite simply besieged by the storm, they were a day and a night without eating or drinking, most of their animals dead, many of themselves dead, many blinded by the driving hail and the glare of the snow, many crippled in their extremities, many stiff, numb, and immobilized with cold, though still in possession of all their senses.

Alexander saw a nation in which they bury their fruit trees in winter to protect them from the frost.

On the subject of clothing, the king of Mexico changed his clothes four times a day and never put them on again, using his cast-offs for his continual liberalities and rewards; likewise neither pot, nor dish, nor any kitchen or table utensil was ever put before him twice.

Questions

1. Does Montaigne persuade you that "all things that live, are naturally equipped with sufficient covering to defend themselves"? Or at least entice you to peer around the "barrier of custom"?

2. At the beginning of his essay, what feature of the "lately discovered nations" causes him to be "wondering"? (He refers to the native inhabitants of the Americas; "Indian" means those of India or the East Indies.)

3. Does the author's shift from Plato to Poles, near the middle of his essay, seem too random? Do his historical references keep your interest?

4. Do the last few paragraphs stick to the subject? If not, would you agree that since they are charming and not too far from the subject, the digressions are forgivable?

5. Montaigne's original text made no use of paragraphs. Does the editor make divisions at satisfactory points?

"Nomads at Work"

This editorial appeared in the *Christian Science Monitor* on October 14, 1994. It explores a socioeconomic trend that may affect you.

NOMADS AT WORK

When businesses wish to promote a warm and fuzzy image in television ads, they still describe themselves in old-fashioned terms as a family. If they are not, in fact, a dysfunctional family, they seem ready at least to resemble an empty nest these days.

The corporate workplace as a sustained community is being deconstructed by layoffs and downsizing. At the extreme, displaced white-collar workers are becoming a species of itinerant laborers.

A whole new vocabulary has developed to describe the tenuous connections between employees and their employers. Welcome to the floating world of temps, contract workers, leased employees, and just plain free-lancers—a world in which business executives are as likely to be transients as are their former secretaries.

An example of how former rocks of Gibraltar are turning into skipping stones: Xerox has been striking deals in which the giant corporation takes over the mail rooms and print shops of other companies, making them units of Xerox. At the same time, Xerox eliminated its own telecommunications division, outsourcing (to use the new jargon) the operation to Electronic Data Systems—which just happens to be a unit of General Motors.

A state-of-the-art business can have as many outsourced employees as a state-of-the-art automobile has outsourced components. These organizational reshufflings may well prove to be short-lived, to be succeeded by further improvisations.

Observers of this merry-go-round warn that white-collar workers of the future, from the chief executive down, can count on only three to five years in one position—and that's if their performance is first-rate.

So far economists are putting a positive spin on things, making a virtue of adaptability. A broken business family is not the equivalent of a broken family. But the destabilizing of the workplace needs to be considered more seriously, more thoughtfully. It's not enough to hire stress counselors—contract workers no doubt—and assume the problem has been met.

Shared responsibilities and shared rewards, a common purpose, a mutual loyalty—these bonds nurture men and women at work as well as in the home. It would be a sad irony if, just when the family is being reacknowledged as fundamental to society's well-being, the business family should be heedlessly dismembered, leaving the workplace an assembly line of strangers.

Questions

1. Would you describe the mask of this editorial as constructively skeptical? Angrily cynical? Something else?

2. Is the thesis "Workers are becoming nomads?" Or "The destabilizing of the workplace needs to be considered more seriously?" Or both combined in a problem-solution sequence?

3. To what extent does this editorial resemble the meditation form?

4. The writer echoes the title-word "nomads" by using synonyms in paragraphs 2 and 3; what are they?

5. Where does the writer make a concession?

Pitts, Leonard, Jr.

Leonard Pitts, Jr., is a syndicated columnist who writes for the *Miami Herald*. This piece reveals touches of a meditation, a personal essay, and an argument on a topical (current) subject.
Printed in the Myrtle Beach, S.C., *Sun News,* 18 May, 1996: p. 10A.

EXPLAINING RACE TO A CHILD
※

My daughter didn't understand black. She insisted that she was tan. Patiently and with a child's faultless logic, she repeated it, even holding up her arm so I could see for myself.

Hampered by the imperfect logic of adults, I fumbled to correct her. No, I explained, you're black.

It was a conversation that could only happen in America, but I knew it had to be done. She had to be prepared for the day one of her friends, in a fit of pique, said some awful word picked up from the grown-ups.

But even so, some small part of me rebelled at the task of explaining race to a child. Was saddened by the reminder that we haven't yet managed to make it irrelevant.

One hundred years ago this week, the Supreme Court codified that failing into a law that, for the next 58 years, gave backbone to Jim Crow. At the center of the case was a man named Homer Plessy who wound up in a jail while trying to get to Covington, a small town in Louisiana.

The facts of the case were simple. On June 7, 1892, Plessy bought a first-class ticket on the East Louisiana Railway and took a seat in a whites-only coach. In the language of the day, Plessy was an octoroon—one-eighth black.

That was one-eighth too much. He was arrested and charged with violating a Louisiana statute requiring separate accommodations for blacks and whites.

In its ruling, the high court upheld the concept of "equal but separate" facilities. Justices said it was a "fallacy" to think this meant government was calling blacks inferior.

Of course, that's precisely what it meant.

The Plessy case was historic, but it really only sanctioned what was already ingrained in American life. Blacks and whites had never lived side by side in the years before the ruling. For that matter, they haven't been neighbors in the 42 years since the decision was overturned, in the Brown v. Board of Education case.

Some people don't see the problem. Some wonder what is gained when black and white live together. Better to discuss the things that are lost: ignorance and fear.

We trade that weight for wings. We gain a sense of nation that doesn't depend on war or crisis for lifeblood. We draw strength from the fact that we all sing "America" with different accents and dance it with different rhythms.

In theory, at least. We are not yet there in practice. Not even now, a century after the Supreme Court rebuked Homer Plessy, a generation after the Court said we must find a way to live together.

Which is why I felt a little sad at having to wear my little girl down with adult illogic to protect her from the cruelties that are yet to come.

I watch her sometimes as she plays, running across the lawn in a giggling flock of brown and blond children. And I know that while nothing has changed for her, everything, irrevocably, has. That Plessy's lesson is rushing at her, that it will take her innocence, pull her out of the moment of idyll.

And that it will make her forget what it was like to rush laughing across the lawn in the days when she was tan.

Questions

1. What connection does Pitts see between his daughter and Homer Plessy?
2. What distinction does Pitts make between tan and black?
3. Does Pitts state a thesis? Imply one? If so, what might it be?
4. To you, does his perspective as a father add credibility and power? Or detract from what might have been a more objective look?
5. How does the mood of this essay compare to that of "How It Feels to Be Colored Me," by Zora Neale Hurston?

Plato (*ca.* 428–348 or 347)

In this dialogue the great Greek philosopher depicts his teacher, Socrates, in conversation with Phaedrus, who was also a historical person. The subject is the rhetorical art needed by an orator.

From *The Dialogues of Plato*, trans. B. Jowett, 2 vols. (New York: Random, 1937), 1: 233–82. Introduction by Raphael Demos.

FROM *PHAEDRUS*

Socrates. . . . I should like to tell you generally, as far as is in my power, how a man ought to proceed according to rules of art.

Phaedrus. Let me hear.

Socrates. Oratory is the art of enchanting the soul, and therefore he who would be an orator has to learn the differences of human souls— they are so many and of such a nature, and from them come the differences between man and man. Having proceeded thus far in his analysis, he will next divide speeches into their different classes: — "Such and such persons," he will say, "are affected by this or that kind of speech in this or that way," and he will tell you why. The pupil must have a good theoretical notion of them first, and then he must have experience of them in actual life, and be able to follow them with all his senses about him, or he will never get beyond the precepts of his masters. But when he understands what persons are persuaded by what arguments, and sees the person about whom he was speaking in the abstract actually before him, and knows that it is he, and can say to himself, "This is the man or this is the character who ought to have a certain argument applied to him in order to convince him of a certain opinion;" —he who knows all this, and knows also when he should speak and when he should refrain, and when he should use pithy sayings, pathetic appeals, sensational effects, and all the other modes of speech which he has learned;—when, I say, he knows the times and seasons of all these things, then, and not till then, he is a perfect master of his art; but if he fail in any of these points, whether in speaking or teaching or writing them, and yet declares that he speaks by rules of art, he who says "I don't believe you" has the better of him. Well, the teacher will say, is this, Phaedrus and Socrates, your account of the so-called art of rhetoric, or am I to look for another?

Phaedrus. He must take this, Socrates, for there is no possibility of another, and yet the creation of such an art is not easy. (274–75)

Questions

1. Although there is not much interplay between characters in this excerpt, what strengths can the dialogue have over the monologue used by most writing? For exploration? For explanation? For persuasion?
2. What elements could writing adapt from dialogue?

Robinson, Michael H.

Robinson is the director of the National Zoological Park in Washington, D.C. This piece demonstrates the power of verbal symbols to enable reflection, explanation, and persuasion. It appeared as a regular column of *Smithsonian* magazine in 1992 (23.4: 22–24+.)

PHENOMENA, COMMENT AND NOTES

✳

In-flight musings lead to the verdict that our fine feathered friends are not as "birdbrained" as we thought.

I was recently on a nonstop flight from Sydney, Australia, to Los Angeles—the ultimate in voluntary confinement and habitat deprivation. All the best efforts of the airline's in-flight entertainment, beverage and meal service, and efficient flight attendants could not prevent me from ultimately lapsing into depressive ennui. Even the latest Reginald Hill detective story, with Dalziel and Pascoe in full cry, did not stave off the doldrums. So, as always when boredom sets in, I slept.

Every now and again I slipped into that state of reverie where thoughts creep in unannounced. I thought about birds and what *they* might think about on long flights. After all, some birds migrate from pole to pole: that's a lot farther than my boring flight. Is it "flap, flap, glide, look at the stars, check the mental compass, flap, flap, glide, adjust for that wind from starboard, oh my, this is boring"? Probably not. For birds, long-distance flying must be virtually automatic. Flapping, making trim adjustments, varying the wingtip slots, compensating for drift and other behaviors must be like our own mental involvement in swimming, surfing, driving, horseback riding or hang gliding, where conscious control is minimal once the learning stage is passed. Driving a car in city traffic is a fearsomely complex process, but while doing it we listen to music, sing along or even (in my case) "write" mental essays. Do birds fantasize while flying?

These thoughts were clearly wild or perhaps delusional, but then I started thinking about intelligence in animals, cognition and consciousness. The epithet "birdbrain" is meant as condemnation: but are birds really stupid? Do they learn? Can they think? What about the size of the bird's brain?

The issue of brain size is not a simple one. For a start, most birds are small-brained because most birds are small. The physiology and mechanics of muscle-powered flight has restricted the size of birds. The biggest flying birds with the biggest brains—but not the greatest mental capabilities—are the earthbound ratites: flightless striders and runners such as ostriches, rheas, cassowaries and kiwis.

When all is said and done, absolute brain size is not the measure of "braininess." Big bodies need more control tissue but not necessarily more thinking power. Thinking power makes for big brains in small bodies. The real test is the proportion of brain size to body mass (weight). Weight for weight, comparisons do index "intelligence." But even this kind of comparison can be misleading. Flying birds are built for lightness, with hollow bones and generally low-mass structural components. This skews the brain-body comparison in their favor. The flightless birds score lower than the flying birds on relative brain size. Flight-related lightness of structure in birds also affects comparisons with other vertebrates. Bearing in mind this positive bias, it is true that the brains of birds overlap those of many mammals, although not the primates.

Birds group with the mammals in their distinct separation from the fishes and reptiles. In proportion to body weight, the bird brain is 5 to 20 times larger than the reptile brain. Thus reptiles, successful as they are, rank distinctly lower than mammals and birds. "Fish-brain" and "lizard head" are much more appropriate derogatory epithets than "birdbrain."

The dinosaurs, from which the birds are descended, don't fare any better than other reptiles when it comes to brains. Some, of course, had huge masses of nerve tissue in the sacral (hip) region. Some wag claimed that this enabled them "to think a *posteriori* as well as a *priori*." However, the sacral nerve mass was probably responsible for the control of the hindparts, distant from the head, and not for higher functions. It would be fun, though, if we could accept the possibility of dinosaurian afterthoughts. For all these reasons, alas, as an insult "birdbrained" does not stand the biological test. The avian brain is not of inferior relative size. Or at least it passes muster for relative size compared with rabbits, cats, dogs and other nonprimates.

Certain families of birds are distinguished by their lower-than-average brain-body ratio. Ostriches, gallinaceous birds (chickens and the like) and pigeons have the lowest relative brain weights, while the parrot and crow families score high. No wonder the raven quoth "Nevermore."

But what about brains in the sense of "brightness," "intelligence" or "cleverness"? All these terms have an immediate meaning for us but are extraordinarily difficult to define. If called upon to define them most of us would quote examples. We would refer to people or behaviors that exemplify the possession of these attributes or define their opposites. "Stupidity" is a good catchall opposite. For most of us it is an inability to solve problems or to learn.

In practical terms, for most people, stupidity is exemplified in inflexible persistence in inappropriate courses of behavior. When I try to open the almost identical door of the apartment on the floor vertically below mine, that is unthinking behavior. If I persist and then kick the door down, that is stupidity. If I examine the door and realize my mistake, that is intelligence. This is an operational definition.

Are birds stupid? Most definitely not. They have some quite remarkable learning abilities. My friend Juan Delius, an ethologist with a strong interest in both neurophysiology and experimental psychology, has spent much of his life studying the ability of pigeons to learn complex discriminations and solve problems. One of his discoveries is that pigeons can be taught to distinguish bilaterally symmetrical patterns from bilateral images that are nonsymmetrical. After conditioning they can distinguish between patterns that they have never seen before, when the only variable is in symmetry. Abandoning scientific caution, one could conclude that during the training the birds had developed a "concept" of symmetry. Certainly Delius uses the word in this connection. To me that suggests a

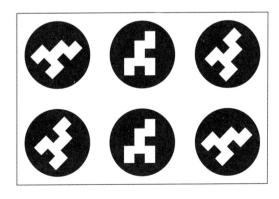

quite complex degree of cleverness. The ability to form concepts is surely a hallmark of intelligence.

Delius and his coworkers also found that pigeons can be taught to solve inversion problems faster and more reliably than many humans can. Inversion problems are those that involve recognizing a complex figure when it is inverted (or rotated) and distinguishing it from its similarly inverted mirror image. Thus the letter E can be rotated through 45, 90 and 180 degrees before returning to its normal orientation. We can quickly recognize these inversions from the back-to-front E. However, we have much more difficulty in spotting inversions of unfamiliar objects.

Test yourself using the illustration above. Trained pigeons can do these tasks quickly and reliably. In real life it must be useful for a pigeon to recognize its loft from whatever angle it may see it as it navigates homeward. Navigation is another function of the pigeon brain involving complex powers of computation—but that is another story. There seems little doubt that some birds have an unnamed number concept. They can count, at least up to seven. Erle Stanley Gardner, prolific creator of Perry Mason, titled one of his detective stories *Crows Can't Count,* but they can. (Look for it under Gardner's pseudonym "A. A. Fair.")

Many birds do many things with minimal learning. They seem to be hardwired to fly, build nests and so on. Complex learning has been recognized, however, in a wide variety of circumstances ranging through singing, parent recognition, chick recognition, mate recognition and species recognition. Some bird species learn song dialects but not the basic patterns of the songs, their basic "tunes." Among the song learners there are species that learn dialects when young and do not use them until they are mature. There is good evidence that some gull species learn the personal call of their parents while they are still developing in the egg. Playing recorded birdcalls to incubating eggs has proved this.

Even more interesting is the phenomenon of imprinting. Many ducklings and goslings learn to recognize their parents (and their species' characteristics) in a short period of intensive learning while very young. This is an economical and efficient process. Such imprinting works well in nature because the young birds respond to the appropriate objects, their parents. Human interference, however, can produce a totally inappropriate response. A young goose can be provided with a proximal non-goose to follow and imprint upon. Goslings will imprint on crouching, quacking and waddling humans, and follow them around as if they were geese. Such imprinting on a pseudoparent may affect the animal long after its infancy. The bizarre result may be that when the gosling becomes a goose or gander, it may make sexual advances to humans rather than to its own species (*Smithsonian,* April 1990). We wise humans might dismiss such behavior as stupid, but it is really a pointed example of learning that is tailored to natural needs and is not profligate or energetically wasteful.

Returning to my in-flight musings, birds may or may not fantasize, but they certainly do not deserve condemnation for their brains. There's a piece of doggerel: "Happy little moron, doesn't give a damn. / Thankfully I'm not a moron; oh dear, perhaps I am!" We should think about our own capacities and recognize that we are blind to many of our inadequacies. Would we, or could we, know if there were some parts of our behavior that were unalterable by learning? I doubt it. Or what if, for some kinds of learning, there were a sensitive period after which we were imprinted, doomed forever to respond to an irrelevant stimulus? We may discover our limitations only by studying our cohabitants of this planet that we disregard and mutilate so often.

Questions

1. To your way of responding, does Robinson fully amalgamate his exploration, explanation, and persuasion?
2. What kind of audience does the writer assume for this piece? How zoologically expert? Why do you think so?
3. Can you distinguish the two main phases of Robinson's argument, each one comprising a series of paragraphs?
4. What does Robinson think is implied by a pigeon's ability to recognize complex figures when they are inverted? Do you agree?
5. To what extent would Robinson's definition of *stupidity* as "inflexible persistence in inappropriate courses of behavior" apply to the cavemanlike neighbor as portrayed in Robert Frost's "Mending Wall?"

Roosevelt, Franklin D. (1882–1945)

It was incontestably an invasion when, 449 years after Columbus landed from Europe, airborne marauders from Asia attacked U.S. territory.

Responding quickly, President Franklin Delano Roosevelt delivered a speech to the Congress. A deliberative oration, a type that urges the

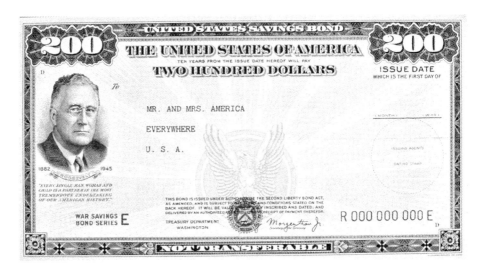

WAR BOND WITH FDR'S PORTRAIT ON IT

body politic to take a certain course of action, it led up to a request that Congress declare war. Roosevelt, despite and probably because of the supercharged atmosphere, composed a text that systematically laid out facts and logically drew a conclusion from them. Minus his patrician accent and commanding voice, this bare transcript highlights his verbal craftsmanship.

Originally printed in the *Congressional Record,* 77th Congress, 1st Session, Volume 87, Part 9, pp. 9504–9505, December 8, 1941.

SPEECH TO CONGRESS

Yesterday, December 7, 1941—a date which will live in infamy—the United States of America was suddenly and deliberately attacked by naval and air forces of the Empire of Japan.

The United States was at peace with that nation and, at the solicitation of Japan, was still in conversation with its government and its Emperor, looking toward the maintenance of peace in the Pacific. Indeed, one hour after Japanese air squadrons had commenced bombing in Oahu, the Japanese Ambassador to the United States and his colleague delivered to the Secretary of State a formal reply to a recent American message. While this reply stated that it seemed useless to continue the existing diplomatic negotiations, it contained no threat or hint of war or armed attack.

It will be recorded that the distance of Hawaii from Japan makes it obvious that the attack was deliberately planned many days or even weeks ago. During the intervening time the Japanese government had deliberately sought to deceive the United States by false statements and expressions of hope for continued peace.

The attack yesterday on the Hawaiian Islands has caused severe damage to American naval and military forces. Very many American lives have been lost. In addition, American ships have been reported torpedoed on the high seas between San Francisco and Honolulu.

Yesterday the Japanese government also launched an attack against Malaya.

Last night Japanese forces attacked Hong Kong.

Last night Japanese forces attacked Guam.

Last night Japanese forces attacked the Philippine Islands.

Last night the Japanese attacked Wake Island.

This morning the Japanese attacked Midway Island.

Japan has, therefore, undertaken a surprise offensive extending throughout the Pacific area. The facts of yesterday speak for themselves. The people of the United States have already formed their opinions and well understand the implications to the very life and safety of our nation.

As Commander-in-Chief of the Army and Navy I have directed that all measures be taken for our defense.

Always will we remember the character of the onslaught against us.

No matter how long it may take us to overcome this premeditated invasion, the American people in their righteous might will win through to absolute victory.

I believe I interpret the will of the Congress and of the people when I assert that we will not only defend ourselves to the uttermost but will make very certain that this form of treachery shall never endanger us again.

Hostilities exist. There is no blinking at the fact that our people, our territory, and our interests are in grave danger.

With confidence in our armed forces—with the unbounded determination of our people—we will gain the inevitable triumph—so help us God.

I ask that the Congress declare that since the unprovoked and dastardly attack by Japan on Sunday, December 7, a state of war has existed between the United States and the Japanese Empire.

Questions

1. Since there was little or no resistance to overcome in his audience, what purpose(s) might Roosevelt have had in mind for the indirect sequence?

2. Roosevelt uses repetition of initial words dramatically in "Last night. . . . Last night. . . ." This technique was named "anaphora" by Greek rhetoricians. Where is it used by the advertisement shown in Figure 7.1? To you, does the technique seem to recall oratory?

Ruffin, Kimberly N.

As a graduate student at the University of Illinois-Chicago, Ms. Ruffin wrote this commentary for *Essence* Magazine, whose primary readership is African-American females. Volume 26, number 4 (August 1995): 130. Copyright Essence Communications, Inc., 1995.

Do You Hear What I Hear?

✳

"Flexxxx, time to have sex!" is what my 7-year-old cousin Tina belted out as she danced provocatively through the living room. I was embarrassed by her radio sing-along and her adult dance style. But before I could come up with a response, her older brother, Lil' Ray, rushed into the room urging us to turn to the local rap music station.

This "listening session" prompted me to contemplate the ongoing debate about what has been demonized in the media as hard-core, or "gangsta," rap. The critics of hard-core rap loudly and aptly assert that it promotes violent images to our youths. It is time, however, that we also challenge the air-worthiness of sex-obsessed R&B and dance-hall reggae material played on today's radio stations. The references to lickin', pumpin', sweatin', freakin', sexin', tastin', lovin', bumpin', feelin', rubbin' and grindin' are much more plentiful, more popular and arguably more debilitating than hard-core rap material. If the current playlists of Black popular-music radio stations were representative of Black life, it would appear that most of us had sex all day long!

The outcry against sexually explicit lyrics has a long tradition in African-American history. When "down-home blues" was the nemesis of the moment during the 1920's, certain sectors of the community rose up in arms about the supposed moral decay resulting from sex-drenched lyrical content.

Today many Black organizations have banned (and even bulldozed) certain gangsta-rap releases to spread consumer awareness.

Unfortunately, confining "hot" songs to late-night Quiet Storm shows would probably be as ineffective as Prohibition was in the fight to curb alcohol consumption.

I am not suggesting that sexuality be silenced for social asceticism. But is it too much to ask that popular Black radio play thematically diverse music that reflects the complexity of our lives?

Many contemporary artists are proving that celebrating Black survival on wax can be accomplished, and with mass appeal. Des'ree's recent anthem of self-respect, "You Gotta Be," hit number five on the Billboard charts. Earlier this year, Queen Latifah won a Grammy for Best Rap Solo Performance for "U.N.I.T.Y."—her call for collective responsibility.

Likewise, Arrested Development's recent single, "I Need Some Time to Ease My Mind," rocks the beat while emphasizing the importance of mental health. The Sounds of Blackness call for a strong connection to spirituality in their song "I Believe." And rapper KRS-ONE promotes social advancement through hip-hop with his concept of "edutainment."

With violence against women as well as teenage pregnancy on the rise in our community, Black women should be able to envision their self-worth beyond their sexuality. Black men need to understand that controlling women's lives is no way to be a man. Both of these ideals can be cultivated through music that advances a nonobsessive and nonviolent view of sex and romance.

In isolation, the lyrical content of Top 40 songs may seem harmless, but because these songs echo themes of sexual domination in our culture, they become the sound track of our lives. Meanwhile, many progressive songs remain buried on artists' releases, never to be heard on radio. Yet there is hope: A simple phone call to your local "request line" for an uplifting song every now and then can make an impact.

As consumers we should ask that more attention be paid to music celebrating a full range of our experiences, for our children and for ourselves. Our need for music that validates a wide spectrum of our lives does not end with childhood.

African-Americans of all ages need to hear life affirming songs that prove Nikki Giovanni's contention that "Black love is Black wealth." After all, Black love does extend beyond what happens between the sheets!

Questions

1. How do paragraphs 1 and 2 resemble the beginning of a Meditation as described in Chapter 2? What would be lost if Ruffin, instead of describing the family scene, had begun with sentence 5 ("The critics of hard-core rap . . .")?
2. What is her thesis? What change does she recommend?
3. What does she assume about her audience by using a few difficult words (e.g., *debilitating, nemesis,* and *asceticism*)?
4. What function does she envision for music in the paragraph on violence and teenage pregnancy?
5. Does her "sound track" metaphor (in the paragraph beginning "In isolation . . .") seem apt?

Smith, Ronald V. (student)

Can people still enjoy an almost extinct form of mass media, the silent movie? Yes, according to the persuasive drift of this explanation. Like any a good personal essay it has a personal "voice"—perhaps ironical, considering the topic.

THE ART OF WATCHING SILENT FILMS

✳

Viewing silent movies can be rather annoying—after all, there are so many subtitles to read. And there are so many good movies with sound tracks. But the old-time silent movies can be something different to do, and they can be a good social experience. A few techniques will help the watcher get more out of them.

If you can sit through a two-hour Hollywood movie without falling asleep; or if you are the type of person who can sit through a long church service without dozing in the pew; or if you can cross-stitch or needlepoint for hours; or if paint-by-number is your hobby—then you are a good candidate for patience. If you fidget during a half-hour sitcom, better leave these types of art films alone.

It is important in silent film that the film be of the correct projection speed. It wasn't until the Seventies and Eighties that cinema studios even remembered that the silent film crews used a different camera speed. Usually, when silents were first transferred, the film ran so fast that even the greatest tragedies were still comical to look at. That funny fluttering that is typical of the wrong projection speed did not occur in early cinema. The Kinetograph (as it was called then) ran at a speed of 46 frames per second. This was later reduced, with the shutter, to 15–18 frames per second and this resulted in no flutter.

It is well advised to watch these genre films with a friend or many friends. These types of films rely on heavy symbolism—for example, a black-clad figure usually suggested death. Without friends around, this symbolism may be missed by the single viewer. Symbolism isn't always an easy target to grasp. Any previous knowledge of symbolism is a plus. Art films are fraught with symbolism that can be talked about.

These films also rely on heavy audience participation. People used to "cut up" during these films all the time—these films were hardly silent! *Rocky Horror Picture Show* is not unique—it had nothing on the silents. Don't feel bad about stopping the movie to discuss something; with VCR's this is easy to do. In fact, most foreign films are usually rented and it is doubtful that you'll ever see a silent film on the big screen anymore.

Any knowledge of art is also important. You will see cities and backgrounds that are so expressionistic they will boggle the senses. These expressionistic works tend to reflect feelings of despair and anxiety, and tormented or exalted states of mind. In them, images of the real world are transformed so that they correspond with these feelings or states of mind by subjective, often intense coloring, distortion of form, strong lines and dramatic contrasts. These devices were used as money was often times not available, so artisans were used to mark out pseudo-villages or towns. Germany was most famous for its expressionistic sets and the films, *The Cabinet of Dr. Caligari* and *Metropolis* being the most commonly used examples. Some art background gives more pleasure to viewing these make-believe cities and buildings. After all, these are "art films," so termed by the artisans who invented them.

There will be times during a silent film that there will be no title cards, yet the characters are still talking. What are they saying? That is for the audience to decide. Many times the language will be simple gestures to convey meaning and definition. Body talk was quite useful to silent film stars; Zasu Pitts was probably the most prolific. Also there will be scenes on top of scenes and fancy editing was done to strongly portray the mood or tone of the scene.

If you laboriously say "I'm going to **have** to watch a silent film," then the event may become boring and laborious. And if you don't like the original silent's soundtrack, usually a solo organ accompaniment, then turn off the television's volume. Put on whatever type of music you enjoy in the background. Approach the event with patience and popcorn: you might like it so much you'll come back for more.

Questions

1. In a revision, Ronald Smith added details in at least two areas of this paper, projection speeds and expressionism. Does this information improve clarity? Do you understand both sections? Should the writer acknowledge any sources?

2. Does Smith "project" this explanation at the right speed? In other words, does he present information in small enough increments for the brain to process it?

Stanton, Jamie L. (student)

From pain to perception: A meditation undertaken on the scratchy carpet.

FALLING SHORT

—✳—

The cinder block wall feels cold against my sweating back while the scratchy carpet pokes at my hot, bare legs. I can feel a slight thud as the ball is smashed off the rear wall by a sturdy racquet. Its sounds echo off the faces of the six-sided box and into the hall, which is quiet except for my embarrassing sobs. The boys continue to play with the same intensity, the same drive, I had until a few moments ago. Now I sit shivering, sprained ankle and bruised ego throbbing, crying tears of anguish against a cold wall.

Why do I go on doing this to myself? Is the fun of a good game really worth all the injuries? Are the games really fun or is it the challenge I'm after? I can remember when Uncle George put up the basketball hoop in our yard; competition has been thriving in my life ever since. I always wanted to be the best—the best athlete, the best student, the best friend.

However, I never quite reached the heights of which I dreamed. I fell just short of valedictorian, most valuable player, and being someone's best friend. Yet I was still the best—the best I could be.

I often wonder what goals have slipped from the grasps of those who were valedictorians and most valuable players and "best friends." There has to be something they've wanted and lost. But I would like to believe that those people do not let their missed goals get in their way. Rather, they set new goals and keep striving despite life's misfortunes. The achievers don't feel sorry for themselves and sit around thinking about what could have or should have been. They get up and make other things happen. And whatever they do, they give it all they've got.

Then what makes these people so special? Doesn't everyone live this way, to life's fullest? No? What a shame. Those who don't, have to live with knowing that they could have done better. They will always sit and wonder, "What if I had really tried?" Until those people understand the idea that anything worth doing is worth doing right, they will continue to drown in "What if's," and their wasted potential is certainly a pitiful sight.

On the other hand, if people do give their all and yet fail, they can rest assured in the fact that they did their best and don't have to worry over "What if?"

Whether people give up or keep trying to reach their goals is up to them. But if they live by the motto, "a winner never quits and a quitter never wins," I don't think they'll feel much like giving in.

So why don't I get back to the game. After all, it's just a little sprain I got while trying my best.

Thrash, Kyle (student)

Notice a tension between foreboding title and lighthearted tone.

INFERNO

———*———

This story begins on Sunday, October 30. My sister, Alison, myself, and our friend Chris were arriving at a party thrown by my friend Damon. Walking up to the backyard we passed several of our friends—Supergirl, General Lee, bellydancers, aliens, and Mr. Furley. Damon's backyard is very large. It starts next to the road with about a hundred feet of grass, containing a jungle gym, followed by a pool area with patio. Everyone was gathered around the pool, with a thicker concentration surrounding the keg. Like proper party animals, we bee-lined it to the keg. Much to our pleasure, the keg was full of nice, ice cold Icehouse, our favorite.

Before we could get settled, I noticed someone starting a fire over in the grass area. The person, realizing it was a sorry attempt, grabbed one of those red, plastic gasoline containers and doused the tiny flames. This yielded spectacular results. What was once a patch of smoke was now a raging fire—including the creator's hand and the gas container held by it. The person, who I now realized was Tony, threw the container down and extinguished his hand. The can, however, remained burning.

By this time everyone was yelling at Tony to put the gas container out; it was really burning by now. Tony turned around, grabbed it, and tossed it into the pool. The container was now floating around, full of gas and shooting flames. People were beginning to get scared. The container would eventually melt and expose the gas to open flames. What to do?! As the container floated around the pool, shooting flames and charring the edges, our friend Collin decided, out of drunkenness I imagine, to poke it with a stick. The little poke punctured the container and unleashed the gasoline. As the gas spread over the pool, the flames followed.

Half the pool was now a certifiable inferno, shooting flames up to about ten feet and generating heat that drove everyone away from the patio. The fire also created some of the most toxic smoke I have ever inhaled. Only the bravest party animal dared make a run for the keg.

I retreated to the house, like most everyone else, and continued to party. I sat next to the kitchen window and watched the fire from a safe distance. After twenty minutes the inferno was reduced to a small, flaming glob of plastic, floating around the pool. A weird film of gas and melted plastic coated the pool. The icky film, combined with the charred edges, made for a realistic toxic sludge costume for the pool.

Questions

1. Does the "costume" metaphor in the last sentence help to make art from chaos? By contrast, how would this literal version work: "The icky film . . . made toxic sludge"?

2. In a revision of "Inferno," how could Kyle give the reader more raw information about the shape, height, color, and motion of the flames?

3. Where could the author present some dialogue?

4. If the gas can has just been thrown into the pool and is now floating, does Kyle need to add "around the pool"? If the heat is driving everyone away, does he need to call it "unbearable"?

5. Can you isolate four different mistakes with fire that heat up the story?

Walker, Gary E., and Diana Jo Wilson (students)

The novel *Little Women*, by Louisa May Alcott, was published in 1869. In 1994 the third movie version of the book appeared, and a novelization of the film was published for middle school readers. The author was Laurie Lawlor.

Having read an excerpt from this novelization, two students in Advanced Composition rewrote part of the original story that corresponded to it (pp. 165–66). Alcott had set this phase of the book in the autumn. For the original segment of the novel, see Alcott, above.

HEAT IN THE ATTIC

Jo was very uncomfortable in the garret. The long July afternoons spread out with the sun beating on the roof of the attic all day long, warming her little space to an almost unbearable temperature. Each day she could be found working feverishly on her papers, sprawled on the sofa with her bodice undone to catch the cooling breeze that gently circulated from the high window.

This day was the hottest day of the summer and Jo felt that the garret could easily substitute for an oven, implying of course that she herself could substitute for the bread dough, a sentiment that was once again echoed as she slowly wiped the perspiration from her forehead. Jo put aside her writing for the moment and leisurely rose from the sofa. She moved toward the window where she stood upon the small wooden stool beneath it, hoping to catch a soft wind that would provide her with some measure of relief, but the air which greeted her was still, resonating with the same heat which mercilessly strove to drive her mad.

Her eyes panned across the scene before her, briefly resting on Laurie's house. She noticed the heat rising from his roof and seemed to feel a similar ardor radiating outward from her own body. Once again Jo laced up her bodice, sounding a sigh of frustration.

"Why can't women be like men?" she said to herself. "They're lucky. They get to wear loose-fitting shirts and trousers; while we women must try and survive the heat in these ridiculous petticoats and ruffles."

At that moment, Jo walked toward the dusted mirror in the corner of the garret as she simultaneously buttoned the last button on her white cotton dress. She needed to check her appearance before leaving her hideaway.

While Jo wiped her forehead again she noticed reflected in the mirror an antique water basin sitting upon her mother's sewing desk.

"Ah-ha!" she thought, "that's what will beat this heat," and quickly ran downstairs to the kitchen. Once she got there she purloined a bucket from the pantry and hung it over the spout of the black iron water pump. The kitchen, while cooler than the garret, was still terribly warm, and Jo pumped the long handle furiously, the water spurting out of the spout in bursts to quickly fill the bucket to overflowing.

Jo looked around the kitchen briefly, finding a clean hand towel which she tucked in the tie of her apron before lifting the bucket out of the sink and trundling it unevenly back up to the attic. There she tried ever so hard to be careful pouring the cold water into the basin, but despite her best efforts she managed to slosh a generous portion onto the floor. She started to clean it up, only to stand amazed as the water quickly dried up, soaking into the parched wood and evaporating into the hot, dusty air.

Jo dipped a corner of the hand towel into the cold water and daubed the moisture on her fevered brow. She sighed with disappointment as it failed to make an impression on the heat which suffused her, seemingly trapped beneath the thick layers of her clothing to torment her. Jo came to an internal decision, realizing that what she was about to do controverted the social mores of her family, and locked the garret door.

Returning to the washbasin, Jo delicately unfastened the buttons of her dress, folding it neatly on the sewing table. This done, her two petticoats soon joined it, along with her shoes and stockings, leaving her clad in only her bloomers and a tight-fitting camisole which mounted to a lacy frill at her neck and shoulders. She again doused the cloth in the cold well water, wringing it out over her upturned face with a slow twist that dripped the water across the sun-dappled cheeks and down her chin. Jo swabbed the water over her, feeling the much needed relief from the confines of her clothes and the oppressive heat. Refreshed, she returned to her writing.

She channeled this new energy into the lives of her characters, instilling them with a life which, heretofore, they had lacked. They became organic, possessed of an individuality and intelligence which seemed to have nothing at all to do with her, and everything to do with them. She rushed toward the climax of her story, her mind forming tantalizing images of the hero (who looked for all the world like Laurie) that elicited girlish giggles from her as her pen scratched across the paper.

As she penned the last lines, she became aware of the fact that she had grown unbearably hot again, though the heat was accompanied on this occasion by a strong flushing of her skin. She began to wonder if she didn't have the beginnings of a case of heatstroke. She walked, somewhat unsteady, to the sewing table to bring back the bucket of revitalizing water.

Jo filled the basin and seated herself, leaning back against the arm of the sofa, to stretch out in the intense sunbeam which streamed through the attic's single round window. She filled her cloth again and wrung it out, quickly this time, opening her mouth to catch the water. Suddenly a thrush landed with an abrupt back-paddling of air on the sill of the window, startling her. Her mouth contracted in an O of surprise and water squirted out in a thick stream.

Jo laughed heartily at her appearance and, in that moment, disaster struck. One of her arms, let fall where it would in her mirth, landed on the edge of the basin which tipped over suddenly into her lap, soaking her bloomers and the tails of her camisole.

She jumped up from the couch in a shock, struggling with her soaking clothes. First the camisole dropped to the floor with a wet flap, then, after a pitched battle, the bloomers followed dropping rivulets of lukewarm water onto her bare feet and the boards beneath them. Jo looked up with an exasperated expression on her face. What would she tell her mother?

Suddenly she was struck by the sight of what she thought, at first, was another woman in the garret with her. Her fears subsided just as quickly when she realized it was only her reflection in the full-length dressing mirror. For a moment she was unable to move, captivated by the almost unique sight of her naked body. Standing, as she was, in the full sunbeam, she cut an exquisite figure, her auburn hair pulled back into a single tail and her long, white limbs brought into sharp relief.

Questions

1. Does the interplay among kinds of heat—meteorological, sexual, and creative—seem artful to you?

2. Which images, whether sensory or figurative, seem most powerful?

3. The writers occasionally supply information that should be obvious from the context—for example, "warming her little space to an almost unbearable *temperature*" instead of "warming her little space unbearably." Can you underline phrasing that you would compress or cut in a revision so as to heighten intensity? (Do you agree with the student who thought that the last sentence in the paragraph beginning "Jo dipped a corner" should be condensed to "Jo locked the garret door"?)

4. Where could the writers go into more detail, if anywhere?

5. What is the significance of Jo's particular style of clothing?

Will, George F.

A syndicated columnist, George Will wrote this essay shortly after an earthquake struck the San Francisco area in 1989.

Although Will forecasts a discussion of three "lessons," he declines to announce each as it comes up, thus preserving a sense of seamless thought.

The column was reprinted in *Suddenly: the American Idea Abroad and at Home* (New York: Free Press, 1990): 11–12.

TEARING THE SOCIAL THREADS

※

San Francisco's geography is histrionic—its fogs can be as spectacular as the vistas they obscure—and its geology is downright dangerous. On Tuesday (October 17) that geology taught the nation three lessons. They concern the predictability of some surprises, the sovereignty of nature and the web of dependencies that define civic life.

The earth's shell is composed of numerous plates from 45 to 95 miles thick, slowly migrating. North America—The United Plates of America, as a geologist calls it—is united only for now. This "collage of wandering fragments" (geologists are phrasemakers) may disperse to form new aggregations in a few hundred million years.

Meanwhile, California straddles two plates, one moving south, the other north. No good can come of this. Sudden slippages between plates produce quakes, and not only in the West.

Quakes around New Year, 1811–12, near New Madrid, Missouri, reached perhaps 8.8 on today's Richter scale. They reversed the flow of the Mississippi, altered its course, caused waves in the Earth several feet high and rang church bells in Boston. Last November, a 6.0 quake hit rural Quebec. In 1983, a 6.5 quake shattered Coalinga, California. The scale is logarithmic: San Francisco's 1906 quake (8.3) was 90 times more powerful than Coalinga's and less powerful than Alaska's 1964 quake (8.4).

There are between 2,500 and 10,000 measurable tremors during a normal day on this fidgety planet. (Instruments can measure ground movements the size of an oxygen molecule.) Big quakes are rare. They also are certainties.

Earth sciences predicted the 1980 eruption of Mount St. Helens and six months ago **Science** magazine examined evidence that "dangerous quakes are closing in on the San Francisco area." A 1976 quake in China killed 400,000, but in 1975 the evacuation of a Chinese city in response to a correct prediction saved an estimated 100,000 lives. As a predictive science, seismology is still developing, but it suggests that a big quake is highly likely in eastern America within 30 years.

Tuesday's quake should concentrate minds. One-tenth of all Americans live in California. One-quarter of the semiconductor industry is in one county near the San Andreas fault. About 47,000 Americans die each year in motor vehicle accidents, the equivalent of a major plane crash every day. An 8-strength quake—smaller than 1906, larger than 1989—could kill that many in 15 minutes. Only 60 people died when Charleston, South Carolina, shook for eight minutes in 1886, but people then did not live in high-rise structures over natural gas lines and downwind from chemical plants.

An earthquake once shook the Western mind. It struck Lisbon on All Saints' Day, 1755, killing thousands in churches and thousands more who, fleeing to the seashore, were drowned by a tidal wave. It was as though nature were muttering "Oh, really? Says who?" in response to mankind's expanding sense of mastery. The quake was an exclamation point inserted arbitrarily into the Age of Reason, raising doubts about the beneficence of the universe and God's enthusiasm for the Enlightenment.

In this secular age, when the phrase "acts of God" denotes only disasters, we still can learn lessons from them. One of the striking vignettes from television coverage of the aftermath of San Francisco's quake was a policeman exhorting citizens to "go home and prepare for 72 hours without services." Perhaps no electricity, no gas, no running water for three days. Of course mankind lived for millennia without any of those. Today, however, our well-being depends on a network of many systems too easily taken for granted.

The words *civic, civil, citizen* have a common root. They originally pertained to residents of cities. It is in these complex creations—cities—that we see the truth of the phrase "social fabric." Any community, but especially a modern city, is a rich weave of diverse threads. The strength of each thread is derived from its relation to the rest. All the threads can snap or unravel when the fabric is ripped by jagged events. San Francisco's fabric has been strained but not torn.

From any catastrophe some good can come. It is no bad thing to be reminded—the world relentlessly sees to this—of the fragility of all social arrangements. Americans, for whom individualism is instinctive, need periodic reminders that their individual pursuits of happiness are utterly dependent upon the functioning of civic, collective community institutions—government—and upon habits of civility of the sort San Franciscans showed in their crisis. An earthquake is a tough teacher but it tells the truth.

Questions

1. Bursting with geological facts and numbers, this piece is still an essay. Where does it give you a sense of the author's personality. In vocabulary? In breadth of reference? In values?

2. Can you set off the three main sections by putting a bracket in the margin next to each?

3. Why do you think Will has used this particular order for his "lessons"?

4. Will repeats key words or ideas to tighten the connection between his first paragraph and the body of the essay. What word or idea in the introduction do these words echo:

   "geologist" (paragraph 2)
   "certainties" (paragraph 5)
   "predicted" (paragraph 6)
   "nature" (paragraph 8)
   "network" (paragraph 9)
   "civic," "fabric," and "weave" (paragraph 10)
   "dependent" (paragraph 11)?

5. Does the following assertion seem to endorse Will's third lesson?

There seems to be a growing realization that a society that values individual fulfillment above all else is a scary place to live—for adults as well as children. The web of obligation, commitment and responsibility—call it family—is our true safety net.

Joanne Jacobs, San Jose, C.A., *Mercury News*. Quoted in *The Charlotte* (North Carolina) *Observer* 1 December 1996: C-1.

CREDITS

Page 6: Excerpt from interview of Janie B. Johnson by Horry County Oral History Project.

Page 15: Excerpt from "Quetzalcóatl," in *Micropaedia*. Reprinted with permission from *Encyclopaedia Britannica*, 15th edition, © 1990 by Encyclopaedia Britannica, Inc.

Page 17: Excerpt, program note in the Pacific Film Archive series, "Classic Mexican Cinema," *University Art Museum and Pacific Film Archive; Calendar,* January/February 1994; University of California at Berkeley; © Regents of the University of California.

Page 17: Fig. 1.1, "Santa" (Rafael Calderon, 1932), Movie Poster, Courtesy of the Academy of Motion Picture Arts and Sciences.

Page 19: Excerpt from *Andele, the Mexican-Kiowa captive: a story of real life among the Indians* by J.J. Methvin, University of New Mexico Press, 1996. Originally published *Andele, or, The Mexican-Kiowa Captive.* Louisville, KY.: Pentecostal Herald Press, 1899.

Page 41: "Talking Dust Bowl" (Talking Dust Blues). Words and music by Woody Guthrie, 1960 (Renewed), 1963 (Renewed), Ludlow Music Inc., New York, New York. Used by permission.

Page 49: Excerpt from Donald C. Stewart, "The Meditation," in *The Versatile Writer,* © 1986 by D.C. Heath and Company. Reprinted by permission of Houghton Mifflin Company.

Page 50: "Multiple Identity: The Healthy, Happy Human Being Wears Many Masks," by Kenneth J. Gergen. Reprinted with permission from *Psychology Today Magazine,* copyright © 1972 (Sussex Publishers, Inc.).

Page 58: Fig. 2.2, Wooden mask with abalone inlay. Ft. Rupert. Kwakiutl tribe (Northwest Coast). Acquired by Emmons in 1929. H 41.6 cm. × w 30.5 cm. © Steve Myers 1988 A.M.N.H. 16.1 (1872).

Pages 58, 245: Excerpt from Ellen Goodman, "Planning on the Luxury of Rest," Boston Globe, 1985. © 1985, Washington Post Writers Group. Reprinted with permission.

Page 59: "Reflections on a Visit to the Burke Museum, University of Washington, Seattle," by Gail Tremblay, is reprinted from *Indian Singing in Twentieth Century America* by Gail Tremblay (1990) by permission of the publisher, CALYX Books.

Page 65: Excerpt from Ellen Goodman, "Gentle Communication," *Boston Globe,* 3rd ed. 1 August 1985: 15. © 1985, Washington Post Writers Group. Reprinted with permission.

Page 76: Fig. 3.2, The Miller—detail from the Ellesmere MS of *The Canterbury Tales.* Geoffrey Chaucer 1342–1400 English. The Huntington—San Marino, CA.

Page 79–80: Paul Rice, *"Dear Christopher,"* in *Dear Christopher: Letters to Christopher Columbus by Contemporary Native Americans,* eds. Darryl Wilson and Barry Joyce, 62–63, Native American Studies, University of California, Riverside, 1992.

Page 91: Excerpts from "Valium" entry, from *Physicians' Desk Reference®*, pp. 2182, 2183. © *Physicians' Desk Reference®* 50th edition, 1996 published by Medical Economics, Montvale, New Jersey 07645. Reprinted by permission. All rights reserved.

Pages 64, 84: Excerpt from Charles Brashear, "Aesthetic Form in Familiar Essays," CCCC 22 (1971). Copyright 1971 by the National Council of Teachers of English. Reprinted with permission.

Page 89: Excerpt from Lynn K. Stoner, *Latinas of the Americas: A Source Book.* Vol. 363, Garland Reference Library of Social Science, New York 1989.

Page 96: Excerpt from Thomas G. Hollinger, *Microscopic Anatomy,* Gold Standard Multimedia, University of Florida, Gainesville, 1995.

Pages 101, 113: Excerpt from *Modern Video Production: Tools, Techniques, Applications* by Carl Hausman with Philip J. Palombo. Copyright © 1993 by HarperCollins College Publishers. Reprinted by permission of Addison-Wesley Educational Publishers, Inc.

Page 114–15: Excerpt reprinted with the permission of Rawson Associates/Scribner, a Division of Simon & Schuster from *Letitia Baldrige's New Complete Guide to Executive Manners* by Letitia Baldrige. Copyright © 1985, 1993 Letitia Baldrige.

Page 126: "Rastafari for I and for I," by Gregory Salter, from "The Loudest Island in the World: Jamaica, Home of the Reggae Beat." In *World Music: The Rough Guide.* Edited by Simon Broughton, Mark Ellingham, David Muddyman, and Richard Trillo. London: Rough Guides, 1994: 521–38.

Page 127: Photograph of "Grounation" CD produced by The Mystic Revelation of Rastafari. Used with permission.

Page 144: Authors' abstract of article, "What About Dad? Fathers of Children Born to School-Age Mothers," by Nancy Larson, Jon M. Hussey, Mary Rogers Gillmore, and Lewayne D. Gilchrist, *Families in Society: The Journal of Contemporary Human Services,* May 1996.

Page 147: From *American: A Prophecy* by Jerome Rothenberg and George Quasha. Copyright © 1973 by Jerome Rothenberg and George Quasha. Reprinted by permission of Random House Inc.

Page 152: Excerpt from *The Trail of Tears* by Gloria Jahoda, © 1975 by Gloria Jahoda. Reprinted by permission of Henry Holt & Co., Inc.

INDEX

Double-voice (or double-entry) format:
  "Catholic School," Melissa M. Bjorkland, 226–28
  as heuristic, 12
  as technique for paper, 79, 119
Dylan, Bob, 41
Dyer, John, "The Fleece: A Poem," 120–21, 147

Easyriders, 180, 181
Edge-Man Cards and Collectibles, The, 92, 153, 154 (figure)
Elgin, Kathleen, 39
e-mail, 67, 84
Encyclopaedia Britannica, xxi
Essay, informal, 63–79, 120
Explain, 83–97
  as basic aim, xviii
  motivating reader, 86, 113, 135
  and persuasion, 87, 152, 165
  title and first paragraph as lighthouses, 87–88 (incl. figure)
  See also Audience, Exposition, Memorandum as paradigm, Methods of development, Organization, Paragraphs, Teaching a skill, Visual emphasis techniques, Visual illustrations
Explore, 9–14
  as basic aim, 11
  and indirect persuasion, 193
Exposition, Other, 123–49
  types, 85

FAIR (The Federation for Immigration Reform), 169
Family:
  and bread, 108
  dads, need for, 164–67
  father writing to Ann Landers, 168
  and gang membership, 206
  grandmother, 80
  and immigration, 173
  Ireland, Northern, 203
  Latin American, 89
  letter to parents, 190–91; reply, 211
  meditation upon, 46–49
  on motorcycle, 165, 185 (figure)
  "Numbers of Fatherless Kids Takes a Huge Leap," 167
  social web as, 302
  stepfamily (video), 84
  as theme of *Stretch,* xix
  Tilly, Chris, 166
  as topic of paper, 57, 118, 143, 183, 208
  See also "Annie Mae," D.J. Greene,

67–69; "Anthony's War Time," L.A.Occhipinti, 129–31; "California Unwed Mom Count," A. Bancroft, 222–23; "Designer Genes," S. Kape, 264–68; "Explaining Race to a Child," L. Pitts, Jr., 283–84; "Gentle Communication," E. Goodman, 65–66; "Heritage," M. Gonzales, Jr., 70–71; "Isn't She Lovely?" Anonymous, 51–53; "Lacretia," C. Greene, 252–53; "Laugh, Sherry!", S. Murrell, 28; "Light Dawning," 19–22; *nigger: An Autobiography,* D. Gregory, 253–56; "Nomads at Work," 282; "Pleasant Hill," S.O. McCall, 271; "Talking Dust Bowl," Woody Guthrie, 41–42; Untitled Poem, C. Mendez, 274–75.
"Far Side, The" (figure), 35
Figures of speech:
  in "How It Feels to Be Colored Me," Zora Neale Hurston, 261, 262
  metaphor, 34–35, 78, 81, 177, 206, 296
  in persuasion, 209
  simile, 38
  in writing versus speaking, 5
Film:
  "The Art of Watching Silent Films," Ronald V. Smith, 293–94
  Dances with Wolves, 198
  Fantasia, 17
  Goodbye, Columbus, 197
  as heuristic, 13
  as propaganda, 105
  Santa, 17, 18
  scores, 39, 256
  as topic for writing, 186, 230
Five-paragraph theme, 64, 73, 272–73
"For Better or For Worse," 2 (figure)
Forms of discourse:
  advertisement:
    on Internet, 153, 154 (figure)
    in print, 142, 193, 194 (figure), 211
  advice column, 168
  brochure, 85, 184
  case study, 86
  chain letter, 218
  contract, 84, 147
  declaration, or proclamation, 210, 211. See also Roosevelt, Franklin D.
  editorial, 169, 282
  essay examination, 85
  job description, 117
  laboratory report, 85

Rosengarten, Theodore, 109
Rothenberg, Jerome, and George Quasha, eds., *America a Prophecy,* 148
Ruff, James, 34
Ruffin, Kimberly, "Do You Hear What I Hear," 128, 291–93

Sale, Kirkpatrick, *The Conquest of Paradise,* 197
Salter, Gregory, "Rastafari for I and for I," from "The Loudest Island in the World: Jamaica, Home of the Reggae Beat." *World Music: the Rough Guide.* 87, 126–28, 134, 136, 212
"Santa," 17 (figure), 22
Schaffner, Amy Lang, 30
Schlette, Constance, 33, 34
Sentences:
    anaphora, 209, 291
    "be," overuse of, 119, 145–46
    first in story, 31
    fragments, 8, 36, 78, 209, 212, 271
    grammatical subject, 28
    length, 28, 36, 38, 78, 138
    run-ons, 78
    "topic," 87, 89, 90, 177, 249
    transitional, 78, 90, 177, 185, 251
Shaw, Harold, *Dictionary of American Pop/Rock,* 40
Sizer, Theodore, *Horace's Compromise: The Dilemma of the American High School,* 44
Slover, Pippa D., 31
Slugoski, Charlene, xx
Smith, Frank, *Understanding Reading,* 50, 113
Smith, Ronald V., "The Art of Watching Silent Films," 112, 120, 293–94
Smithsonian Magazine, 285
Socrates. See Plato
Soldier's Handbook, 113
Spanish language, 3, 4, 24, 70–72, 142, 274–75
Speaking:
    books on tape, 16
    extemporaneous speeches (with notes), xx
    for group cohesion, 128
    as heuristic, 12
    and reading, 50
    and storytelling:
        flavor of speech in writing, 36, 253–55, 278
        oral delivery, 39

on telephone, 64–66, 193
versus writing, 5–8
and written explanation, 85, 98–99
See also Roosevelt, Franklin D.
Spelling, 79
Stanton, Jamie L., "Falling Short," 295
Statistics, 95
Steinbeck, John, *Grapes of Wrath,* 42
Stewart, Donald C., "The Meditation," in *The Versatile Writer,* 49
Stoner, K. Lynn, *Latinas of the Americas: A Source Book,* 88
Story (5–43):
    dialogue, 28, 34, 244, 256, 270, 297
    elements of, 42–43, 253
    in essays, 73, 261
    in explanation, 94
    narrative mode:
        dramatized, 20, 33, 256
        generalized, 256
        summarized, 20, 33
    oral telling, 39
    in persuasion, 157, 193, 210
    research for, 38–39, 244
    scenes, 22
    speech "zing," 36
    as "stretch," xviii
    structure of, 18 (figure), 19–22, 25, 38, 253
    within story, 253
    symbol, 108
    with thesis, 256
    types of, 216
    See also Dialogue
Stretching, types of, 93
Sun News, The [Myrtle Beach, S.C.], 178, 188, 222
Synonyms, 283

Taylor, Colin, *Myths of the North American Indians,* 122
Teaching a Skill (98–122):
    chronologically or logically, 100
    with double-entry instructions, 119
    as informal essay, 120
    with ironic instructions, 119
    oral versus written, 98–99
    with two-column script, 120
Themes in *Stretch,* xix–xx
Thesis. See Persuasion
Thrash, Kyle, "Inferno," 35, 296–97
Tilly, Chris, and Randy Albelda, "It's Not Working: Why Many Single Mothers Can't Work Their Way out of Poverty," 167
Tinter, Elissa, and Jan Hall, 147